Poultry Science and Practice

A Textbook

as Per Revised VCI Syllabus for Veterinary Students

Poultry Science and Practice

A Textbook

as Per Revised VCI Syllabus for Veterinary Students

Nilotpal Ghosh

BVSc & AH, MVSc (APM), PhD, FNAPM

Associate Professor and Head
Department of Animal Science
Bidhan Chandra Krishi Viswavidyalaya
Mohanpur, Nadia, West Bengal, India

CBS

CBS Publishers & Distributors Pvt Ltd

New Delhi • Bengaluru • Chennai • Kochi • Mumbai • Pune
Hyderabad • Kolkata • Nagpur • Patna • Vijayawada

Poultry Science and Practice
A Textbook

ISBN: 978-81-239-2544-8

Copyright © Author and Publisher

First Edition: 2015

Published by Satish Kumar Jain and produced by Varun Jain for

CBS Publishers & Distributors Pvt Ltd

4819/XI Prahlad Street, 24 Ansari Road, Daryaganj, New Delhi 110 002, India.
Ph: 23289259, 23266861, 23266867   Website: www.cbspd.com
Fax: 011-23243014   e-mail: delhi@cbspd.com; cbspubs@airtelmail.in.
Corporate Office: 204 FIE, Industrial Area, Patparganj, Delhi 110 092
Ph: 4934 4934   Fax: 4934 4935   e-mail: publishing@cbspd.com; publicity@cbspd.com

Branches

- **Bengaluru:** Seema House 2975, 17th Cross, K.R. Road,
  Banasankari 2nd Stage, Bengaluru 560 070, Karnataka
  Ph: +91-80-26771678/79   Fax: +91-80-26771680   e-mail: bangalore@cbspd.com
- **Chennai:** 20, West Park Road, Shenoy Nagar, Chennai 600 030, Tamil Nadu
  Ph: +91-44-26260666, 26208620   Fax: +91-44-42032115   e-mail: chennai@cbspd.com
- **Kochi:** 36/14 Kalluvilakam, Lissie Hospital Road, Kochi 682 018, Kerala
  Ph: +91-484-4059061-65   Fax: +91-484-4059065   e-mail: kochi@cbspd.com
- **Mumbai:** 83-C, Dr E Moses Road, Worli, Mumbai-400018, Maharashtra
  Ph: +91-22-24902340/41   Fax: +91-22-24902342   e-mail: mumbai@cbspd.com
- **Pune:** Bhuruk Prestige, Sr. No. 52/12/2+1+3/2 Narhe, Haveli
  (Near Katraj-Dehu Road Bypass), Pune 411 041, Maharashtra
  Ph: +91-20-64704058/59, 32392277   Fax: +91-20-24300160   e-mail: pune@cbspd.com

Representatives

- **Hyderabad**   0-9885175004
- **Nagpur**   0-9021734563
- **Vijayawada**   0-9000660880
- **Kolkata**   0-9831437309, 0-9051152362
- **Patna**   0-9334159340

Printed at : Swastik Packagings, 506 F.I.E. Patparganj, Delhi - 92

to

Prof DN Maitra
my esteemed teacher

Aporna
my wife

Archisman
my son

Foreword

The poultry production in our country has witnessed significant progress over the years primarily due to research and development thrust of government and organised private sectors. Compared to the other livestock sectors, poultry production in India is more scientific, better organised and continuously progressing towards modernisation. At present India ranks third in egg production in the world after China and the USA, with the total annual egg production of about 66.45 billion and fifth in broiler production with 2.47 million tonnes of broiler meat. Currently, it is growing at the rate of 6 percent per annum in egg production and 12 percent per annum in broiler production. Here poultry production has emerged as an industry, and this sector of livestock industry is already employing in excess of 7 million persons in various activities and can generate a huge number of new jobs per year with the present growth rate. This sector alone contributes about 0.5 percent of the India's GDP and 10 percent of the livestock GDP, and it is becoming a significant contributor to the Indian economy. It may be mentioned here that China is the number 1 country in the world so far in egg and chicken production. However, in China, most of the poultry is in the form of backyard poultry or in unorganised sector which is not overdependent upon the imported germplasm. It is also true in case of Bangladesh and Vietnam where two-thirds of the total egg production comes from rural poultry, while in India, the situation is just the reverse. So in India, apart from expanding high input intensive poultry production system under organised sector, reorienting and strengthening of rural poultry can be an important tool for improving living standards, poverty alleviation and nutritional security of the people belonging to lower strata of the society.

Veterinary Council of India's "Minimum Standards of Veterinary Education—Degree Course (BVSc & AH) Regulations, 2008" rightly gave extra emphasis on poultry science education in undergraduate veterinary curricula by introducing two separate courses, viz. 'Avian Production Management' and 'Commercial Poultry Production and Hatchery Management'.

This book entitled *Poultry Science and Practice: A Textbook* written by Dr Nilotpal Ghosh is unique of its kind as it covers the entire syllabus of two courses framed by the VCI. The basics as well as all the applied aspects of poultry production, including fowl, duck, quail, turkey, Guinea fowl, emu and goose, have been nicely highlighted in the single volume. It is written in a simple language, and a large number of objective as well as subjective questions at the end of each chapter will help the students to prepare for their examinations. I hope because of its contents and style of presentation, this book would become quite popular amongst students, teachers, animal husbandry extension personnel, progressive poultry keepers and persons working in the field of poultry husbandry. The efforts of the author deserve appreciation.

D. K. Bagh.

D.K. Bagchi
Ex-Vice Chancellor
Bidhan Chandra Krishi Viswavidyalaya
Mohanpur, Nadia, West Bengal

Preface

This book *Poultry Science and Practice: A Textbook* is actually composed of two parts, viz. Part I: Avian Production Management and Part II: Commercial Poultry Production and Hatchery Management.

This book has been prepared by strictly covering the revised syllabus of two courses (LPM-211 and LPM-221) for BVSc and AH students, framed by the Veterinary Council of India, the apex body for veterinary education in India. Such a type of VCI syllabus-oriented textbook is rarely available in India. The text material is presented in a simple and lucid language.

The information is up-to-date and given in concise form and in such a manner that the book can be used as a substitute for class notes. A large number of objective as well as subjective questions given at the end of each chapter is an additional attraction of the book, as the students can prepare themselves for the composite annual examination under VCI pattern.

For the use of this book in practical fields, all the relevant points in poultry production including chicken, duck, quail, turkey, Guinea fowl, emu and goose have been highlighted in this text. Besides, the poultry drug index indicating medicines and vaccines available in the market for maintenance of poultry health, helps a lot to the neovets and practising poultry specialists.

Who will be benefited?

This book is primarily meant for veterinary students of India. It will also help the concerned teachers/demonstrators of all veterinary colleges/universities in India for offering this course.

This book will also be useful for veterinarians, livestock development officers, animal husbandry extension personnel and progressive poultry farmers in India and other tropical countries.

Nilotpal Ghosh

Acknowledgments

It is my immense pleasure that this book has ultimately come to light. The information received from various sources is gratefully acknowledged. Bibliography has been given at the end of this book to give due credit to the authors. I extend my thanks to my teachers, relatives, friends and colleagues for their inspiration and motivation. My acknowledgment would be incomplete, if I do not mention the name of my reverend teachers Prof DN Maitra, Prof L Mandal and Prof G Choudhuri, without whose blessings and encouragement I could not have completed this work. I also convey my regards to my teachers Prof SC Majumdar, Prof SK Roy, Prof AK Samanta, Prof S Pan and Prof R Samanta, who nurtured me during my masters degree study and research.

My sincere thanks are due to Mr SK Jain, Mr YN Arjuna and their team at CBS Publishers & Distributors, New Delhi, for publishing this title. I will welcome any suggestion and observation from students, teachers and other readers which would help in bringing out a revised and improved version of this title. Suggestions may please be sent to my e-mail address: gnilotpal@yahoo.com.

Nilotpal Ghosh

Contents

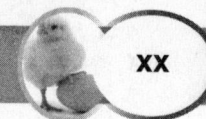

Abbreviations

AICRP	All India Coordinated Research Project
ALC	Avian Leucosis Complex
APF	Animal Protein Factor
APM	Animal Production and Management
BVSc & AH	Bachelor of Veterinary Science and Animal Husbandry
BBB	Broad Breasted Bronze
BBW	Broad Breasted White
BIS	Bureau of Indian Standards
BWD	Bacillary White Diarrhoea
Ca	Calcium
$Ca(OH)_2$	Calcium Hydroxide
CARI	Central Avian Research Institute
CF	Crude Fibre
CP	Crude Protein
CPBF	Central Poultry Breeding Farm
CPDO	Central Poultry Development Organisation
CRD	Chronic Respiratory Disease
DAHD	Department of Animal Husbandry and Dairying (Now Department of Animal Husbandry, Dairying and Fishery)
DM	Dry Matter
DOC	Day-Old Chick
EDS	Egg Drop Syndrome
ESI	Egg Shape Index
FAO	Food and Agriculture Organisation
FAOSTAT	Statistics Division of Food and Agriculture Organisation
FCR	Feed Conversion Ratio
g	Gram
GDP	Gross Domestic Product
GI tract	Gastrointestinal Tract
GI weld	Galvanised Iron Weld
GNC	Groundnut Cake
HCl	Hydrochloric Acid
HDL	High-Density Lipoprotein
HDP	Hen Day Production
HHP	Hen Housed Production
HU	Haugh Unit
I/M	Intramuscular
IBD	Infectious Bursal Disease
ICAR	Indian Council of Agricultural Research
ICMR	Indian Council of Medical Research
IFOAM	International Federation of Organic Agriculture Movements
ITK	Indigenous Technological Knowledge
JAS	Japan Agricultural Standard
K_2O	Potassium Oxide
KAU	Kerala Agricultural University

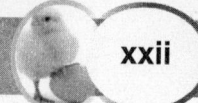
kcal	Kilocalories
kg	Kilogram
$KMnO_4$	Potassium Permanganate
KVAFSU	Karnataka Veterinary, Animal and Fishery Sciences University
LPM	Livestock Production Management
lux	SI unit of illuminance and luminous emittance, measuring luminous flux per unit area. It is equal to one lumen per square metre.
MD	Marek's Disease
ME	Metabolisable Energy
Mn	Manganese
NABARD	National Bank for Agriculture and Rural Development
NaCl	Sodium Chloride (common salt)
NAFED	National Agricultural Cooperative Marketing Federation of India Ltd
NBAGR	National Bureau of Animal Genetic Resources
NDDB	National Dairy Development Board
NDF	Neutral Detergent Fibre
NECC	National Egg Coordination Committee
NFE	Nitrogen-Free Extract
NSOP	National Standards for Organic Production
NSPs	Non-Starch Polysaccharides
P	Phosphorus
P_2O_5	Phosphorus Pentoxide
PDP	Project Directorate on Poultry
PDRC	Poultry Diagnostic Research Centre
PEF	Performance Efficiency Factor
PEI	Performance Efficiency Index
PPLO	Pleuropneumonia-like Organism
PSI	Pound-force per Square Inch/Pound per Square Inch
RD	Ranikhet Disease
RH	Relative Humidity
RIL	Routine Inclusion Level
RIR	Rhode Island Red
RNA	Ribonucleic Acid
RSPPTC	Random Sample Poultry Performance Testing Centre
S/C	Subcutaneous
SDS	Sudden Death Syndrome
TANUVAS/ TANVASU	Tamil Nadu Veterinary and Animal Sciences University
UAS, Bengaluru	University of Agricultural Sciences, Bengaluru
UK	United Kingdom
UP	Uttar Pradesh
USA/US	United States of America
USDA	United States Department of Agriculture
UT	Union Territories
VCI	Veterinary Council of India
WAMP	Week A Month Programme
WHO	World Health Organisation
WLH	White Leghorn
WTO	World Trade Organisation
Zn	Zinc

PART I

Avian Production Management

1

Introduction— Indian Poultry Industry

1.1 WHAT IS POULTRY?

The birds which are reared for production of meat and/or eggs for the benefit of human beings are called poultry. It is a broad term, and includes number of avian species, viz. fowl/chicken, duck, quail, turkey, Guinea fowl, pea fowl, goose, pheasant, ostrich, emu, *etc*. In India, poultry industry is primarily chicken oriented. More than 90% of Indian poultry birds are chicken. So in India, 'poultry' and 'chicken' are used mostly as synonymous terms.

1.2 IMPORTANCE OF POULTRY

Contribution of poultry in the country's economy is enormous. The role of poultry in enhancement of family nutrition status of poor farmers as well as income generation and self-employment is well-recognised. The salient features of importance of poultry rearing are as follows:

- **Source of high quality protein food items and their market demands**

Poultry is the source of high quality animal protein food items, viz. egg and meat. Both the food items are nutritious and tasty, and regarded as protective food to human beings. Egg is commonly called 'a complete planned food of natural origin'. Egg is the only food item available in the market which cannot be adulterated. Market demand of both the egg and chicken is well-established. These are comparatively cheap. Poultry meat has no religious taboo.

- **Source of income**

Unemployment problem in our country is in increasing trend. Nowadays, it is very hard to get a job either in government or non-government sectors. So many people particularly in villages take poultry rearing as a profession for generating sole income of the family. Poultry can be taken as a business on small scale or large scale basis. It is a very good income generating option for the small and marginal farmers. There are facilities of getting loan for this business.

The **primary business avenues** in relation to poultry are:

   i. **Layer farming**—for egg production with chicken or duck.
   ii. **Broiler farming**—for meat production with chicken, quail, turkey, *etc*.
   iii. **Hatchery enterprise**—for chick or duckling production by hatching of eggs.

Poultry rearing can be taken as a source of subsidiary income also in case of low income families particularly marginal farmers and landless labourers.

Poultry farming provides self employment to unemployed educated youth, and it can solve the problem of unemployment and under employment in our country.

[*See Chapter 15*]

- **Quick return in poultry business**

Quick return of invested money is an important characteristic of poultry rearing. For example, in case of hatchery enterprise, return is possible within 21 days as the incubation period of chicken egg is only 21 days. Broiler birds are generally kept in farm only for 42 days. In case of layer farming, chickens start to lay eggs at 18–20 weeks of age. Quails start to laying eggs at the age of 6 weeks only. Income from poultry farming is round the year.

- **Less requirement of space**

Owing to the small size, birds require very small floor space to live and grow. A poultry shed measuring 25 ft × 10 ft can accommodate about 210–250 broiler chickens (i.e. 1–1.2 sq ft per bird only) under deep litter system. In case of layer under deep litter system, space requirement is more to some extent (1.75–2 sq ft per bird). However, in cage rearing system the space requirement is again less.

- **Less requirement of physical labour**

There is no requirement of heavy physical labour in poultry rearing. Retired persons, female and young members of a farmer's family may be involved in various poultry management practices. Thus complete utilisation of family labour is possible in this business.

- **Farmers need not to be highly educated** to operate the poultry business.

- **Investment in starting a poultry farm is comparatively less**

Feed is the major item of expenditure (about 70%) in poultry rearing. Feed conversion efficiency in broiler chicken production (1.7–2.0) is less in comparison to other meat animals like pig (3.0–3.5) or cattle (5.0).

- **Risk is less in poultry farming**

In case of large scale poultry farms scientific methods of rearing that are already standardized and available can be followed. Proper vaccination and other medication usually reduce the risk in this business. Besides this, the poultry farms can be insured against the possible risk, if any, through the subsidiaries of General Insurance Corporation of India like National Insurance Co Ltd, New India Insurance Co Ltd, Oriental Insurance Co Ltd and United India Insurance Co Ltd.

- **Impact of environmental factors (like draught, heavy rain, *etc.*) on performance of poultry business is less** in comparison to many agricultural operations like crop or vegetable production.

- **Poultry manure is a valuable fertiliser**

In poultry, faeces and urine are mixed together and voided as droppings. So the poultry excreta or poultry manure is very rich in fertiliser value. It contains 1.0–1.8%

nitrogen, 1.4–1.8% phosphorus pentoxide (P_2O_5) and 0.8–0.9% potassium oxide (K_2O). Poultry manure may be used to improve the quality of soil for better crop production as well as in aquaculture. The comparative manurial value of poultry droppings and other animal excreta is given in Table 1.1. Poultry droppings can be used as an ingredient of ruminant feed after processing, and also for production of biogas.

Table 1.1: Manurial value of various animal excreta (in %)

Animal excreta	N	P_2O_5	K_2O
Poultry droppings	1.0–1.8	1.4–1.8	0.8–0.9
Cattle dung	0.3–0.4	0.1–0.2	0.1–0.3
Sheep dung	0.5–0.6	0.4–0.5	0.3–1.0
Goat dung	0.7–0.8	0.6–0.7	0.8–1.2
Night soil	1.0–1.6	0.8–1.2	0.2–0.6

On an average, a laying hen produces about 60 kg fresh droppings per year, with a dry matter content of approximately 20–25%, i.e. 12–15 kg dry droppings are produced annually by a laying hen. However, quantity of droppings produced by birds may vary due to several factors including differences in feed and water intake. Poultry feathers are used for making sophisticated and fancy products.

1.3 POULTRY INDUSTRY DEVELOPMENT IN INDIA

1.3.1 Some Milestones

India and its neighbouring countries are considered to be the origin of poultry birds. It is believed that the modern breeds of domestic fowl (*Gallus domesticus*) have originated from the Indian red jungle fowl (*Gallus gallus*). However, the scientific poultry keeping in India was initiated by the **Christian Missionaries** in the beginning of 20th century, improved breeds of poultry were introduced in India from their countries. Side by side during the World War II, army authorities started setting up a number of farms with improved egg type poultry birds to meet the demand of eggs for defence personnel. Such activity helped a lot in popularising scientific poultry farming in the surrounding areas. Commercial poultry farming was started through organised efforts during the **1st Five-Year Plan** period (1951–55). During this plan ₹ 2.5 crores was spent on poultry development. Thirty-three extension centres were established under poultry development programmes to supply improved/exotic breeds of chicken to interested farmers.

During the **2nd Five-Year Plan (1956–61)** ₹ 2.8 crores was spent for poultry development programmes in India. An All India Poultry Development Project was initiated. Government of India established 4 regional **Central Poultry Breeding Farms (CPBF)** at Bengaluru (Hessarghata), Mumbai, Chandigarh and Bhubaneswar. Day-old chicks of White Leghorn and Rhode Island Red were imported from the USA in 1956, as foundation stock for extending high quality acclimatized stock to the farmers. The **period between 2nd and 4th Five-Year Plans were considered as the turning point** for poultry development in India, the fund allocations were ₹ 4.6 crores in 3rd plan (1961–66) and ₹ 11.5 crores in 4th plan (1969–74). During these subsequent Five-Year Plans the importance of poultry development was increased, more fund was incurred to develop this sector of Animal Husbandry. Besides, the government efforts, the private sector has contributed significantly to produce high quality commercial breeding stocks, poultry equipments, compounded feed, healthcare products and disease diagnostic facilities. Good genetic stocks, equipments and machinery, medicines and vaccines and skilled manpower are now available in India. But there is a need to improve processing, preservation and marketing of poultry and poultry products.

1.3.2 The Institutes/Organisations Promoting Poultry in India

The following institutes/organisations contribute a lot towards development of poultry in India:

- **Central Avian Research Institute (CARI)**

A premier institute in the field of poultry research, education, extension and training in India, was established in 1979 under the control of Indian Council of Agricultural Research (ICAR). Its headquarter is at Izatnagar, Bareilly in Uttar Pradesh. This institute provides the necessary training and extension support in all disciplines of Poultry Science for promoting productivity and profitability of Indian Poultry Industry. The institute also has played a pioneering role in transforming backyard poultry farming into several billion rupees agroindustry. Some of the best germplasms of avian species in the country are maintained here. For example, egg type pure line like *White Leghorn*, egg type commercial stock like *CARI-Priya, CARI-Sonali* and dual purpose *CARI-Devendra*, meat type pure lines, meat type commercial line like *CARIBRO-Veshal* (white), *CARIBRO-Dhanraja* (coloured), *CARIBRO-Mrityunjay* (for hot and dry region), *CARIBRO-Tropicana* (for hot and humid region), indigenous stock like *Aseel, Frizzle, Kadaknath, Naked neck, UPCARI, HITCARI, CARI-Nirbheek* and *CARI-Shyama* birds, large variety of turkeys like *Broad Breasted White*, broiler quail line like *CARI Uttam, CARI Ujjawal* and *CARI Sweta*, egg type quail like *CARI Pearl*, and Guinea fowl like *GUNCARI, etc.*

- **Project Directorate on Poultry, Hyderabad**

Andhra Pradesh is an important organization under the control of ICAR working for the development of poultry in India. The Coordination unit of All India Coordinated Research Project (AICRP) on Poultry Breeding (under ICAR) was upgraded to the status of a Directorate during the last part of VII plan and named as "Project Directorate on Poultry (PDP)". The Directorate was established at its present location in Acharya NG Ranga Agricultural University campus, Hyderabad in 1988. The research programmes carried out under AICRP made significant progress in developing high yielding layer and broiler strains since its inception. Besides, the Directorate has evolved synthetic strains, viz. *Vanaraja* and *Gramapriya* for free range backyard farming in rural and tribal areas and *Krishibro* for small scale intensive broiler farming. Keeping in view the growing demands and the challenges that the Directorate has to face in future, various programmes have been prepared with a visionary approach.

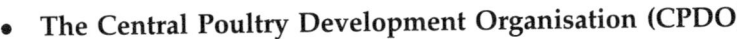

- **The Central Poultry Development Organisation (CPDO)**

Under Ministry of Agriculture, Department of Animal Husbandry, Dairying and Fisheries, Government of India, was formed to meet the requirements for poultry development in various parts of our country. During the X plan, it was decided to club all the existing 13 Central Poultry Development Organisations regionwise into 4 Centres so as to confer the poultry developmental activities in a single window system. These four Central Poultry Development Organizations (CPDOs) are located at Bengaluru (Southern Region), Bhubaneswar (Eastern Region), Chandigarh (Northern Region) and Mumbai (Western Region). The CPDO (Southern Region) was formed after merging and restructuring of the Central Poultry Units located at Hessarghata, Bengaluru, viz. Central Poultry Training Institute, Central Poultry Breeding Farm, Central Duck Breeding Farm, Random Sample Poultry Performance Testing Centre, during June 2003.

The primary functions of these CPDOs are:

i. **Making available quality chicks:** The CPDOs multiply and supply identified low input technology poultry stocks to all states of their respective regions for their rural poultry development programmes. These organizations procure breeding stock of low input technology developed by the ICAR, State Agriculture Universities (SAU), Private Sectors, NGOs, *etc.*

ii. **Diversification programme:** Under this programme, duck (Southern and Eastern regions), Japanese quail (Western and Northern regions), turkey (Southern and Western regions) and Guinea fowl (Eastern region) have been introduced to boost the poultry industry. Emu farming was started at CPDO (Southern region) as a pilot project for popularising this amazing bird in India.

iii. **Strengthening of feed quality monitoring wing:** The feed analytical laboratories are concentrating their activities on analysis of various feed/feed ingredients and developing least cost feed formulation, based on locally available ingredients for poultry.

iv. **Training programme:** Need-based and flexible training programmes are conducted at all the CPDOs to meet the requirement of trainers, farmers, women beneficiaries, various public and private sector poultry organisations, NGOs, banks, cooperative foreign trainees, *etc.*

v. **Random sample tests:** Four Random Sample Poultry Performance Testing Centres (RSPPTC) at Bengaluru, Mumbai, Bhubaneswar and Gurgaon have conducted egg-laying and broiler tests and provided useful information to poultry farmers, hatcheries and breeding organisations about performance of various participating layers and broiler stocks in the country (both from public/private sector organizations). Presently, the Random Sample Poultry Performance Testing Centre located at Gurgaon (Haryana) is the only centre at the national level to test various stocks of poultry available in the country. The other 3 centres are merged with the respective CPDO. The tests are conducted under uniform environment and standard management practices for assessing the production performance of layers and broilers. Presently, 1 layer and 2 broiler tests are conducted each year.

During 2011–12, the CPDOs have supplied about 1.47 lakhs parent stock, 0.99 lakh ducklings, 15.29 lakhs commercial chicks, 14.12 lakhs chicken duck hatching eggs, and 5.58 lakhs turkey poults/Guinea fowl keets/Japanese quail. These organisations also analysed about 3,814 feed samples and trained about 3,109 persons during the year.

- Indian Council of Agricultural Research (ICAR) initiated **All India Coordinated Research Project (AICRP) on Poultry Breeding** during IV Plan (1970). The objective of the project was to produce superior genetic stock of layers and broilers to achieve self-reliance in poultry production. Initially, AICRP on Poultry Breeding was started at IVRI, Izatnagar, UP and operated till 1997, then it was shifted to CARI, Izatnagar. Now the main centre is at Hyderabad, Andhra Pradesh with a network of research centres located at different State Agricultural Universities (SAU) and ICAR institutes.

- **A Centre for Advanced Studies in Poultry Science** was established in November, 1985 to coordinate the research activities in the disciplines of Poultry Science at College of Veterinary and Animal Sciences, Kerala Agricultural University, Mannuthy 680651, Kerala. Another Centre for Advanced Studies in Poultry Science is at Veterinary College and Research Institute, Tamil Nadu and Veterinary and Animal Sciences University, Namakkal-637 002, Tamil Nadu.

- **Poultry development:** It is a centrally sponsored scheme for states/UTs with an outlay of ₹ 52.50 crores during 2012–13, with 3 separate components, namely:
  - a. Assistance to State Poultry Farms (₹ 10.00 crores)
  - b. Rural Backyard Poultry Development (₹ 40.00 crores)
  - c. Poultry Estates (₹ 2.50 crores)

The componentwise specifications and pattern of assistance are as follows:

  - a. **Assistance to State Poultry Farms:** The assistance provided is 100% in case of the north-east states including Sikkim and 80% in respect of other States. The limit of assistance provided is ₹ 85.00 lakhs for each farm. One time assistance is provided to strengthen farms located in different states/UTs in terms of hatchery, brooding and rearing houses, laying houses for birds with provision for feed mill and their quality monitoring and in-house disease diagnostic facilities and feed analysis laboratory.

  - b. **Rural Backyard Poultry Development:** Granted to State Governments and is fully funded by government of India except for mother units and pheriwalas, which will be provided to NABARD. This scheme beneficiary will farmers' families, belonging to BPL category only and will be implemented in all states/UTs.

c. **Poultry Estates:** Two poultry estates are decided to be established on pilot basis, in low commercial activity states/regions, viz. Bihar, Chhattisgarh, Jharkhand, Gujarat, Madhya Pradesh, Odisha, Uttarakhand, some districts of Uttar Pradesh and West Bengal, Vidharba region of Maharashtra and north-eastern states in the field of poultry. Grant is being provided to states for infrastructure development on 75:25 centre to state sharing basis and 100% grant to NABARD for other components, except establishment of poultry units and other input services which will be supported by providing interest free loan to the extent of 50% of cost. Two estates have already been approved at Sikkim and Odisha on pilot basis. Further proposals can be examined only after the outcome of these 2 estates.

- The **veterinary colleges** under agriculture/veterinary universities also played an important role in poultry development in India.

1.4 POULTRY STATISTICS IN INDIA

The poultry production in the country has made significant progress over the years due to research and development thrust of government and organised private sectors. Compared with the rest of the livestock sector, poultry industry in India is more scientific, better organised and continuously progressing towards modernisation. India has 649 million poultry birds (18th All India Livestock Census, 2007; Table 1.3). Tamil Nadu, Andhra Pradesh and West Bengal lead in the country in poultry population (Table 1.4). The annual per capita consumption of eggs in India is 55 and that of poultry meat is 1.97 kg (2011–12, Table 1.6). However, these figures are low in comparison to many developed countries like the USA, Denmark, the UK, the Netherlands, *etc*. The world's average figures are 124 eggs and 12.62 kg meat (FAO, 2009). On the other hand, the recommended minimum per capita consumption is 180 eggs and 11.0 kg of poultry meat (as per recommendation of National Institute of Nutrition). To meet these requirements the volume of layer and broiler industry should reach 5 and 10 times the present volume respectively (PDP Vision, 2030). So the poultry industry has a great potential to expand many folds in our country.

At present, **India ranks among the top 3rd nations in egg production (5%) in the world** after China (37.6%) and the USA (8.5%), and **5th largest producer of chicken meat (2.3%) after the USA (20.3%), China (14.3%), Brazil (12.4%) and Mexico (3.2%) (FAO, 2009).** Currently, it is growing at the rate of 12 per cent per annum in broiler production and 6 per cent per annum in egg production. **Presently India ranks 5th in chicken population and 6th in duck population in the world** (FAOSTAT production data, 2010).

Present poultry indicators along with changes in production and productivity of poultry during last one and a half decade are given in Table 1.2.

Table 1.2: Poultry indicators in India

Performance Indicators	1993	2008
Egg production per hybrid hen (at 72 weeks of age)	300 eggs	320 eggs
Feed/egg (g)	135	125
Economic egg production age (in weeks)	20–72	18–90
Average number of hens per cage house	5,000	25,000
Market age of broilers	56 days	< 40 days
Market weight of broilers	1.5 kg (in 56 days)	2.1 kg (in 40 days)
Feed conversion ratio (FCR) in broilers	2.2	< 1.7
Market body weight of Japanese quail	100 g in 35 days	150 g in 30 days
Egg production in Japanese quail (40 weeks of age)	155 eggs	190 eggs
Commercial emu farms (in nos.)	Not existing	> 1,500 farms

Source: Sasidhar PVK (2009), Poultry Science Education and Human Resource Planning for Poultry Sector. Recommendations of the National Seminar (January 21–22, 2009), Central Avian Research Institute, Izatnagar, India.

Table 1.3: Poultry population in India (in '000)

Particulars	2003	2007*	% change from 2003–2007
Fowls	4,57,399	6,17,734	35.1
Ducks	29,959	27,643	–7.7
Turkeys and other poultry	1,654	3,452	108.7
Total poultry	4,89,012	6,48,829	32.7

Source: 18th Indian Livestock Census 2007. Department of Animal Husbandry, Dairying and Fisheries, Ministry of Agriculture, Government of India, Krishi Bhavan, New Delhi. This census was conducted with 15th October, 2007 as reference date.

* Out of total poultry 95.2% are fowls and the rest 4.8% are duck, turkey, guinea fowl and other poultry birds in India. There is a sharp increase in the fowl population in the country during the period from 2003 to 2007. The fowl population has increased by more than 35% and the total poultry by 32.7% in the country. The population of duck has decreased marginally. Out of total poultry birds, 356 million were in poultry farms (55%) and remaining 293 million were in backyard poultry (45%). West Bengal (21.9%), Andhra Pradesh (12.9%), Assam (9.9%) and Tamil Nadu (9.2%) accounted for 53.9% poultry birds in backyard poultry. Tamil Nadu (28.5%), Andhra Pradesh (24.2%), Maharashtra (12.6%) and Karnataka (8.7%) accounted for 74.0% of total pultry birds in poultry farms.

Table 1.4: Poultry population and per capita egg production in various states/union territories of India according to 18th Indian Livestock Census, 2007.

India and its states, UTs and NCT	Fowl (in thousand nos.)	Duck (in thousand nos.)	Total poultry* (in thousand nos.)	Poultry population of the country (per cent)	Per capita egg production (nos./head/year)**
India	6,17,734	27,643	6,48,829	—	53
Andhra Pradesh	1,23,036	766	1,23,981	19.11	238
Arunachal Pradesh	1,259	90	1,348	0.21	33
Assam	20,609	8,439	29,060	4.48	15
Bihar	10,755	499	11,420	1.76	8
Chhattisgarh	13,838	127	14,246	2.20	52
Goa	504	1	505	0.08	9
Gujarat	13,327	18	13,352	2.06	23
Haryana	28,619	33	28,785	4.44	157
Himachal Pradesh	725	0	810	0.12	15
Jammu and Kashmir	6,487	190	6,683	1.03	66
Jharkhand	10,448	615	11,231	1.73	13
Karnataka	41,845	13	42,068	6.48	52
Kerala	14,219	995	15,686	2.42	49
Madhya Pradesh	7,311	59	7,384	1.14	11
Maharashtra	64,431	34	64,756	9.98	38
Manipur	1,830	559	2,403	0.37	47
Meghalaya	3,026	66	3,093	0.48	39
Mizoram	1,232	7	1,239	0.19	39
Nagaland	2,991	120	3,156	0.49	36
Odisha	19,489	594	20,600	3.17	58
Punjab	10,536	25	10,685	1.65	129
Rajasthan	4,914	27	4,946	0.76	10
Sikkim	157	1	157	0.02	23
Tamil Nadu	1,26,879	1,039	1,28,108	19.74	171
Tripura	2,895	756	3,701	0.57	44
Uttar Pradesh	8,460	270	8,754	1.35	6
Uttarakhand	2,563	25	2,602	0.40	26
West Bengal	73,626	12,160	86,210	13.29	45
Andaman and Nicobar Islands	916	54	979	0.15	137
Chandigarh	129	0	129	0.02	13
Dadra and Nagar Haveli	169	0	170	0.03	20
Daman and Diu	25	0	26	0	7
Delhi	2	0	2	0	0
Lakshadweep	137	26	167	0.03	183
Puducherry	345	35	387	0.06	8

Source: 18th Indian Livestock Census 2007, Department of Animal Husbandry, Dairying and Fisheries, Ministry of Agriculture, Government of India, Krishi Bhavan, New Delhi. This census was conducted with 15th October, 2007 as reference date.

* Besides fowl and duck, total number of poultries also includes other birds like turkey, Guinea fowl, quail, etc.

** 2010–11, as per DAHD Annual Report 2011–12. 0—negligible with respect to thousands.

There is a tremendous growth in poultry population as well as production in India and now it is being considered as an industry in the country (Tables 1.5 and 1.6).

Table 1.5: Poultry population and egg production in India since 1951

Year	Poultry population (million)	Egg production (million)	Per capita egg availability (nos./head/year)
1951	73.50	1,832	5
1956	94.80	1,908	5
1961	114.20	2,881	7
1972	138.50	7,752	14
1982	207.74	10,876	16
1987	275.32	17,310	22
1992	307.07	21,983	26
1997	347.61	27,496	29
2003	489.01	39,823	38
2007	648.83	50,663	45

Source: Various All India Livestock Census reports.

Table 1.6: Egg and poultry meat production statistics in India

Year	Egg production		Poultry meat production	
	Total (nos. in million)	Per capita (nos./annum)	Total ('000 tonnes)	Per capita (kg/annum)
2007–08	53,583	47	1,755	1.54
2008–09	55,562	48	1,884	1.63
2009–10	60,267	51	2,087	1.78
2010–11	63,024	53	2,193	1.85
2011–12	66,449	55	2,470	1.97

Notes: Data for financial year (April–March)
Source: Government of India, Department of Animal Husbandry, Dairying and Fisheries.

India's poultry industry is said to be 5,000 years old, but it is only in the past few decades that it has begun to witness tremendous growth. At present, Indian poultry sector is a vibrant subsector of agriculture. It has shown a dramatic 500-fold growth rate during the last 4 decades, which no other agroindustry has recorded so far. Poultry industry is already employing in excess around 7 million persons in various activities and can generate more than 50,000 new jobs per year with the present growth rate. The share of all livestock and poultry sectors put together to the GDP, is about 3.64%, of which the poultry sector alone contributes about 0.5% of the India's GDP and 10% of the livestock GDP, and it is becoming a significant contributor to Indian economy (Central Statistical Office, M/o Statistics and Programme Implementation, Government of India, 2010–11).

At present, Asia produces about 60% of the total world production of eggs and China is the largest producer of eggs (28,674 thousand tonnes) and poultry meat (10,233 thousand tonnes) [FAOSTAT, 2005; Table 1.7]. It may be mentioned here that in China most of the poultry is in the form of backyard poultry or in unorganised sector which is not overdependent upon the imported germplasm. It is also true in case of Bangladesh and Vietnam where 2/3rd of the total egg production comes from rural poultry, while in India, the situation is just reverse. So in India, apart from expanding high input intensive poultry production system under organised sector, reorienting and strengthening of rural poultry can be an important tool for improving living standard, poverty alleviation and nutritional security of the people belonging to the lower strata of the society.

Table 1.7: Per capita consumption of eggs (nos.) and broiler meat (kg) in selected countries during 2005

Countries	Egg[1]	Broiler meat[2]
Argentina	174	18.54
Brazil	130	37.27
South Africa	107	24.70
India	46	1.72
Iran	133	4.88
Thailand	105	10.54
Canada	188	31.82
France	251	14.24
Hungary	295	27.81
Russian Federation	259	16.45
USA	255	44.24
UK	172	26.76

[1] International Egg Commission (2006)
[2] FAOSTAT (2005)

1.5 COMMON NAMES OF MALE, FEMALE AND YOUNG ONES OF VARIOUS POULTRY SPECIES

Different specific terms are used to denote male, female and young ones of various poultry species (Table 1.8).

Table 1.8: Specific terms for male, female and young ones of various poultry species

Species of poultry	Male	Female	Young
Chicken/fowl	Cock	Hen	Chick
Duck	Drake	Duck	Duckling
Quail	Quail cock	Quail hen	Quail chick
Turkey	Tom turkey	Hen turkey	Poult
Guinea fowl	Male Guinea fowl	Female Guinea fowl	Keet
Goose	Gander	Goose	Gosling
Pigeon	Male pigeon	Female pigeon	Squab
Swan	Male swan	Female swan	Signet

EXERCISE

A. Objective Questions

i. Indicate the correct answer by putting tick (√) mark (multiple choice).

1. The headquarter of CARI is at
   (a) Izatnagar
   (b) Hissar
   (c) Bengaluru
   (d) Hyderabad

2. The Central Poultry Development Organisation (CPDO) is located at
   (a) Bengaluru
   (b) Bhubaneswar
   (c) Chandigarh
   (d) All of these

3. The Project Directorate on Poultry is located at
   (a) Bengaluru
   (b) Bhubaneswar
   (c) Hyderabad
   (d) Izatnagar

4. The Centre for Advanced Studies in Poultry Science is located at
   (a) Mannuthy, Kerala
   (b) Namakkal, Tamil Nadu
   (c) Both a and b
   (d) None of these

5. Presently the four Random Sample Poultry Performance Testing Centres (RSPPTCs) are merged with the respective CPDOs except one which is located at
   (a) Bengaluru
   (b) Mumbai
   (c) Gurgaon
   (d) Bhubaneswar

6. The rank of India in chicken population in the world is
   (a) 3rd
   (b) 5th
   (c) 7th
   (d) 18th

7. Which state leads in poultry population in India?
   (a) Tamil Nadu
   (b) Andhra Pradesh
   (c) West Bengal
   (d) Maharashtra

8. Present per capita availability of eggs in India is
   (a) 33
   (b) 38
   (c) 40
   (d) 55

9. The recommended minimum per capita consumption of egg as per NIN is
   (a) 34
   (b) 46
   (c) 100
   (d) 180

10. *Vanaraja* and *Gramapriya,* the two important synthetic strains, were evolved for free range backyard farming in rural and tribal areas at
    (a) CARI, Izatnagar
    (b) PD on Poultry, Hydearabad
    (c) CPDO, Chandigarh
    (d) None of these

ii. Fill in the blanks.

1. The study of _____ is called Poultry Science and the study of birds is called _____.

2. The term 'poultry' is very often used as synonymous to _____ as it accounts for more than _____% of the total poultry population in India.

3. The new born fowl is called _____ and the new born duck is called _____.

4. Per capita egg consumption is _____ in India, whereas the world average is _____ (write the figures).

5. The full form of CARI is _____.

6. The headquarter of CARI is located at _____.

7. The full form of CPDO is _____.

8. In India, so far poultry population is concerned _____ is next to chicken.

9. _____ (state) leads in poultry production in India.

10. Currently, poultry production is growing at the rate of _____ per cent per annum in broilers and _____ per cent per annum in layers.

iii. Write True (T) or False (F) against each statement.

1. More than 90% of Indian poultry birds are chicken.

2. Poultry sector alone contributes about 2% of the total GDP of India and it is becoming a significant contributor to Indian economy.

3. China is the highest egg producing and second highest chicken meat producing country in the world.

4. Most of the poultry in China is in the form of backyard poultry or in unorganised sector.

5. Per capita egg production in Andhra Pradesh is 238, whereas the Indian average is only 53 (as per 2007 statistics).

6. At present, India ranks among the top 5 nations in egg production in the world.

7. In India, the fowl population has increased by about 4.5% during the period of 2003 to 2007.

8. A synthetic strain of poultry *Krishibro* was evolved for small scale intensive broiler farming at CPDO, Bhubaneswar.

9. On an average a laying hen produces about 60 kg fresh droppings per year.

10. Feed is the major item of expenditure in poultry rearing.

B. Subjective Questions

1. What is poultry? Highlight the importance of poultry farming in alleviating rural poverty in your state. Which state leads in poultry production in India?

2. Discuss in detail about the scope and future prospects of poultry industry in India. Mention the present per capita availability of eggs in India.

3. Write a note on present position of poultry development in India.

4. What do you mean by the term 'poultry'? What changes have come about in the sphere of poultry production in India during the last decade?

5. Write short notes on the following.

    (a) Poultry statistics in India

    (b) CARI

    (c) CPDO

    (d) Poultry manure—a valuable fertiliser

    (e) Random sample test

Answers of the Objective Questions

i. Multiple choice

1. (a) Izatnagar   2. (d) All of these   3. (c) Hyderabad

4. (c) Both a and b   5. (c) Gurgaon   6. (b) 5th

7. (a) Tamil Nadu (as per 18th Census, 2007)   8. (d) 55

9. (d) 180   10. (b) PD on Poultry, Hyderabad

ii. Fill in the blanks

1. poultry birds, ornithology   2. chicken/fowl, 90

3. chick, duckling   4. 55, 124

5. Central Avian Research Institute   6. Izatnagar, Uttar Pradesh

7. Central Poultry Development Organisation   8. duck

9. Tamil Nadu   10. 12, 6

iii. True or False

1. T   2. T   3. T   4. T   5. T

6. T   7. F   8. F   9. T   10. T

2
Breeds and Varieties of Poultry

2.1 CLASSIFICATION OF POULTRY

Poultry may be classified as follows:

i. Poultry is a common term, which includes a number of avian species reared for egg and/or meat. These are chicken or fowl, duck, turkey, quail, Guinea fowl, goose, pheasant, *etc*. The different species of poultry have definite number of chromosomes (2n). For example, chicken has 78 chromosomes, duck 80, turkey 82, Japanese quail 78, Guinea fowl 80, goose 80 and pheasant 82.

ii. Chickens or fowls (popularly known as 'poultry' due to their predominance) are commonly grouped into various classes on the basis of their origins. These are American class (e.g. Rhode Island Red, New Hampshire), English class (e.g. Australorp, Sussex), Mediterranean class (e.g. Leghorn, Minorca) and Asiatic class (e.g. Aseel, Langshan).

iii. Fowls may be classified on the basis of their utilities as (a) egg type (e.g. White Leghorn), (b) meat type (e.g. Cornish), (c) dual type—both egg and meat type (e.g. Rhode Island Red) and (d) game birds (e.g. Red Malay game). The birds of different utility groups have different shapes and depths of their bodies. Egg type (layer) chickens have triangular body, dual purpose chickens have rectangular body, and meat type (broiler) chickens have round body.

iv. They may be classified on the basis of their body weights as (a) heavy breeds (e.g. Rhode Island Red, Sussex) and (b) light breeds (e.g. White Leghorn).

v. They may be classified on the basis of their broodiness as (a) Sitter (e.g. Indian *deshi* birds and (b) non-sitter (e.g. White Leghorn, Minorca).

2.2 ZOOLOGICAL CLASSIFICATION OF VARIOUS POULTRY SPECIES

It is believed that the modern domestic fowls have been originated from red jungle fowl (*Gallus gallus*). India and its neighbouring countries are considered to be the home of this red jungle fowl. The zoological classification of various poultry species is depicted here.

Kingdom: Animalia
Phylum: Chordata (having backbone)
Subphylum: Vertebrata (having spinal column)
Class: Aves (feathered, warm blooded, 4-chambered heart)
Subclass: Neornithes (having no tooth)

Order	Family	Genus and species (scientific name)	Common name
Galliformes (birds with short wings and legs, and toes adapted for scratching and running)	Phasianidae	*Gallus domesticus*	Domestic chicken
		Coturnix japonica	Japanese quail
		Pavo cristatus	Pea fowl
		Phasianus colchicus	Pheasant
	Meleagrididae	*Meleagris gallopavo*	Turkey
	Numididae	*Numida meleagris*	Guinea fowl
Anseriformes (aquatic birds)	Anatidae	*Anas platyrhynchos*	Duck
		Cairina moschata	Muscovy duck
		Anser anser	Goose
Columbiformes	Columbidae	*Columba livia*	Pigeon
Struthioniformes (ratite group)	Casuariidae	*Dromaius novaehollandiae*	Emu
	Struthionidae	*Struthio camelus*	Ostrich

Source: Adopted from Hale, 1962. In: The Behaviour of Domestic Animals. ESE Hafez (edit.) London, Tindall and Cox. and Wikipedia, an internet encyclopedia.

2.3 IDEA ABOUT THE TERMS SPECIES, CLASS, BREED, VARIETY AND STRAIN OF POULTRY

Species: It is a group of living organisms consisting of similar individuals, capable of exchanging genes or interbreeding and is considered as the basic unit of taxonomy. The important poultry species in Indian poultry industry scenario are:

i. Chicken/fowl—*Gallus domesticus* (reared for egg and meat)

ii. Duck—*Anas platyrhynchos* (mainly reared for egg and to some extent meat)

iii. Japanese quail—*Coturnix japonica* (mainly reared for meat and also egg)

iv. Turkey—*Meleagris gallopavo* (mainly reared for meat)

Class: It indicates group of breeds developed in a particular geographical area. Class denotes the place or origin of the breed. The breeds of chicken are mainly classified into 4 classes, viz. American class, English class, Mediterranean class and Asiatic class.

Breed: A group of birds which are similar in shape, size and body conformation, and descendants of common ancestry is known as breed. It largely denotes the shape and size of the birds. All the birds of a breed have more or less same genetic makeup with common morphological and physiological setups. The examples of some breeds of chicken are White Leghorn, Rhode Island Red, New Hampshire, Australorp, Sussex, Aseel, *etc.*

Variety: It is the subdivision of a breed distinguished mainly by colour of plumage and type of comb. In other words, variety denotes the plumage colour and/or type of comb of the birds. For example, Plymouth Rock breed of chicken has 7 varieties, viz. barred, white, buff, silver-penciled, partridge, columbian and blue. Rhode Island Red breed has 2 varieties, viz. single comb and rose comb.

Strain: It indicates a group of birds with some special characters within a breed or variety. It is developed by a breeder by introducing some economic characters like egg size, growth rate, feed efficiency, laying ability, mortality, *etc.* Nowadays strain is more popular than breed. For example, Anak-2000, Hubbard, CARIBRO-91, Vencob, Starbro are some broiler strains of chicken.

2.4 EXTERNAL BODY PARTS OF POULTRY

The knowledge of external body parts of poultry helps in (a) studying the breed characteristics and identifying breeds of poultry, (b) selection and culling of birds (layer vs non-layer), (c) identification of sexes (male vs female), and (d) proper application of poultry husbandry practices.

The terms used to denote different body parts of chicken are:

a. **Head region:** Comb, beak, nostril, eye, ear, ear lobe, wattle

b. **Neck region:** Neck, neck feather (hackle), cape (a feather just after hackle, only present in male)

c. **Body:**

   Back—back, back plumage, saddle (only in male)

   Breast—breast, breast plumage, breast bone (keel)

   Wings—wing, wing front (a feather), wing bow (a feather), flight feathers of wing

   Abdomen—abdomen, abdominal feather (fluff)

   Tail—main tail feather (flight feather of tail), greater sickle feather (only in male), lesser sickle feather

   Legs—thigh, thigh plumage, hock, shank, claw, toes, nails, spur (only in male)

External body parts of chicken and duck are presented in Figs 2.1 and 2.2 respectively.

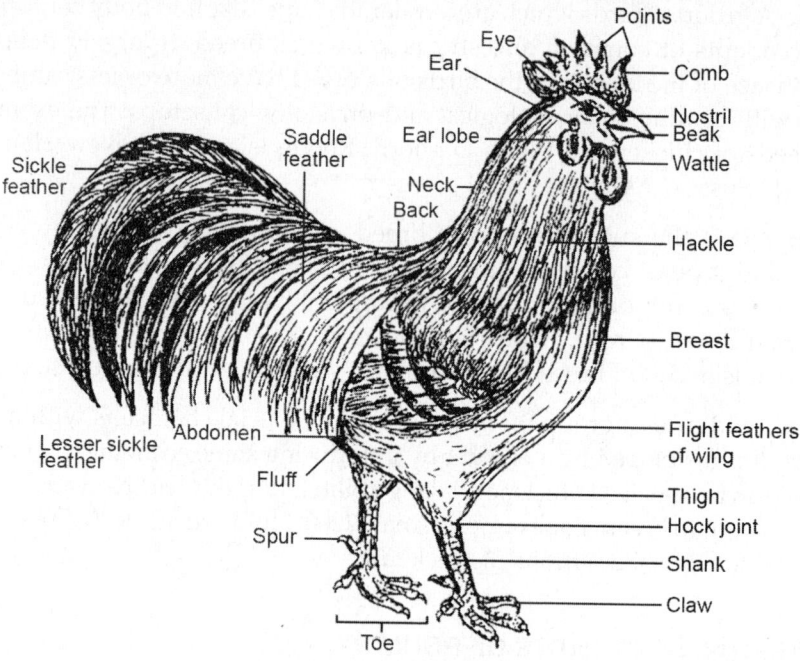

Fig. 2.1: External body parts of a chicken

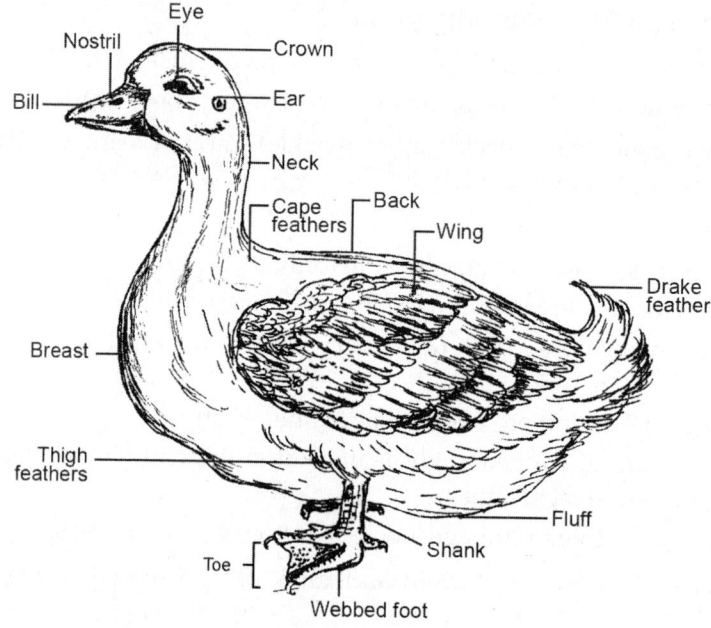

Fig. 2.2: External body parts of a duck

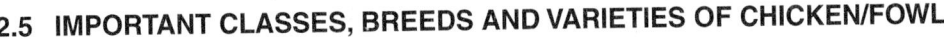

2.5 IMPORTANT CLASSES, BREEDS AND VARIETIES OF CHICKEN/FOWL

All the chicken breeds of the world are classified into 4 classes on the basis of their origins. These are American class, English class, Mediterranean class and Asiatic class. The breeds of each class have some common characteristics. Important breeds and varieties of chickens of the 4 classes are given in Table 2.1 and Fig. 2.3.

Table 2.1: Classes, breeds and varieties of chickens

Class	Breed	Variety
American class [Non-feathered and yellow shank, yellow skin, red ear lobes, brown-shelled egg (except Lamona), specially bred for dual purpose.]	• Rhode Island Red	Single comb and rose comb.
	• New Hampshire	—
	• Plymouth Rock	Barred, white, buff, silver-penciled, partridge, columbian and blue. *The Barred and the white varieties are popular.*
	• Wyandotte	White, buff, black, silver-laced, golden-laced, silver-penciled, columbian and partridge.
English class [Non-feathered shank, white skin (except Cornish which has yellow skin), red ear lobes, brown-shelled egg (except Dorking and Red Cap), primarily meat type breed having excellent fleshing properties.]	• Australorp	—
	• Cornish	White, dark, white-laced red. *White Cornish is the most popular as meat type breed.*
	• Sussex	Light, red and speckled.
	• Orpington	Single comb (white, buff, black and blue).
Mediterranean class [Non-feathered and yellow shank (except Black Minorca in which shank is slate coloured), yellow or white skin, white or creamy white ear lobes, relatively large comb, white-shelled egg, non-broodiness, early maturity, primarily egg type breeds]	• Leghorn	Single comb (white, buff, black, silver, red, black-tailed red, columbian, dark brown and light brown), and rose comb (white, dark brown and light brown). *Single comb white leghorn is the most popular as egg type breed.*
	• Minorca	Single comb (black, white, buff) and rose comb (black, white). *Single comb Black Minorca is the most popular.*
	• Ancona	Single comb and rose comb.

Contd.

Table 2.1: Classes, breeds and varieties of chickens *(Contd.)*

Class	Breed	Variety
Asiatic class [Feathered shank, yellow skin (except Black Langshan in which skin is pinkish white), red ear lobes, brown-shelled egg, generally poor layers, and miscellaneous type breeds. Unfortunately the breeds of this class are on the verge of extinction.]	• Brahma • Cochin (Sanghai fowl) • Langshan	Light, dark and buff. White, black, buff and partridge. White and black.

NB: A number of exotic breeds of chicken are listed in the American Standard of Perfection (published by American Poultry Association), out of these only few are important in India. These are White Leghorn, Rhode Island Red, New Hampshire, Plymouth Rock (barred and white varieties), Australorp and White Cornish.

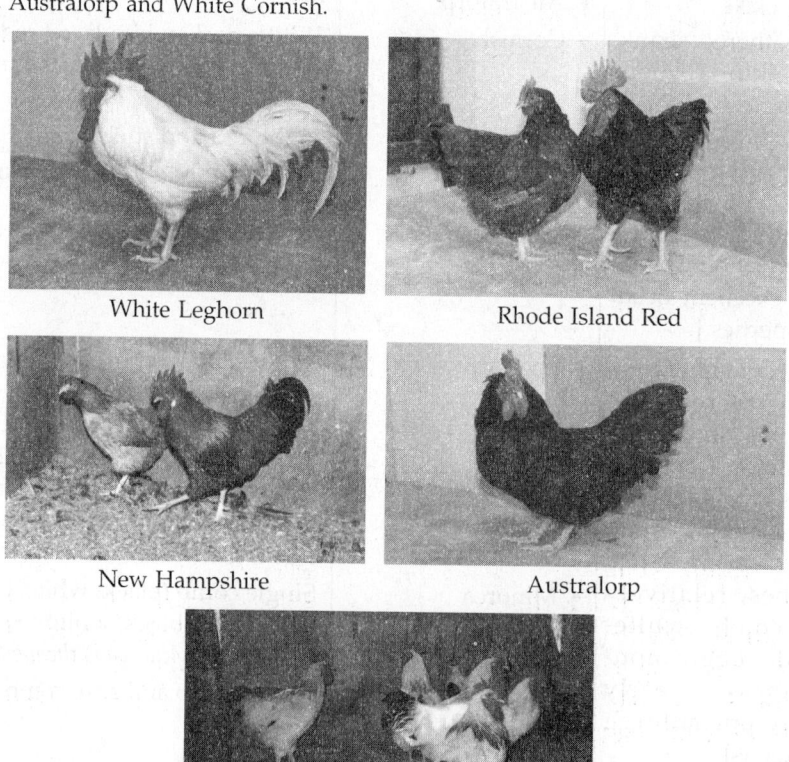

White Leghorn

Rhode Island Red

New Hampshire

Australorp

Light Sussex

Fig. 2.3: Various breeds of chicken

2.5.1 Popular Crosses of Chicken

Nowadays, pure breeds of chicken are not generally used for commercial production of egg or meat. Most of the present day commercial chickens are crosses of different breeds, varieties or strains. They are popularly called hybrid chickens. Single comb White Leghorn is widely used as the genetic base for production of white egg layer crosses and Rhode Island Red, New Hampshire, Australorp, Barred Plymouth Rock and Dahlem Red, *etc.* are used as the genetic base for brown egg layer crosses. White Plymouth Rock is commonly used as female parent line and White Cornish as male parent line for production of meat type (broiler) crosses. However, for production of coloured broiler other breeds are also used. The main advantage of these crosses is that they perform better than their parents due to heterotic effects in them. Some important breed crosses and strain crosses of chickens are given below.

Breed Crosses

1. **Austra-White:** It is a dual purpose cross. The Australorp male is crossed with White Leghorn female to produce this breed cross. Both the sexes are nearly white with occasional black speckles on feathers.

2. **Red-Rock:** The Rhode Island Red (or New Hampshire) male is crossed with Barred Plymouth Rock female to produce this breed cross. The male progenies are barred and females are black. Day-old sexing is possible on the basis of colour pattern only due to sex-linked inheritance.

3. **Rhodo-White:** The Rhode Island Red male is crossed with White Leghorn female to produce this breed cross. White plumage is dominant with occasional blackish feathers.

4. **Sussex-Hampshire:** The Sussex male is crossed with New Hampshire female to produce this breed cross.

Strain Crosses

1. **Broiler strains:** CARIBRO Vishal (CARI), CARIBRO Dhanraja (CARI), Giriraja (UAS, Bengaluru), IBB-83 (UAS, Bengaluru), Hubbard (Kasila Farms, Hyderabad), Vencob (Venco Research and Breeding Farms, Pune), Anak-2000 (Tarakeshwara Hatchery, Nasik), Chabro (CPBF, Chandigarh), *etc.*

2. **Layer strains:** HH-260 (CPBF, Hessarghata), BH-78 (CPBF, Mumbai), CARI Priya (earlier known as ILI-80) (CARI), Kalinga hybrid (CPBF, Bhubaneswar), CARI Sonali (earlier known as CARI GOLDEN-92, CARI), BV-300 and BV-380 (Venkateshwara Hatchery), Starcross-288 (Ranishaver Hatchery), *etc.*

2.5.2 Characteristics of Common Exotic Breeds of Chicken

Rhode Island Red (RIR)

Origin	Its origin is Rhode Island State of America. It was developed by crossing between Brahma or Langshan and the Chittagong fowls in early 1900s. It is a breed of American class.
General appearance	Long rectangular body, broad and deep breast, flat back and massive look. They have 2 varieties—single comb and rose comb, of which single comb variety is more popular.
Plumage colour	Brownish red and well glossed. Main tail feathers and sickle feathers (in male) are black. In females, hackle (neck feather) shows slight black marking at the base.
Standard weight	Cock 3.8 kg, hen 3.0 kg
Skin colour	Yellow
Colour of ear lobe	Reddish
Colour of beak	Blackish
Shank	Yellow coloured, clean
Eggshell colour	Brown
Commercial importance	Dual purpose for egg and meat. They can produce approximately 230 eggs per year. More resistant to diseases than other exotic breeds, used for upgrading the local/*deshi* stock. Slow feathering character is a minus point of this breed. It is very popular in rural areas of tropical countries. This breed is a good choice for small flock owner.

New Hampshire

Origin	Its origin is New Hampshire State of America. It is a breed of American class. This breed was developed from Rhode Island Red (RIR) through selective breeding.
General appearance	Less rectangular than RIR. They have single comb.
Plumage colour	Chestnut red. Main tail feathers are black. In females, lower neck feathers are distinctly tipped with black.
Standard weight	Cock 3.8 kg, hen 3.0 kg
Skin colour	Yellow
Colour of ear lobe	Reddish
Colour of beak	Yellow
Shank	Yellow, clean
Eggshell colour	Brown
Commercial importance	Dual purpose for egg and meat. Early maturity and quick feathering are particular features of this breed.

Plymouth Rock

Origin	This breed was developed by crossing between Domonique and Black Cochin. It is a breed of American class. Out of various varieties, the Barred and the White Plymouth Rocks are popular. The barred variety of the breed was developed in around 1865.
General appearance	Long body with fairly prominent breast, large body size. They have single comb.
Plumage colour	White variety has white plumage. Barred Plymouth Rock has greyish-white plumage. The feathers are crossed by black bars. In males, the black and white bars are of equal length; whereas in females, the black bars are 1½ times wider than the white bars.
Standard weight	Cock 4.3 kg, hen 3.4 kg
Skin colour	Yellow
Colour of ear lobe	Red
Shank	Yellow coloured, clean
Eggshell colour	Brown
Commercial importance	Widely used for development of commercial broiler and synthetic lines.

Wyandotte

Origin	It is a breed of American class.
General appearance	Circular body. They have rose comb.
Plumage colour	Plumage colour depends on the varieties of the breed like white, buff, black, *etc.*
Standard weight	Cock 3.8 kg, hen 3.0 kg
Skin colour	Yellow
Colour of ear lobe	Red
Colour of beak	Yellow
Shank	Yellow coloured, clean
Eggshell colour	Brown
Commercial importance	Dual purpose for egg and meat. It can perform well both in range and intensive conditions.

Australorp

Origin	It was basically developed in Australia from Black Orpington for egg purpose, and after a long time it has been selectively bred in Britain for meat. It is a breed of English class.
General appearance	Very fleshy, body slopes gradually towards tail, deep body, closely feathered, long back, more upright and less massive look. They have single comb.

Plumage colour	Black, plumage is lustrous and greenish black in all the sections of the body. The under colouring is dull black.
Standard weight	Cock 3.8 kg, hen 3.0 kg
Skin colour	White
Colour of ear lobe	Red
Colour of beak	Black
Shank	Black or dark slate coloured, clean
Eggshell colour	Brown
Commercial importance	It is used as a layer or a dual purpose breed. They can maintain themselves in wet and heavy rainfall areas.

Light Sussex

Origin	It was developed around 1900 in the county of Sussex, England. It is a light variety of Sussex breed of English class.
General appearance	Long and deep body with very good fleshing quality, broad shoulder. They have single comb.
Plumage colour	The breed has white plumage with a black tail and black wing tips, its neck is white striped with black and has a very striking appearance.
Standard weight	Cock 4.0 kg, hen 3.0 kg
Skin colour	White
Colour of ear lobe	Red
Colour of beak	Horn coloured
Shank	White coloured, clean
Eggshell colour	Brown
Commercial importance	They have excellent fleshing property. They are comfortable in both free range or confined conditions. Sussex is one of the oldest breeds of chicken that still exists today.

Cornish

Origin	This breed was selectively bred in Cornwell, Britain. It was developed by crossing Aseel/Malay with English Game breed. It is a heavy breed of English class.
General appearance	Closely feathered very compact body distinctly shaped with heavy flesh, broad and deep breast. All birds have pea comb.
Plumage colour	The white, the dark and the white laced red are the 3 colour varieties. White Cornish is the most popular as meat type breed.
Standard weight	Cock 4.5 kg, hen 3.2 kg
Skin colour	Yellow
Colour of ear lobe	Red
Colour of beak	Yellow

Shank	Yellow coloured, clean
Eggshell colour	Brown
Commercial importance	They have excellent fleshing property. It is used for broiler production. It is believed that most of the male lines used for commercial broiler production, probably contain 50% or more Cornish blood.

Orpington

Origin	It was developed in England at the town of Orpington in County Kent during the 1880s. It is a breed of English class.
General appearance	Long, deep and well rounded body with full breast and broad back, very closely feathered. They have single comb. Soft almost fluffy appearance together with their rich colours and gentle contours make them very attractive.
Plumage colour	The colour varieties of this breed are buff, black, white and blue.
Standard weight	Cock 4.5 kg, hen 3.5 kg
Skin colour	White
Colour of ear lobe	Red
Shank	Bluish coloured, clean
Eggshell colour	Brown
Commercial importance	They have excellent fleshing property.

White Leghorn (WLH)

Origin	Its origin is from Leghorn village of Italy. It is a breed of Mediterranean class.
General appearance	Small and very compact, small head with well set comb and wattle, long back, prominent breast, tail lowered down and it is the neatest of all birds. They have single and rose comb, of which single comb White Leghorn is the most popular.
Plumage colour	White, evenly distributed over the entire body surface.
Standard weight	Cock 2.7 kg, hen 2.0 kg
Skin colour	Yellow
Colour of ear lobe	Yellowish white
Colour of beak	Yellow
Shank	Yellow coloured, clean
Eggshell colour	White
Commercial importance	Excellent producer of large white eggs. It has no tendency to deposit body fat and feed consumption is less (around 110 g per day during laying period). It is regarded as the egg laying champion of the world. All the commercial hybrid layers are derived from this breed.

Minorca

Origin	It is a breed of Mediterranean class.
General appearance	It is the largest and heaviest breed of the Mediterranean class. They have long and strong body, large comb and long wattles. They have single comb.
Plumage colour	Black, white or buff as per the respective variety. The black colour is more popular.
Standard weight	Cock 3.5–4.0 kg, hen 2.8–3.0 kg
Skin colour	Black/blue/white
Colour of ear lobe	White
Colour of beak	Black
Shank	Black coloured, clean
Eggshell colour	White
Commercial importance	Egg type bird. It stands second among the egg laying breeds in the world.

Ancona

Origin	Its origin is believed to be the Ancona city of Italy. It is a breed of Mediterranean class.
General appearance	They resemble Leghorn in shape and size. They are small, active and alert. They have single and rose combs.
Plumage colour	Black with white tipped feathers
Standard weight	Cock 2.5 kg, hen 2.0 kg
Skin colour	Yellow
Colour of ear lobe	White
Colour of beak	Yellow
Shank	Yellow coloured, clean
Eggshell colour	White
Commercial importance	Egg type bird

Brahma

Origin	This breed was originated in the Brahmaputra valley. The ancestral type of this breed is known as 'Grey Chittagongs'. It is a breed of Asiatic class.
General appearance	Large massive body with heavy bones, well-feathered. They have pea comb.
Plumage colour	They have 3 varieties—light, dark and buff. Their intricate colour patterns make them show bird.
Standard weight	Cock 5.4 kg, hen 4.3 kg
Skin colour	Yellow
Colour of ear lobe	Red
Colour of beak	Yellow

Shank	Yellow coloured, feathered
Eggshell colour	Tinted brown
Commercial importance	Meat type breed. This breed was exported to America and England during 19th century for development of American/English breeds.

Cochin

Origin	This breed was originated in Sanghai region of China. It is also known as 'Sanghai fowl'. It is a breed of Asiatic class.
General appearance	Large massive body with long and profuse feathering, heavily feathered shank. They have single comb.
Plumage colour	Colour varieties of this breed are buff, black, white and partridge.
Standard weight	Cock 5.0 kg, hen 3.8 kg
Skin colour	Yellow
Colour of ear lobe	Red
Shank	Black coloured, feathered
Eggshell colour	Brown
Commercial importance	Meat type breed

Langshan

Origin	This breed was originated in Langshan region of China. It is a breed of Asiatic class.
General appearance	Circular body, upstanding with high tail carriage. They have single comb.
Plumage colour	White and black are two main varieties of this breed.
Standard weight	Cock 3.8 kg, hen 3.4 kg
Skin colour	Brown/black
Colour of ear lobe	Red
Shank	Yellow coloured, feathered
Eggshell colour	Brown
Commercial importance	Meat type breed

2.5.3 Indigenous Fowl in India

Presently, 15 indigenous breeds of fowl are recognised in India (NBAGR, ICAR, 2012). They are more resistant to many poultry diseases, good foragers, and very good mother for hatching of eggs. Some of them have better meat quality, and some look like Leghorn in shape and size, but poor in layers. Nowadays some of these indigenous breeds are used for development of suitable variety for rural poultry production. The names of the registered indigenous or deshi breeds of fowls in India are Ankaleshwar, Aseel, Busra, Chittagong, Danki, Doathigir, Ghagus, Haringhata Black, Kadaknath, Kalasthi, Kashmiri Favorolla, Miri, Nicobari, Punjab Brown and Tellichery.

A short description of indigenous fowls with their home tracts is presented in Table 2.2.

Table 2.2: Characteristics of indigenous fowls in India

Sl no.	Name of the breed	Home tract	Characteristics	Remarks
1.	Ankaleshwar	Bharuch and Narmada districts of Gujarat	Golden yellow plumage colour in cocks and black golden in hens are common, however, it may vary from a combination of white and light grey to brown and golden. The age at 1st laying is 6 months, annual egg production 75–80, and average body weight at 12 weeks of age is 830 g in male and 750 g in female.	The name is given according to its origin at Ankaleshwar in Bharuch district of Gujarat. Also known as *gowrani*, *gamthi* and *deshi*. It is a dual purpose breed.
2.	Aseel	Andhra Pradesh, Chhattisgarh and Odisha	Biggest in size among indigenous breeds, measures 28 inches from back to toe. Well-known for its high stamina, majestic gait and dogged fighting quality. Standard body weight: Cock 4–5 kg and hen 3–4 kg	Renowned game bird; also known for its delicious and flavoured meat. Its varieties are Noorie (white), Peela (golden yellow), Kagar (black), Yakub (black and red), Chitta (black and white), Sabja (white and golden), Java, Teekar and Reja (light red).
3.	Busra	Gujarat and Maharashtra	There is wide variation in plumage colour. They are small to medium in size. It is deep bodied, light feathered and alert.	They are found in small numbers.
4.	Chittagong	Eastern India, Meghalaya and Tripura (and also in Bangladesh)	Plumage colour may be buff, white, black, grey or dark brown. It is a large bird. The breast is broad and deep. The legs are yellow with fewer feathers. The head is long. Beak is long and yellow. They have small pea comb, red wattles, and usually red ear lobes. Standard body weight: Cock 3.5–4.5 kg and hen 3–4 kg	Also known as *Malay*.

Contd.

Table 2.2: Characteristics of indigenous fowls in India *(Contd.)*

Sl no.	Name of the breed	Home tract	Characteristics	Remarks
5.	**Danki**	Andhra Pradesh	The birds have glossy and lustrous plumage and compressed single comb. The males have long legs and long neck. This breed is fairly heavy. Standard body weight: Cock 3.1 kg and hen 2.2 kg	They are fairly resistant to some of the common poultry diseases, and good fighters.
6.	**Daothigir**	Assam	Stripped or spotted plumage pottern, plumage colour is black interspersed with white feathers, single comb. Average weight: Cock 1.8 kg and hen 1.6 kg. Their annual production is about 60–70 eggs weighing 42–48 g each.	It is mostly reared by Bodo community.
7.	**Ghagus**	Andhra Pradesh and Karnataka	This breed is smaller in size. They have single comb, thick neck and feathered shank. Average weight: Cock 2.2 kg and hen 1.4 kg	They are mostly reared by nomadic tribes, and fairly resistant to common poultry diseases.
8.	**Haringhata Black**	West Bengal	Plumage colour is black; body is small with typical layer type conformation.	The population is declining fast.
9.	**Kadaknath**	Jhabua and Dhar districts in western Madhya Pradesh	Plumage colour varies from silver and gold-spangled to bluish-black without any spangling. It is a small bird. The skin, beak, shank, toe and sole of feet are slate coloured; comb, wattle and tongue are purple. Most of the internal organs show black colouration due to deposition of melanin pigment. Hen lays about 80–95 eggs in a year. Standard body weight: Cock 1.5 kg and hen 1.0 kg	Known as *Kalamasi* because of its black flesh. The flesh is ugly looking, but delicious in taste.
10.	**Kalasthi**	Andhra Pradesh	This breed is smaller in size. Males have long legs and long neck. Plumage colour bluish black, neck is covered with golden feathers. Average weight: Cock 2.5 kg and hen 1.9 kg	They are fairly resistant to some of the common poultry diseases, and good fighters.

Contd.

Table 2.2: Characteristics of indigenous fowls in India *(Contd.)*

Sl no.	Name of the breed	Home tract	Characteristics	Remarks
11.	**Kashmir Favorolla**	Jammu and Kashmir	Body is small. The comb is small and feathered. Average egg weight is 45 g. Plumage colour is mixed shades of black, red, green and gold. Average weight: Cock 1.2 kg	Feathered comb or feathered cap on head is a special character.
12.	**Miri**	Dhemaji, Lakhimpur and Sivasagar districts of Assam	They are small and black. Body weight is 1–1.5 kg. Sometimes frizzle feathers, necked neck and feathered shank are observed. Plumage colour is white and brown.	Mostly reared by Miri tribes.
13.	**Nicobari**	Andaman and Nicobar Islands	This breed is medium in size. They have compact body, short legs, short and thick neck, mostly single comb and pinkish wattles and ear lobes. The breast is bulging in front, tail feathers are medium and saddle feathers are long. It is of 3 colour varieties, viz. black, brown and white. Their annual production is about 120–140 eggs weighing 40–45 g each. Average weight: Cock 1.8 kg and hen 1.3 kg	Also known as *Takniet Hyum* due to their short legs. They are fairly resistant to common poultry diseases like Ranikhet disease and Marek's disease. They are very good scavenging birds.
14.	**Punjab Brown**	Punjab and Haryana	Brown plumage, yellow beak and legs are common. The average weight: Cock 2.2 kg and hen 1.6 kg	It is a meat type breed.
15.	**Tellichery**	Kerala	Body is small; common plumage colour is black to grey with shining bluish tinge. Average weight: Cock 1.6 kg and hen 1.2 kg	The meat is said to have medicinal value.

2.6 BREEDS OF DUCK

Duck breeds are broadly classified into three types, viz.

1. Egg type ducks, e.g. Khaki Campbell, Indian Runner
2. Meat type ducks, e.g. Aylesbury, White Pekin, Rouen, Cayuga, Muscovy duck
3. Ornamental type ducks, e.g. Call, Crested White, Carolina, Mandarin, Black East India

Indian breeds of ducks: There are some special types of ducks available in various parts of our country, however, they may not be called as breed. Nageswari, Sylhet Mete and Pati hans are found in north eastern parts. Kuttand duck is found in Kerala. It has 2 varieties, viz. Chara and Chemballi. Other 2 native ducks are Moti (meat type) and Khaki (egg type).

2.6.1 Characteristics of Common Breeds of Ducks

Khaki Campbell

- This breed of duck was developed in England by crossing between Rouen, Mallard, and Fawn and White Indian Runner. It was developed by Mrs A Campbell in 1901 in England and it has 'khaki' coloured plumage, so named as 'Khaki Campbell'. Campbell duck has 3 varieties, viz. khaki, dark and white; out of which Khaki Campbell is most popular for egg production.
- The average body weight: Duck 2.0–2.2 kg and Drake 2.2–2.4 kg
- Ducks lay about 300 eggs per year with egg size 70 g. They start to lay at the age of 18 weeks.
- They do not require water for swimming. So they can be reared under complete confinement, where there is no facility of pond and range land.

Indian Runner

- Body is well carried up in front and shape is as good as that of penguin. The common popular varieties of this breed are white, white-penciled and fawn. They have a characteristic lean appearance.
- The average body weight: Duck 1.5–2.0 kg and Drake 2.0–2.5 kg
- They can lay 250–300 eggs per year. They are good forager and hardy, and they can maintain themselves in all types of climates and localities.

Aylesbury

- It is a good table duck. Plumage colour is completely white and they produce creamy white meat. Their leg and feet are bright orange and bill is yellow in colour.
- The average body weight: Duck 3.5–4.0 kg and drake 4.5 kg
- Initially large scale duck breeding was carried out in Aylesbury in Buckinghamshire in the UK. So the duck name is 'Aylesbury'.

White Pekin

- It is very popular table duck. Its genetic development was carried out in the USA, but its origin is in China in the year 1873. Plumage colour of this duck is creamy white, bill and legs are deep orange. They lay about 160 eggs in first laying year and they are very fertile.

- The average body weight: Duck 3.5 kg and drake 4.0 kg
- White Pekin was a table delicacy of Chinese Emperors. So they are also known as Emperor Duck.

2.7 VARIETIES OF QUAIL

Quail is recently domesticated species of poultry. It is also called *'Bater'* in Hindi and *'Titir Pakhi'* in Bengali. This bird was firstly used in Japan for production of egg and meat. So it is known as Japanese quail (*Coturnix japonica*). The important varieties of Japanese quail on the basis of plumage colour are:

1. **English White**—feather colour is white with or without few black spots.
2. **British Range**—feather colour is dark.
3. **Pharaoh** (wild type)—feather colour is mixture of black and brown.
4. **Tuxedo**—feather colour of face, neck and entire ventral surface is white and remaining part is black.
5. **Manchurian Golden**—feather colour is golden or light golden.

Many improved varieties of quail are evolved and maintained at CARI, Izatnagar for commercial exploitation of this species of poultry. These improved quail varieties are CARI Uttam (broiler), CARI Pearl (white egger), CARI Ujjwal (white breasted), CARI Sweta (white feathered), CARI Brown (brown feathered) and CARI Sunheri (brown feathered, white breasted).

CARI Uttam is a very good broiler quail which have better body weight (240 g) and feed conversion efficiency (2.60 at 5th week). CARI Pearl is a very good layer quail. Its body weight at 5th week is 140 g, hen lay egg production is 285–295 eggs and hatchability is 70–80%.

2.8 VARIETIES OF TURKEY

Turkey is not a popular species of poultry in India, but in western countries turkey is popular for meat production. Turkeys are not classified as breed. Eight standard varieties are being recognised by American Poultry Association. These are:

1. Bronze (sometimes referred to as Broad Breasted Bronze, BBB)
2. Beltsville Small White (BSW)
3. White Holland (sometimes referred to as Broad Breasted White)
4. Bourbon Red
5. Black
6. Slate
7. Narrangansett
8. Royal Palm

The recent day's turkeys were developed from North American wild turkey. The varieties of turkey differ in plumage colour, size and meat characteristics, but the shape is common in general. Out of the 8 varieties of turkey, BBB and BSW are important from which most of the varieties have been developed.

Broad Breasted Bronze (BBB)

- This is truly not a variety, but a non-standardised commercial strain. The origin of this strain of turkey is in England. Plumage colour is black and they are derived from 'Bronze' wild turkey.
- Sex determination can be done at the age of 12 weeks. The females are having white tipped black feathers at chest region.
- The body weight at marketing age: Females 6–7 kg at 22–25 weeks of age; males 10–14 kg at 27–29 weeks of age

Beltsville Small White (BSW)

- This variety of turkey is originated in Beltsville area of the USA. Plumage colour of this variety is white.
- They are smaller in size. The market weight is 4–5 kg at the age of 14 weeks under standard management practices.

2.9 VARIETIES OF GUINEA FOWL

There are three principal varieties of Guinea fowl available for rearing in India. These are Pearl, Lavender and White. Pearl variety has a purplish grey plumage, regularly dotted or 'pearled' with white. The Lavender Guinea resembles those of Pearl variety except the plumage which is light grey or lavender, regularly dotted with white. The White variety has pure white plumage. Its skin is lighter in colour than that of Pearl variety.

2.10 NEW COLOURED FEATHERED BIRDS DEVELOPED FOR RURAL POULTRY IN INDIA

A few new varieties of chicken have been developed in India for rural poultry farming. They are coloured feathered birds, and their plumage colours are just like our *deshi* birds. They are also called low-input technology birds. Their adaptability to natural feed resources and disease resistance are comparable to the *deshi* birds, but their productivity is better. So they are acceptable in rural and tribal areas of various parts of our country. For development of these new varieties of chicken, few Indian and exotic fowls were mainly used. The Indian breeds are Aseel, Kadaknath, Frizzle fowl, Naked neck and Nicobari fowl and the exotic breeds are White Leghorn, Red Cornish, Black Rock and Dahlem Red. A list of such new varieties of chicken is given in Table 2.3.

Table 2.3: New varieties of chicken for rural poultry farming in India

Sl no.	Name of variety	Type	Developed by
1.	CARI Gold	Egg	Central Avian Research Institute (CARI), Izatnagar, Bareilly, UP
2.	Gramapriya	Egg	Project Directorate on Poultry (PDP), Rajendranagar, Hyderabad 500030, Andhra Pradesh
3.	Gramalakshmi	Egg	Centre for Advance Studies in Poultry Science, College of Veterinary and Animal Sciences, Kerala Agricultural University (KAU), Mannuthy 560024
4.	Kalinga Brown	Egg	Central Poultry Breeding Farm, Bhubaneswar, Odisha
5.	Rajasri	Egg	AICRP on Poultry Improvement, Sri Venkateswara Veterinary University, Rejendranagar, Hyderabad 500030
6.	Swarnadhara	Egg	Department of Poultry Science, Karnataka Veterinary, Animal and Fishery Sciences University (KVAFSU), Hebbal, Bengaluru 560024
7.	CARI Nirbheek	Meat	CARI, Izatnagar
8.	CARI Shyama	Meat	CARI, Izatnagar
9.	Giriraja	Meat	KVAFSU, Bengaluru
10.	Chabro	Meat	PDP, CPDO (NR), Chandigarh
11.	Gramasree	Dual	KAU, Mannuthy
12.	Hitcari	Dual	CARI, Izatnagar
13.	Nandanam	Dual	Poultry Research Station, Nandanam, TANVASU, Chennai 600035
14.	Upcari	Dual	CARI, Izatnagar
15.	Vanaraja	Dual	PDP, Hyderabad
16.	Satpuda desi	Dual	Dr Yashvant Agritech Pvt Ltd, Jalgaon, Maharashtra
17.	Kuroiler	Dual	Kegg Farms, New Delhi
18.	Rainbow Rooster	Dual	Indbro Research and Breeding Farm Pvt Ltd, Hyderabad

Note: The first 15 low-input technology birds are of public sector organisations and last 3 birds are of private sector organisations.

2.11 VARIETIES OF CHICKEN FOR COMMERCIAL POULTRY FARMING IN INDIA

Although a number of poultry breeds are available in India, the Cobb 100 breed owned by Venkateshwara Hatcheries (VH) currently accounts for 60–70% of all broilers in India. The VH supplies its breed to broiler operators in the form of grandparents, parents or day-old chicks (DOCs). At present, all broilers supplied by VH are Cobb 100, relatively older breed based on breeding stock imported from the United States, which are adapted to Indian climatic and disease conditions. The other broiler/breeds present in India are Cobb 400 (a cross between Cobb 500 and Cobb 100), Ross (the UK), Hybro (Netherlands), Hubbard (the US), Avian (the US), and Anak (Israel). The exotic layer breeds available in the Indian market are Babcock (more than 80% of total layer), Hyline, Bovans, Hisex, Lohmann, *etc.* The different brands of hybrid DOCs are marketed by various companies in India (*See Chapter 14, Table 14.9*).

EXERCISE

A. Objective Questions

  i. **Indicate the correct answer by putting tick (√) mark (multiple choice).**

1. The origin of Rhode Island Red breed of poultry is
    (a) America (b) Australia
    (c) England (d) Italy

2. The origin of New Hampshire breed of poultry is
    (a) America (b) Australia
    (c) England (d) Italy

3. The origin of Australorp breed of poultry is
    (a) America (b) Australia
    (c) England (d) Italy

4. The origin of White Leghorn breed of poultry is
    (a) America (b) Australia
    (c) England (d) Italy

5. The origin of Light Sussex breed of poultry is
    (a) America (b) Australia
    (c) England (d) Italy

6. The origin of Aseel breed of poultry is
    (a) Italy (b) Spain
    (c) India (d) China

7. The origin of Cornish breed of poultry is
    (a) America (b) England
    (c) India (d) China

8. Which of the following is the best breed for egg production?
    (a) Plymouth Rock (b) White Cornish
    (c) Light Sussex (d) White Leghorn

9. Which one is not related with others so far colour of eggshell is concerned?
    (a) Cornish (b) New Hampshire
    (c) Australorp (d) Leghorn

10. Which one is a dual purpose breed of poultry?
    (a) Rhode Island Red   (b) White Leghorn
    (c) Cornish   (d) Aseel
11. Which one is an egg type breed of duck?
    (a) Indian Runner   (b) Pekin
    (c) Aylesbury   (d) Crested White
12. Which one is a meat type breed of duck?
    (a) Indian Runner   (b) Khaki Campbell
    (c) Aylesbury   (d) Call
13. Which is not a variety of turkey?
    (a) Broad Breasted Bronze   (b) White Holland
    (c) Crested White   (d) Beltsville Small White
14. Which one is a light breed of fowl?
    (a) Rhode Island Red   (b) New Hampshire
    (c) White Leghorn   (d) Australorp
15. Kalinga Brown, a new variety of poultry for rural poultry farming, is evolved
    at
    (a) CPBF, Chandigarh   (b) CARI, Izatnagar
    (c) CPBF, Bhubaneswar   (d) PD on Poultry, Hyderabad
16. The home tract of Aseel breed of fowl is
    (a) Odisha   (b) Andhra Pradesh
    (c) Haryana   (d) Gujarat
17. Which of the following is known as *Kalamasi* because of its black flesh?
    (a) Aseel   (b) Kadaknath
    (c) Chittagong   (d) Naked neck
18. Austra-White, a crossbred fowl for egg production, developed by crossing
    (a) Australorp male × White Leghorn female
    (b) Australorp male × New Hampshire female
    (c) Australorp male × White Plymouth Rock
    (d) Australorp male × White Cornish
19. The exotic breeds of poultry of American class are specially reared for
    (a) Egg   (b) Meat
    (c) Egg and meat   (d) Broiler
20. The exotic breeds of poultry of English class are specially reared for
    (a) Egg   (b) Meat
    (c) Egg and meat   (d) Broiler
21. The poultry breeds of Mediterranean class are specially considered for pro-
    duction of
    (a) Egg   (b) Meat
    (c) Egg and meat   (d) Broiler

22. Best broilers can be produced by crossing between
    (a) White Leghorn and White Plymouth Rock
    (b) Rhode Island Red and White Leghorn
    (c) White Cornish and White Plymouth Rock
    (d) White Cornish and Minorca

23. Australorp breed of poultry was developed in Australia from
    (a) Light Sussex
    (b) Black Orpington
    (c) Barred Plymouth Rock
    (d) Black Minorca

24. Which of the following breeds of poultry belongs to American class?
    (a) White Leghorn
    (b) New Hampshire
    (c) Langshan
    (d) Sussex

25. Which of the following breeds of poultry belongs to English class?
    (a) White Leghorn
    (b) New Hampshire
    (c) Langshan
    (d) Sussex

26. Which of the following is the best breed for broiler production?
    (a) Plymouth Rock
    (b) Langshan
    (c) Light Sussex
    (d) Rhode Island Red

27. Which of the following poultry breeds does not lay brown shelled eggs?
    (a) Leghorn
    (b) Australorp
    (c) Brahma
    (d) Rhode Island Red

28. The poultry bird Rhode Island Red has the following features.
    1. It belongs to American class.
    2. Shank is heavily feathered.
    3. Single and rose comb are two varieties.
    4. It lays brown shelled egg.
    Select the correct answer from the code below:
    Code (a) 1, 2, 3 and 4 are correct
    (b) 1, 2 and 3 are correct
    (c) 1, 3 and 4 are correct
    (d) 1, 2 and 4 are correct

29. White Leghorn bird can be identified by the following points.
    1. Its scientific name is *Gallus gallus*.
    2. It is the best egg producing breed of fowl.
    3. It has red comb and white ear lobe.
    4. Single comb of male erects at five regular points.
    Select the correct answer from the code below:
    Code (a) 1, 2, 3 and 4 are correct
    (b) 1, 2 and 3 are correct
    (c) 2, 3 and 4 are correct
    (d) 1, 2 and 4 are correct

30. Match List I with List II and select the correct answer using the code given below the lists.

List I	List II
A. The largest fowl breed	1. Light Sussex
B. White skin coloured bird	2. RIR
C. Dual purpose chicken breed	3. Aseel
D. Indian game bird	4. Brahma

Code (a)
A	B	C	D
2	1	4	3

(b)
A	B	C	D
2	3	4	1

(c)
A	B	C	D
4	1	2	3

(d)
A	B	C	D
1	2	3	4

ii. Fill in the Blanks.

1. *Gallus domesticus* is the scientific name of _____, and _____ is the scientific name of duck.
2. The scientific name of chicken is _____.
3. The scientific name of duck is _____.
4. The scientific name of quail is _____.
5. The scientific name of turkey is _____.
6. _____ breed of duck can be reared without the source of water for swimming.
7. _____ is a good egg type breed of chicken.
8. _____ is a good dual purpose breed of chicken.
9. White Leghorn belongs to _____ class of poultry.
10. New Hampshire/Rhode Island Red belongs to _____ class of poultry.
11. Australorp belongs to _____ class of poultry.
12. Plymouth Rock belongs to _____ class of poultry.
13. Sussex belongs to _____ class of poultry.
14. Cornish belongs to _____ class of poultry.
15. Chickens of _____ class always lay white shelled eggs.
16. New Hampshire breed was developed from _____ breed of poultry.
17. Pekin is a/an _____ type duck and _____ is an egg type duck.
18. The origin of Rhode Island Red breed is _____.
19. The origin of New Hampshire breed of poultry is _____.
20. The origin of White Leghorn breed of poultry is _____.
21. The origin of Australorp breed of poultry is _____.
22. The origin of Light Sussex breed of poultry is _____.
23. _____ is a very good egg type duck.

24. _____ is a meat type duck.
25. Manchurian golden is a variety of _____.
26. Broad Breasted Bronze is a variety of _____.
27. The home tract of Aseel breed of chicken is _____.
28. _____ is a variety of Guinea fowl.
29. Vanaraja is a/an _____ purpose new variety of poultry developed at PD on Poultry, Rajendranagar for rural poultry farming.
30. _____ is a dual purpose new variety of poultry developed at Central Avian Research Institute, Izatnagar for rural poultry farming.

iii. Write True (T) or False (F) against each statement.

1. Chickens of Mediterranean class always lay white shelled eggs.
2. Rhode Island Red, New Hampshire and Plymouth Rock breeds of poultry are under American class.
3. Australorp, Light Sussex and White Cornish breeds of poultry are under English class.
4. Leghorn, Minorca and Ancona breeds of poultry are under Mediterranean class.
5. Brahma, Cochin and Langshan breeds of poultry are under Asiatic class.
6. Australorp breed of poultry was developed from Black Orpington.
7. New Hampshire breed of poultry was developed from Rhode Island Red.
8. Rhode Island Red is a dual purpose breed of poultry.
9. Khaki Campbell is a very good meat type duck.
10. Aylesbury is a good egg type duck.
11. White Leghorn is the most popular breed of Mediterranean class.
12. Triangular body shape is desirable in case of layer type poultry.
13. Round body shape is desirable in case of meat type poultry.
14. Spur is only present in male fowl.
15. Saddle feathers are only present in female chicken.

B. Subjective Questions

1. What is the scientific name of chicken? From where do chickens originate?
2. What is poultry? Name four important poultry species along with their scientific names.
3. Classify poultry. Mention the common breeds of poultry including duck, quail, turkey and guinea fowl (two in each case).
4. Classify the breeds of chickens on the basis of their origin with suitable examples. Name three popular strains from each of layer and broiler, which have been developed in government sectors in India.
5. Write in tabular form different classes of fowl along with their main characteristics, breeds and important varieties.

6. Mention three important breeds of chicken of English class. Describe the characteristic features of any one of them.

7. Mention three important breeds of chicken of American class. Describe the characteristic features of any one of them.

8. Mention three important breeds of chicken of Mediterranean class. Which one is the best and why? Describe its characteristic features.

9. Describe the characteristics of White Leghorn and Rhode Island Red breeds of chickens along with their classes and purpose of rearing.

10. Write short notes on the following.
    (a) White Leghorn
    (b) Rhode Island Red
    (c) Khaki Campbell
    (d) Aseel
    (e) Indigenous fowls of India
    (f) BBB
    (g) New coloured feathered birds developed for rural poultry

Answers of the Objective Questions

i. Multiple choice

1. (a) America
2. (a) America
3. (b) Australia
4. (d) Italy
5. (c) England
6. (c) India
7. (b) England
8. (d) White Leghorn
9. (d) Leghorn
10. (a) Rhode Island Red
11. (a) Indian Runner
12. (c) Aylesbury
13. (c) Crested White
14. (c) White Leghorn
15. (c) CPBF, Bhubaneswar
16. (b) Andhra Pradesh
17. (b) Kadaknath
18. (a) Australorp male × White Leghorn female
19. (c) Egg and meat
20. (b) Meat
21. (a) Egg
22. (c) White Cornish and White Plymouth Rock
23. (b) Black Orpington
24. (b) New Hampshire
25. (d) Sussex
26. (a) Plymouth Rock
27. (a) Leghorn
28. (c) 1, 3 and 4 are correct
29. (c) 2, 3 and 4 are correct
30. (c)

ii. Fill in the blanks

1. chicken, *Anas platyrhynchos*
2. *Gallus domesticus*
3. *Anas platyrhynchos*
4. *Coturnix coturnix japonica*
5. *Meleagris gallopavo*
6. Khaki Campbell
7. White Leghorn
8. RIR/New Hampshire/Australorp
9. Mediterranean
10. American
11. English
12. American
13. English
14. English

15. Mediterranean   16. Rhode Island Red/RIR
17. meat, Khaki Campbell
18. Rhode Island State of America/Indian Runner
19. New Hampshire State of America   20. Italy
21. Australia   22. England
23. Khaki Campbell/Indian Runner   24. Aylesbury/Pekin
25. Japanese quail   26. turkey   27. Andhra Pradesh
28. Pearl/Lavender/White
29. Dual   30. Hitcari/Upcari

iii. True or False

1. T	2. T	3. T	4. T	5. T
6. T	7. T	8. T	9. F	10. F
11. T	12. T	13. T	14. T	15. F

3

Reproduction in Fowl and Egg

3.1 REPRODUCTION IN FOWL

The avian reproductive system is heterosexual and has separate male and female individuals. The male contributes its half of the genetic constitution and remaining half is contributed by the female to their offsprings. The yolk contains ovum which is referred as blastoderm. It is released from the ovary and moves into the oviduct. In the first part of oviduct called infundibulum, the ovum is fertilised by the sperm which already came from the male counterpart. The female and male reproductive systems are discussed here.

3.2 FEMALE REPRODUCTIVE SYSTEM

Female reproductive system of chicken consists of 2 ovaries and 2 oviducts at the time of hatching, but in adults generally left ovary and its oviduct are developed and functional. The right one presents as functionless rudiment.

The ovary is located at the upper part of abdominal cavity below last 2 ribs and at the anterior end of left kidney. Ova at different stages of maturity are found in the ovary of a laying hen. In mature stage, shape of the ovary is just like a bunch of grapes, and size varies from 3–5 g (broody hen) to 50–52 g (laying hen).

Oviduct consists of 5 major parts or sections (Fig. 3.1), viz. infundibulum or funnel (9 cm), magnum or albumen secreting portion (33 cm), isthmus or shell membrane secreting portion (10 cm), uterus or shell gland (12 cm) and vagina (12 cm). (the measures within parenthesis are in case of laying hen.) The total length of oviduct in case of laying hen is approximately 76 cm, and in non-laying hen it is about 15 cm only. Egg is formed in the female reproductive system of chicken.

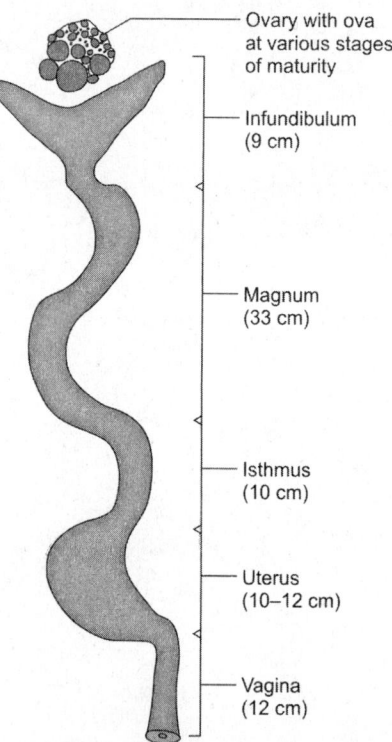

Fig. 3.1: Female reproductive system of chicken

3.3 MALE REPRODUCTIVE SYSTEM

Male reproductive system of chicken consists of a pair of testis, vas deferens and papillae or rudimentary copulatory organ (Fig. 3.2). Fowls do not have a penis which is found in other animals.

The testes are bean-shaped yellowish-white bodies and located against the backbone at the anterior end of kidneys. The left testis is often larger than the right.

Vas deferens are narrow convoluted ducts arise from the inner border of each testis and conveys spermatozoa and seminal fluid from testis to the cloaca. Papillae or rudimentary copulatory organ is located at the median ventral portion of the cloaca. It introduces spermatozoa into the oviduct through the cloaca of the female at the time of mating.

In testis twisted tubes called seminiferous tubules are present. In seminiferous tubules **the sperms** are produced. One cubic millimetre of semen of chicken produced by the male contains on an average of 3–5 million sperms. The chicken sperm has a long pointed head with a long tail. The testes also produce hormones called **androgens** that influence the development of secondary sex characteristics such as comb growth, male behaviour and mating.

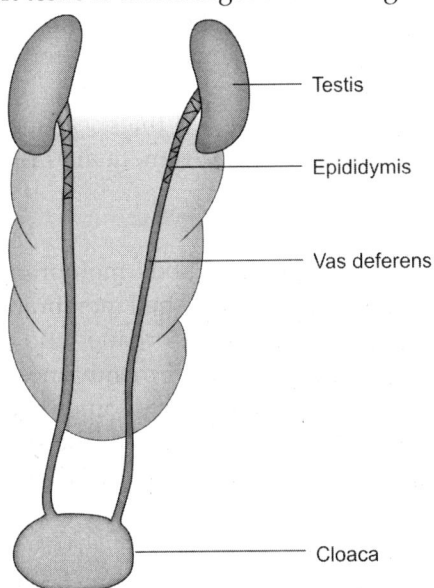

Fig. 3.2: Male reproductive system of chicken

3.4 STRUCTURE OF EGG

3.4.1 Parts of An Egg

The egg consists of 4 main parts, viz. (i) shell, (ii) shell membrane, (iii) albumen or egg white and (iv) yolk (Fig. 3.3).

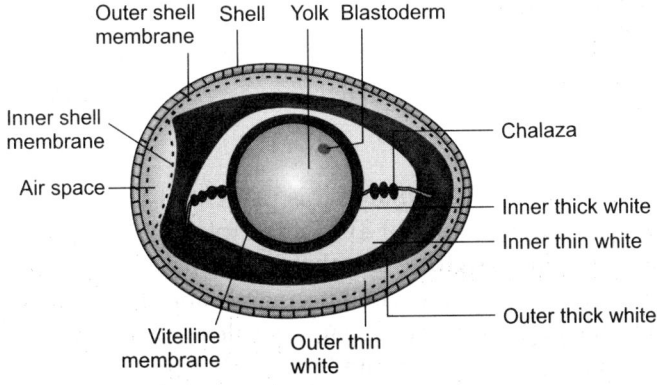

Fig. 3.3: Parts of an egg

Eggshell

The shell is the hard outermost covering of an egg. The colour of eggshell may be white or brown depending on the class or breed of chicken (poultry breeds of Mediterranean class always lay white shelled egg, and breeds of other classes lay brown shelled egg). The eggshell is composed of calcium carbonate (94%), magnesium carbonate (1%), calcium phosphate (1%) and organic matter (chiefly protein, 4%). The shell has numerous pores (about 1,700 to 7,500) on it, which help in gaseous exchange required for embryo development. The shell is covered by a thin transparent protein coating, called **cuticle**. It gives natural protection to the shell pores. The shell thickness may vary among different avian species (chicken 0.31 mm, duck 0.32 mm, quail 0.13 mm and turkey 0.41 mm).

Shell membrane

Next to shell are 2 shell membranes, viz. outer shell membrane and inner shell membrane. Both the shell membranes are attached firmly to each other throughout the egg except at the broader end of egg where **air space** or **air cell** is formed in between the two shell membranes. The depth of the air cell of freshly laid egg is 1–3 mm. The thickness of outer and inner shell membranes are 0.04–0.07 mm and 0.01–0.02 mm, respectively. The shell and shell membranes are non-edible parts of an egg and constitute about 11% of the total egg weight.

Albumen or egg white

The albumen consists of 4 layers, viz. outer thin white, outer thick white, inner thin white and inner thick white. The inner thick white layer of albumen is also known as **chalaziferous layer**. Two thick spiral band-like structures emerge from this layer, known as **chalazae**. They hold the yolk in position. The albumen accounts for about 58% of the total egg weight.

The four different types of albumen or egg white in the normal egg are as follows:

Albumen type	%
Chalaziferous layer and chalazae	2.7
Inner thin white	17.3
Outer thick white	57.0
Outer thin white	23.0

Yolk

The rounded yellowish coloured material is present at the centre of the egg, it is called egg yolk. It accounts for about 31% of the total egg weight. Yolk is enclosed by a thin membrane called **vitelline membrane**. A small whitish disc-like structure is present on yolk just below the vitelline membrane. It is called **germinal disc** (blastoderm in fertile egg and blastodisc in infertile egg). The diameter of germinal disc is 4.5 mm in fertile egg and 3.5 mm in infertile egg.

The composition of the yolk material is as follows:

Component	%
Water	48.0
Protein	17.5
Fat	32.5
Carbohydrate	1.0
Other compounds	1.0

3.4.2 Chemical Composition of Egg

Egg is one of the nature's most perfectly balanced foods, containing quality protein, all vitamins (except vitamin C) and minerals essential for good health. Today's large sized egg contains only a moderate amount of fat, about 5 g only in egg yolk (out of which 1.5 g is saturated), 213 mg of cholesterol and 80 kilocalories of energy. Eggs can easily fit into one's daily fat limit. One standard sized chicken egg has the following composition (NECC, www.e2necc.com, Table 3.1).

Table 3.1: Composition of one standard sized chicken egg

Parameters	Quantity
Other compounds	1.0
Energy value	80 Kcal
Protein	6.3 g
Carbohydrates	0.6 g
Total fat	5.0 g
— monounsaturated fat	2.0 g
— polyunsaturated fat	0.7 g
— saturated fat	1.5 g
Cholesterol	213 mg
Sodium	63 mg

Egg proteins have been considered as the standard against which all other food proteins are measured because of its ideal protein composition. The biological values of proteins in various common food items are given in Table 3.2.

Table 3.2: Biological values of proteins in common food items

Food items	Biological values
Egg (whole)	94
Milk	85
Fish	76
Meat	75
Soybean	73
Rice (polished)	64
Wheat (whole)	64
Corn	60

While the egg white is free of fat and cholesterol, yolk contains 213 mg of cholesterol (approximately 22% less cholesterol than previously thought) and 5 g of total fat. Only 1.5 g of the yolk's fat is saturated, the kind of fat that is most likely to increase blood cholesterol level. In fact, compared with dietary cholesterol, saturated fat exerts 4 times stronger influence on blood cholesterol level. Published research actually showed an increase in the HDL or the good cholesterol level of subjects who added an egg everyday to their diet [Farrel *et al.* (1998). American J Clin Nutr. 68: 538–544]. The egg white contains more than half of the egg's total protein, niacin, riboflavin, chlorine, magnesium, potassium, sodium, and sulphur and all the egg's zinc. Egg yolk contains fat-soluble vitamins A, D, and E. Egg yolk is one of the few foods that naturally contains vitamin D. It also provides vitamin B_{12} and folic acid, and the minerals like iron, calcium, copper and phosphorus.

Gross composition and chemical composition of eggs of various poultry species are presented in Tables 3.3 and 3.4.

Table 3.3: Gross composition of egg of various poultry species

Species of poultry	Total egg weight (g)	Yolk (%)	Albumen (%)	Shell and shell membranes (%)
Chicken	58	31	58	11
Duck	70	35	53	12
Quail	10	32	48	20
Turkey	85	32	56	12
Guinea fowl	40	35	52	13
Goose	200	35	53	12
Pigeon	17	18	74	08

Table 3.4: Chemical composition of egg of various poultry species (per 100 g edible portion, without shell and shell membranes)

Species of poultry	Water (mL)	Protein (g)	Fat (g)	Carbohydrate (g)	Mineral (g)	Energy (Kcal)
Chicken	74.0	12.5	11.5	1.0	1.0	163
Duck	70.5	13.0	14.5	0.8	1.2	190
Quail	73.5	13.3	11.0	1.1	1.1	160
Turkey	72.6	13.1	11.8	1.7	0.8	170
Guinea fowl	72.8	13.5	12.0	0.8	0.9	170
Goose	70.4	13.9	13.3	1.5	1.1	185
Pigeon	72.8	13.8	12.0	0.8	0.9	170

3.5 HOW EGG IS FORMED?

Egg is formed in the female reproductive system of poultry. The left ovary and its oviduct are well-developed in adult birds and engaged in egg formation (*See* Fig. 3.1).

The normal egg consists of the following major parts:

1. Yolk carrying the ovum—produced by the ovary
2. Albumen or egg white—produced mainly in the magnum

3. Shell membranes—produced in the isthmus
4. Shell—produced in the uterus or shell gland

Out of these 4 major parts of an egg, yolk is contributed by the ovary, while the other parts of eggs are contributed by various parts of the oviduct.

Yolk is released from the **ovary** and is engulfed by the infundibulum. It remains here for about 18 minutes and fertilisation takes place here, if the female is mated by its male counterpart. Whether fertilised or not, it then goes to the next part **magnum**, remains there for about 2 hours 54 minutes and **egg white** is added here. The developing egg then goes to the next part **isthmus**, stays there for about 1 hour 14 minutes and **shell membranes** are added. Then the developing egg goes to the next part **uterus or shell gland**, remains there for maximum period of about 20 hours 40 minutes and **eggshell** is formed here by means of calcification. At first shell formation occurs slowly, increases to a rate of up to 300 mg/hour over a duration of 15 hours and then it again slows down during the last 2 hours before oviposition. The colour of the shell is also formed here about 5 hours before the laying of egg. The shell pigments are primarily protoporphyrin and billiverdin. Then the fully formed shelled egg passes through the last part of the oviduct called vagina. Functions of various parts of oviduct in relation to egg formation are depicted in Table 3.5.

Table 3.5: Functions of oviduct in relation to egg formation

Parts of oviduct	Approximate length (cm)	Average duration spent in the part	Main functions
Infundibulum	9.0	18 minutes	Engulfs yolk released by the ovary. Fertilisation takes place here, if hen mated with male.
Magnum	33.0	2 hours 54 minutes	Secretion of egg white or albumen
Isthmus	10.0	1 hour 14 minutes	Secretion of two shell membranes, water and mineral salts
Uterus	12.0	20 hours 40 minutes	Secretion of shell matrix, pigment, cuticle, and also thin albumen
Vagina	12.0	Without spending much more time	It is the passage of egg laying.

Notes:
- Approximate time taken for formation of an egg (i.e. the time interval between releasing of yolk from ovary and laying of the fully formed egg) is usually around 25 hours.
- Egg laying cycle of poultry is very characteristic. Hen lays eggs consecutively for few days followed by 'no egg' period, then again egg laying period. This egg laying period is known as **clutch size** and no egg period is known as **pause size**. In hybrid poultry, clutch size is more and pause size is less and *vice versa* in *deshi* poultry.

- Generally 14 to 75 minutes after oviposition (laying of egg), the next ovulation (release of yolk from ovary) takes place.
- Egg formation is a natural phenomenon to female poultry. Hen lays eggs with or without mating with its male counterpart. But for production of fertile eggs (used for hatching), female birds must be mated with male and for good fertile eggs females should be mated at least once a week.
- The release of yolk carrying ovum from the ovary is called **ovulation**, and the release of shelled egg or fully formed egg from the reproductive system of hen through the vent is called **oviposition**.

3.6 TYPES OF ABNORMAL EGG

1. **Egg with double yolk:** Double yolk is due to simultaneous development and ovulation of 2 ova, and is more common in pullets. Double yolked eggs never hatch mostly, though it is larger in size than normal egg.

2. **Presence of blood spot and/or meat spot in egg:** It may be a characteristic of an individual hen. It generally occurs due to nutritional and management faults including low level of vitamin A.

3. **Thin shell or shell-less egg:** Shell quality depends on the levels of calcium, phosphorus, manganese and vitamin D in layers' diet. Respiratory diseases and hot environmental temperature may increase the incidence of thin-shelled egg.

4. **Foreign matter in egg like worms,** e.g. Prosthogonimus may infest ovary and when it passes through the egg formation stages, it is embodied in the egg.

5. **An egg within an egg:** After completion of the formation of an egg in the uterus, sometimes it may be forced back to infundibulum due to reverse peristaltic movement, and again passes through the egg formation stages.

6. **Rotten new-laid egg:** This may be due to over-fat hen or hen with oviduct disease, vent gleet, *etc.* The fully formed egg stays in the oviduct and becomes rotten.

7. **Pale yolk:** Alfalfa meal, yellow maize and other xanthophyll-containing feed ingredients may affect the yellow colour. It occurs primarily due to lack of xanthophyll and carotene pigment.

8. **Off-flavour in an egg:** It is a management fault and occurs mainly due to poor quality of fish meal, or high level of fish meal and fish oil.

3.7 GRADING OF EGG

Grading of eggs is sorting of eggs into different categories on the basis of some parameters like weight and internal quality. It aids in facilitating uniform packing and pricing and quality assurance to the consumers. It encourages the production of quality eggs and helps in reducing wastage. Easier market price reporting, easier advertising and establishment of brand names of the quality product are some of the other advantages of grading.

Indian standards (BIS/Agmark standards) for various grades of table eggs:

According to Indian standards (Bureau of Indian Standards), eggs are graded on the basis of weight and internal quality. The various grade designations of tabled eggs are given in the following 2 tables (Tables 3.6 and 3.7).

Table 3.6: Grade designation of tabled eggs based on weight

Grade	Weight per egg (g)	Weight per dozen eggs (g)
Extra large	60 and above	715 and above
Large	53 to 59	631 to 714
Medium	45 to 52	535 to 630
Small	38 to 44	456 to 534

Table 3.7: Grade designation of tabled eggs based on quality

Quality factors	Grade A	Grade B
Shell	Clean, sound, unbroken, normal shapes	Clean to moderately stained, sound, but slightly abnormal.
Air cell	4 mm or less in depth, practically regular	8 mm or less in depth, may be free and slightly bubbly.
Egg white	Clear and reasonably firm	Clear, may be slightly weak.
Yolk	Fairly well-centred, practically free from defects, outline indistinct	May be slightly off-centred, outline slightly visible.

3.8 PRESERVATION OF EGG

There are various methods of preserving eggs for short as well as long duration. The preservation methods are described under two broad headings as follows:

1. **Methods for preserving less number of eggs (home preservation)**

a. **Using earthen pot**

The principle of this method is to keep the eggs at low temperature. The eggs can be kept in an earthen pot embedded in soil having sand bed, which is sprinkled with water. This method is being used in the rural areas to preserve the eggs in small number for few days.

b. **Immersion in liquids**

Various liquids like lime water, water glass, *etc.* are used to preserve the eggs for a short period.

Lime water method: 1 kg of quick lime is taken in a pot and 1 L of boiling water is added to it. The mixture is brought to room temperature, and 4–5 L of cold water and 225 g of common salt (NaCl) are added to it. After settling down, the solution is strained through a cloth. The eggs are immersed in this clear liquid and kept for 16–18 hours. Then, they are taken out and dried at room temperature. Eggs can be preserved for 3–4 weeks by this method. The preservative effect of lime water is partly due to its alkalinity. Besides this, it deposits a thin film of calcium carbonate on the eggshell leading to sealing of the pores.

Water glass method: In this method sodium silicate is used instead of lime water. Sodium silicate is also known as water glass, so the name of this method is water glass method. A solution is prepared by dissolving 1 part of sodium silicate in 10 parts of water. The eggs are immersed in this solution for overnight. The eggs can be preserved for about 1 month by this method. In this method, a thin film of silica (sand) is deposited on the eggshell leading to sealing of the pores.

c. **Oil coating method**

Mineral oil (food grade, and colourless, odourless, less viscous and free from fluorescent materials) is sprayed over the eggs or eggs are dipped in this oil, which forms a thin film on the surface of shell leading to sealing of the pores. The eggs are to be treated as early as possible after laying to retain better internal quality.

d. **Low temperature method (eggs in refrigerator)**

Few number of eggs can be preserved by keeping them in refrigerator for few days for home consumption purpose. But in this method eggs should not be kept for more than 10 days.

2. **Methods for preserving large number of eggs (commercial preservation)**

a. **Cold storage method**

Fresh eggs are stored by this method. Storing period will be more, if eggs are oil coated prior to load in the cold store.

The temperature and relative humidity (RH), which are to be maintained in the cold store are as follows:

For short-term preservation	For long-term preservation
Temperature: 12.5–15.5 °C (55–60 °F)	Temperature: –10 °C (14 ± 1 °F)
Relative humidity: 70–80%	Relative humidity: 80–90%

Oil coated eggs can be preserved for 8 months when stored at 14 °C and RH 90%, whereas up to 6 months only if eggs are not coated with oil.

b. **Thermostabilisation method**

Eggs are immersed in warm water at 54 °C for 15 minutes or 56 °C for 10 minutes or at 60 °C for 5 minutes.

This heating process stabilizes the thick portion of albumen which reduces the evaporation of moisture from internal parts of eggs, and such eggs retain their fresh appearance for longer period.

c. **Pasteurisation method**

The eggs are immersed in warm water at 63 °C for 2.5 minutes or at 64 °C for 1.5–2 minutes. This destroys the microbes present on the surface of the eggs. This process is known as pasteurisation of eggs.

d. **Dehydration (egg powder)**

Eggs may be preserved as egg powder which is used in bakery products, confectionaries and other food products.

EXERCISE

A. Objective Questions

i. **Indicate the correct answer by putting tick (√) mark (multiple choice).**

1. Egg albumin is formed in
   - (a) Infundibulum
   - (b) Isthmus
   - (c) Magnum
   - (d) Uterus

2. Eggshell is formed in
   - (a) Ovary
   - (b) Isthmus
   - (c) Uterus
   - (d) Cloaca

3. Egg white is mainly composed of
   - (a) Carbohydrate
   - (b) Protein
   - (c) Fat
   - (d) Calcium carbonate

4. Eggshell is mainly composed of
   - (a) Carbohydrate
   - (b) Protein
   - (c) Calcium phosphate
   - (d) Calcium carbonate

5. Approximate length of oviduct in laying hen is
   - (a) 33 cm
   - (b) 10 cm
   - (c) 76 cm
   - (d) 96 cm

6. Chalaziferous layer is also known as
   - (a) Outer thick white
   - (b) Outer thin white
   - (c) Inner thick white
   - (d) Inner thin white

7. Time taken for formation of an egg is
   - (a) 12 hours
   - (b) 16 hours
   - (c) 25 hours
   - (d) 21 hours

8. Shell membrane is formed in which part of the oviduct?
   - (a) Infundibulum
   - (b) Magnum
   - (c) Isthmus
   - (d) Uterus

9. Yellow colour of yolk of 'deshi egg' is due to the presence of
   - (a) Vitamin A
   - (b) Vitamin E
   - (c) Carotene
   - (d) Riboflavin

10. Chalaziferous layer of egg is a part of
    - (a) Yolk
    - (b) Albumin
    - (c) Eggshell
    - (d) Shell membrane

11. Expulsion of egg from the oviduct is known as
    - (a) Ovulation
    - (b) Oviposition
    - (c) Culling
    - (d) Incubation

12. How much fat is present in yolk?
    - (a) 0%
    - (b) 17.5%
    - (c) 32.5%
    - (d) 48.0%

13. How much protein is present in yolk?

    (a) 0%   (b) 17.5%

    (c) 32.5%   (d) 48.0%

14. What is the correct sequence of events in egg formation?

    1. Oviposition

    2. Ovulation

    3. Shell formation

    4. Shell membrane formation

    5. Egg white formation

Select the correct answer from the code below:

Code (a) 1, 2, 3, 4, 5   (b) 2, 5, 4, 1, 3

     (c) 1, 5, 4, 3, 2   (d) 2, 5, 4, 3, 1

15. A developing egg remains for specific time at each part of oviduct during egg formation as follows:

    1. 20 hours 40 minutes at uterus

    2. 1 hour 14 minutes at isthmus

    3. 18 minutes at vagina

    4. 2 hours 54 minutes at magnum

Select the correct answer from the code below:

Code (a) 1, 2, 3 and 4 are correct   (b) 1, 2 and 3 are correct

     (c) 1, 3 and 4 are correct   (d) 1, 2 and 4 are correct

ii. Fill in the blanks.

1. Egg albumen makes about _____% of total egg weight.

2. Yolk makes about _____% of total egg weight.

3. Eggshell and shell membranes make about _____% of total egg weight.

4. _____ and _____ are the two edible parts of an egg.

5. _____ and _____ are the two non-edible parts of an egg.

6. It takes about _____ hours to form a chicken egg.

7. The approximate length of oviduct in laying hen is _____.

8. Magnum is _____ secreting portion of oviduct.

9. Isthmus is _____ secreting portion of oviduct.

10. Uterus is _____ secreting portion of oviduct.

11. The eggshell is mainly composed of _____.

12. Egg contains almost all vitamins excepting _____.

13. The average protein content of chicken egg is _____%.

14. The average fat content of chicken egg is _____%.

15. The average water content of chicken egg is _____ .

iii. **Write True (T) or False (F) against each statement.**
  1. Air cell is present at the broader end of egg.
  2. In poultry, only right ovary is developed and functional at laying stage.
  3. Egg white is mainly composed of carbohydrate.
  4. Egg is very rich in iron and vitamin C.
  5. Egg is a good source of iron and phosphorus.
  6. Air cell is an indicator of freshness of egg.
  7. Magnum is the largest part of oviduct where developing egg remains maximum time.
  8. Uterus is the largest part of oviduct where developing egg remains maximum time.
  9. In non-laying hen the length of oviduct is about 15 cm only.
  10. The release of fully formed egg from the reproductive system of hen through the vent is called ovulation.

B. Subjective Questions

  1. With the help of schematic diagram, describe in brief the parts of reproductive system of hen. How an egg is formed in this system?
  2. Describe the male reproductive system of fowl with the help of schematic diagram.
  3. What are the parts of an egg?
  4. What do you mean by 'clutch size' and 'pause size'?
  5. What is the importance of egg in human nutrition?
  6. What is the function of magnum in egg formation?
  7. What is composition of eggshell?
  8. What is chalaziferous layer?
  9. Will incubation of double yolked egg result in 'twin chickens'?
  10. Write short notes on the following.
      (a) Oviduct
      (b) Structure of chicken egg
      (c) Formation of egg
      (d) Nutritive value of egg
      (e) Edible parts of an egg
      (f) Oviposition

Answers of the Objective Questions

  i. **Multiple choice**

  1. (c) Magnum   2. (c) Uterus   3. (b) Protein
  4. (d) Calcium carbonate 5. (c) 76 cm   6. (c) Inner thick white
  7. (c) 25 hours   8. (c) Isthmus   9. (c) Carotene

10. (b) Albumin   11. (b) Oviposition   12. (c) 32.5%

13. (b) 17.5%   14. (d) 2, 5, 4, 3, 1   15. (d) 1, 2 and 4 are correct

ii. Fill in the blanks

1. 58   2. 31   3. 11

4. Albumen/egg white, yolk   5. Shell, shell membrane

6. 25   7. 76 cm   8. albumen/egg white

9. shell membrane   10. shell   11. calcium carbonate

12. vitamin C   13. 12.5   14. 11.5

15. 74.0

iii. True or False

1. T   2. F   3. F   4. F   5. T

6. T   7. F   8. F   9. T   10. F

4

Economic Traits of Poultry

4.1 IMPORTANT ECONOMIC TRAITS OF POULTRY

The important traits of poultry are egg production, their weight and quality, growth, feed consumption and its efficiency, fertility and hatchability, plumage characteristics and comb types. The traits are genetically controlled and divided into 2 groups, viz. qualitative traits and quantitative traits. Qualitative traits are controlled by one or a few pairs of genes and are least influenced by environmental factors. Examples of qualitative traits of poultry are comb type, plumage pattern and colour, shank colour, curling of feathers, *etc*. Quantitative traits are controlled by many pairs of genes and are markedly influenced by environmental factors or non-genetic factors like feeding, management, disease exposure, climate, *etc*. Most of the economic traits in poultry are quantitative in nature. Examples of quantitative traits are egg production, their weight, fertility and hatchability, body weight, feed efficiency, viability, *etc*.

The important traits of poultry are discussed in the following sections.

4.1.1 Egg Production

Egg production is the most important economic trait in poultry. Recently a hybrid chicken can lay as early as at 18 weeks of age. The peak production reaches at about 5–6 weeks after the first lay, stays for few weeks and then gradually declines. In chicken generally 1 year laying is considered as economical. So hybrid layers are kept in the farm for about 72 weeks with 300–320 eggs per year. Recently they are kept in the farm up to 90 weeks of age with economic production level.

Number of eggs produced in a laying cycle depends on several factors. These are age at sexual maturity (when she lays her first egg), persistency (length of laying cycle), intensity of lay (rate of egg production), number of pauses (i.e. no egg period), and number and duration of broody period. Egg production is generally measured as number (no.) of eggs, and expressed as hen house egg production (HHP) or hen day egg production (HDP). HHP is calculated by dividing the total number of eggs produced by the number of hens housed at the beginning of the laying period. HDP is calculated by dividing the number of eggs on a particular day by the number of birds on that day, or by dividing the total number of eggs produced by the number of hens on the basis of functional day, considering the mortality of the birds. Egg production is an inherited trait and can be improved by selection.

4.1.2 Egg Quality

Egg quality means the inherent characteristics of an egg which determine its degree of excellence and which are liked by customers. Some important egg quality parameters are egg size/egg weight and shape, shell colour, its condition and thickness, their strength and porosity and the quality of albumen, yolk and air cell quality, *etc.* Most of the egg quality traits are highly heritable and respond to selection quickly. These egg quality parameters are discussed below.

A. External qualities of eggs

1. **Egg size/Egg weight**

   The terms 'egg size' and 'egg weight' are used synonymously. The weight of egg of different species of poultry is given in table form.

Species of poultry	Egg weight (g)
Chicken	55–60
Duck	65–70
Quail (Japanese)	10
Turkey	80–85
Guinea fowl	30–40
Goose	140–220
Emu	475–650

   Heavy breeds lay large sized eggs and light breeds lay smaller eggs. Early matured birds may lay small sized eggs. Other factors that affect egg size are nutrition, environment, health condition of birds, system of housing, *etc.* The egg size is measured simply with the help of egg weighing balance. It is a highly heritable trait and can be improved by selection.

2. **Egg shape**

   Normal shape of an egg is oval. Slight abnormality in the shape of an egg (like elongated, flat, round, conical, *etc.*) is not preferred by consumers, because they thought abnormal eggs are laid by diseased birds. Besides this, bad shaped eggs are not suitable for hatching purpose. The egg shape is measured by Vernier Caliper in terms of egg shape index (ESI). The length and breadth of an egg are to be measured near to 0.1 mm and the breadth-length ratio is to be multiplied by 100 to get ESI.

   $$\text{ESI} = \frac{\text{Breadth of egg}}{\text{Length of egg}} \times 100$$

   The higher egg shape index indicates round shape and lower index indicates elongated egg. The optimum shape indices of eggs of various poultry species are—chicken egg 74, duck egg 72 and quail egg 78.

3. **Shell colour**

   The shell colour of egg is characteristic to the breeds of poultry. The breeds of Mediterranean class (e.g. White Leghorn, Minorca, Ancona) always lays white shelled eggs. The breeds of American class (e.g. New Hampshire) and English class (e.g. Australorp, Sussex) always lay brown shelled eggs. Quail eggs are tinted with different colours (nowadays quail strains are produced which lay white shelled eggs.). The shell of duck egg is more transparent than chicken egg. The shell colour is simply observed by visual scoring. The colour of egg, whether white or brown, does not matter, but brightness of colour is definitely preferred by the consumers. Dull or stained colour of eggshell is not preferred by the consumers.

Note: The shell colour of egg has nothing to do with its quality. So it is not included in the USDA egg standards.

4. **Shell conditions (cleanliness and soundness)**

The shell should be clean and sound.

Shell cleanliness: It is judged by visual observation. On the basis of degree of cleanliness, the eggs are classified into 4 groups, viz. clean, slightly stained, moderately stained and dirty.

Clean egg: The shell is totally free from foreign material including stains.

Slightly stained egg: The shell is free from dirt, but having slight stains covering up to 1/16th of its surface area.

Moderately stained egg: The shell is free from dirt, but having moderate degree of stains covering up to 1/4th of its surface area.

Dirty egg: The shell has both dirt and stains covering more than 1/4th of its surface area.

Shell soundness: A sound egg means an egg with intact and unbroken shell. An unsound egg may be cracked (having hairline crack on shell), leaking (having crack on shell and shell membranes leading to oozing of egg contents) and smashed (having crushed shell). Cracked egg is of poor quality, and leaking and smashed eggs are considered in the category of loss (according to USDA grading of eggs). Soundness of shell may be judged by tapping 2 eggs together near the ear. A clear sound indicates sound shell, while dull sound indicates that one or both the eggs may have cracked shell. Leaking and smashed eggs may be identified by visual observation. For identification of hairline crack on shell, candling is to be done.

5. **Shell thickness and strength**

Shell thickness, specific gravity of intact egg, and percentage of shell present in an egg are important parameters for evaluating the strength of shell. Shell strength is an economically important trait as weak shelled eggs may cause considerable losses during handling and transport for marketing purpose due to breakage.

Shell thickness: Shell thickness and shell strength are directly proportional and positively correlated. Shell thickness can be measured with the help of screw gauge. A piece of eggshell is to be inserted in the screw gauge and reading is taken directly from the measuring scale. Normal shell thickness of chicken egg varies from 0.30 to 0.50 mm.

Specific gravity of intact egg: It can be determined by brine flotation technique. The eggs are allowed to float in a series of brine solutions with known specific gravities ranging from 1.062 to 1.102, with difference of 0.004 between each other. The specific gravity of the solution in which egg just floats will be the specific gravity of that egg. The normal specific gravity of chicken egg is 1.062 to 1.090. Higher specific gravity indicates thick shell and *vice versa*, because the specific gravity of inner contents of egg is nearly same in all eggs.

Percentage of shell present in the egg: It acts as an indicator of shell strength. In this technique the shell membranes are removed after treating the shell with 2.5% sodium hydroxide solution for 5 minutes. Then shell is washed and dried for 24 hours at 100 °C in a thermostatically controlled oven. Further on the dried shell is weighed and divided by the weight of the whole egg and converted into percentage. Normally, shell of chicken egg constitutes about 11% of the total egg by weight.

6. **Shell porosity**

   Optimum number of pores should be present in the eggshell. Eggshells with poor porosity as well as more porosity are not desirable, because in first case (less porous shell), less evaporation of moisture and less gaseous exchange will takes place leading to entrance of microorganisms and deterioration of egg quality and in second case (more porous shell), more evaporation of moisture occurs leading to weight loss of egg during storage. The shell porosity can be measured by taking weight of egg under standard conditions. Eggs kept in the incubator at 37 °C and 60% relative humidity for 14 days shows 15 to 18 per cent loss in weight and indicates normal porosity (about 7,500 pores in a normal sized egg).

B. Internal qualities of eggs

Internal egg qualities include conditions of air cell, albumen and yolk. These parameters can be evaluated by both subjective and objective methods. Subjective methods are followed for evaluation of intact eggs by means of candling for commercial purpose, while the objective methods are mainly followed for research purpose.

1. **Evaluation of internal qualities of intact eggs by candling:**

   By means of candling of eggs, i.e. passing white light through the egg contents, shadow is cast by the yolk and air cell. The shadow indicates about the size of air cell, position of yolk, condition of vitelline membrane and condition of albumen. Normal conditions of internal quality parameters of eggs and their observation by means of candling:

   Air cell: Height in freshly laid egg is 3.2 mm and placed at the broader end of egg. It can be observed by candling.

   Yolk: Centrally placed, outline invisible, free from blood spot or meat spot (i.e. free from shadow of foreign bodies). It may be centrally placed or off centred. Vitelline membrane may be weak, if shadow of yolk is flattened.

   Albumen: Clear, thick and completely firm, free from blood spot or meat spot. If shadow of yolk is darker and it moves freely, it indicates thinning of thick albumen.

2. **Evaluation of internal qualities of egg after breaking:**

   i. **Air cell depth:** Depth of air cell is to be measured with the help of scale. Air cell depths of eggs of various ages are:

Freshly laid egg	3.2 mm
3 days old egg	6.4 mm
8 days old egg	9.5 mm
15 days old egg	15.9 mm

    Depth of air cell up to 4 mm is graded as 'A' and up to 8 mm as 'B'.

  ii. **Yolk index:** The yolk index is measured to know the quality of egg yolk. Yolk index is the ratio between height and width of the yolk. The height of yolk is measured by spherometer at the highest point, and width is measured by vernier caliper at right angle across the yolk.

$$\text{Yolk index} = \frac{\text{Height of yolk}}{\text{Width of yolk}}$$

    Yolk index indicates the firmness of yolk and how high it stands when broken on a flat surface. A good quality egg should have yolk index of 0.33 or more. Yolk index value less than 0.33 indicates deterioration in quality of yolk.

 iii. **Albumen index:** Albumen index is the ratio of height and width of thick white.

$$\text{Albumen index} = \frac{\text{Height of thick white}}{\text{Width of thick white}}$$

    Height of thick white at the highest point is measured by spherometer and width is measured by vernier caliper at long and short axes and average value is worked out. A good quality egg should have albumen index value of 0.1 or more. Albumen index value less than 0.1 indicates deterioration in quality of thick white (albumen).

  iv. **Haugh unit:** This is the most widely used method for evaluating albumen quality. This method was originally proposed by Raymond Haugh in 1937.

$$HU = 100 \log\left(h - \frac{\sqrt{G\left(30W^{0.37} - 100\right)}}{100} + 1.9 \right)$$

    where
        HU = Haugh unit
        h = Height of albumen in millimetres
        W = Weight of egg in grams
    and G = 32.2 (gravitational constant)

    The simplified formula of the Haugh unit is

$$HU = 100 \times \log_{10}\left(h - 1.7\, w^{0.37} + 7.6\right)$$

    The higher the HU score the better is the egg quality. The HU of good quality egg is 70.

  v. **pH of egg:** The pH of egg contents (i.e. albumen and yolk) can be measured by pH paper. The normal pH of albumen is 7.2 (slightly alkaline) and yolk is 6.6 (slightly acidic). Any deviation from normal values of pH indicates deterioration of egg quality.

4.1.3 Growth Rate

The growth rate is an important trait in broiler birds. Large body weight in broiler and small or intermediate body weight in layers are preferred. Marketing age of broiler chickens is gradually reduced and feed efficiency is improved, over the years. The marketing age has been reduced from 11 weeks in 1953 to less than 6 weeks in 2008. It is possible due to the improvement of growth rate through the application of genetic principles and providing better feeding and management. This trait is moderate to highly heritable and can be improved by simple mass selection.

4.1.4 Feed Consumption and Feed Efficiency

Feed efficiency is the ratio of feed consumption to weight gain in broilers. Sometimes, it is called FCR (feed conversion ratio). In broilers, it is measured as an amount of feed consumed in kg/kg of weight gained. In layers, it is measured as an amount of feed consumed in kg per dozen of eggs laid or as an amount of feed consumed in kg per kg egg mass produced. The feed efficiency trait has been improved considerably in recent years. The FCR of broiler chicken has been improved from 3.5 in 1953 to about 1.7 or less in 2008. Feed efficiency of birds is a moderate heritable trait.

4.1.5 Fertility and Hatchability

Fertility and hatchability are mostly used synonymously and are expressed as percentage in relation to the number of egg sets. Sometimes hatchability is expressed as percentage in relation to number of fertile egg sets. Fertility and hatchability of a flock depends on several factors. Breed, strain, family and individual variation are noticed in relation to fertility and hatchability. Breeding methods also influence these traits. Inbreeding decreases these while outbreeding increases. Age of bird, nutritional status, environment, disease and management practices affect both fertility and hatchability. Breeders' ration should be fortified with vitamins (A, E, pantothenic acid, biotin) and minerals (Ca, P, Na, Mn, Zn and iodine) for obtaining better fertility. High temperature in the breeder house (more than 30 °C) is not good for obtaining better fertility and hence the hatchability. Sex ratio should be narrow for heavy breeds than light breeds. A sex ratio of 1:10 in broilers and 1:15–16 in layers are considered as optimum. Preferential mating by male and females also reduces fertility. To avoid this, artificial insemination is suggested. In case of artificial insemination, semen volume and sperm concentration are important consideration. About 100 million sperms should be introduced in female reproductive tract for obtaining desired fertility. Flocks laying in high rate of lay have better fertility and hatchability than poor producing flocks. The other factors that affect hatchability are size and shape of egg, eggshell condition, storage of eggs before incubation, incubator and hatchery environment, *etc*. Both fertility and hatchability are low heritable traits and can be improved by adopting appropriate breeding methods and good hatchery management.

4.1.6 Plumage Characteristics

The light horny waterproof structure forming on the external covering of birds is called plumage. In other words, collective feathered covering of a bird is called plumage. It provides protection, insulation, and adornment to the birds. The pattern, colour and arrangement of feathers are also known as plumage. The pattern and colour of plumage vary between species and subspecies and can also vary between different age groups, sexes and seasons. Within species there can also be a number of different colours of plumage. Differences in plumage are used by ornithologists and birdwatchers in order to distinguish between species and to collect species specific information. Many birds (like ducks) have bright, colourful plumage and exhibiting strong sexual dimorphism to attract the females. There are hereditary as well as non-hereditary variations in plumage. The common feather patterns of poultry are plain, laced, penciled, spangled, barred, partridge and ticked. The type of feathers may be smooth, frizzled or silky. The common feather colours are white, black, brown, blue, buff, partridge, silver, gold, variegated, *etc.*

4.1.7 Comb Types

Chickens have various types of comb. The important comb types are single comb, rose comb, pea comb, walnut comb, *etc.* White Leghorn and Rhode Island Red (RIR) breeds of chickens have both rose comb and single comb. Cornish breed of chicken has only pea comb. There are only 2 genes responsible for comb types— rose comb (R) and pea comb (P). A chicken with a rose comb will have at least 1 copy of (R) gene and a chicken with a pea type comb will have at least 1 copy of (P) gene. If neither the (R) nor the (P) is present, the chicken will have a straight comb. A walnut comb is a combination of the rose and pea type combs. There are modifying genes which may be responsible for variation of comb type. There are 16 possibilities of gene combination for comb type and is an example of non-allelic interaction. Chicken breeds are differentiated from each other on the basis of comb type. For example, RIR breed has two varieties, viz. single comb RIR and rose comb RIR.

EXERCISE

A. Objective Questions

i. Indicate the correct answer by putting tick (√) mark (mumtiple choice).

1. The egg weight of guinea fowl is
   - (a) 80–85 g
   - (b) 65–70 g
   - (c) 30–40 g
   - (d) 140–220 g

2. The egg weight of chicken is
   - (a) 80–85 g
   - (b) 65–70 g
   - (c) 55–60 g
   - (d) 10–15 g

3. The egg weight of quail is
   - (a) 70 g
   - (b) 60 g
   - (c) 40 g
   - (d) 10 g

4. Recently a good quality hybrid chicken can lay its first egg at the age of
    (a) 18 weeks   (b) 22 weeks
    (c) 24 weeks   (d) 26 weeks

5. Which of the following breeds lay white shelled egg?
    (a) White Leghorn   (b) Minorca
    (c) Ancona   (d) All of these

6. The optimum sex ratio in broiler breeders is
    (a) 1:5   (b) 1:10
    (c) 1:15   (d) 1:18

7. Which of the following pairs of traits are negatively correlated?
    (a) First egg production—annual egg production (in layer)
    (b) Fertility—growth rate (in broiler)
    (c) Feed efficiency—growth rate (in broiler)
    (d) None of these

8. The body weight of chicken is a polygenic trait and is influenced by
    (a) Epistatic genes   (b) Additive genes
    (c) Recessive genes   (d) Modifying genes

9. Comb type in poultry is an example of
    (a) Dominant gene action   (b) Allelic interaction
    (c) Non-allelic interaction   (d) None of these

10. Which of the following breeds has pea comb?
    (a) Rhode Island Red   (b) Cornish
    (c) Plymouth Rock   (d) Australorp

ii. Fill in the blanks.

1. A hybrid chicken can lay as early as at _____ weeks of age.
2. _____ is measured as an amount of feed consumed in kg per kg of weight gained.
3. Comb type is a _____ trait in poultry.
4. Plumage pattern is a _____ trait of poultry.
5. Egg weight is a _____ trait in poultry.

iii. Write True (T) or False (F) against each statement.

1. Qualitative traits are controlled by one or a few pairs of genes.
2. Quantitative traits are controlled by many pairs of genes, and markedly influenced by environmental factors.
3. Hatchability is a qualitative trait in poultry.
4. Comb type is a qualitative trait in poultry.
5. In case of chicken, peak production of eggs reaches at about 5–6 weeks after the first lay.
6. Preferential mating by male and female increases fertility.

7. Small or intermediate body weight in layer type chickens is preferred.
8. Feeding efficiency of birds is a moderately heritable trait.
9. Hatchability is a slow heritable trait and can be improved by adopting appropriate hatchery management.
10. Egg production is an inherited trait and can be improved by selection.

B. Subjective Questions

1. Enlist the important economic traits of poultry. Describe in short any 3 of them.
2. At what age do chickens begin to lay eggs?
3. Write short notes on the following.
    (a) Plumage characteristics
    (b) Comb type
    (c) FCR
    (d) Egg quality

Answers of the Objective Questions

i. Multiple choice

1. (c) 30–40 g
2. (c) 55–60 g
3. (d) 10 g
4. (a) 18 weeks
5. (d) All of these
6. (b) 1:10
7. (c) Feed efficiency—growth rate (in broiler)
8. (b) Additive genes
9. (c) Non-allelic interaction
10. (b) Cornish

ii. Fill in the blanks

1. 18
2. FCR
3. qualitative
4. qualitative
5. quantitative

iii. True or False

1. T
2. T
3. F
4. T
5. T
6. F
7. T
8. T
9. T
10. T

5

Systems of Poultry Keeping

5.1 DIFFERENT SYSTEMS OF POULTRY KEEPING

Generally 4 types of housing systems are found for keeping poultry. These are:
  i. Free range or extensive system
  ii. Semi-intensive system
  iii. Folding unit system
  iv. Intensive system

Intensive system is again of 2 types, viz. deep litter system and cage system.

5.1.1 Free Range System

It is the oldest method of poultry rearing. It is also known as scavenging system of management for raising poultry. In this system, birds are kept free during day time and take shelter in a house during night. Rearing of birds in this system is apparently profitable as birds find appreciable amount of feed in the surroundings free of cost during day time. However, this method is not suitable for commercial purpose.

5.1.2 Semi-intensive System

This system of poultry rearing is partly free range type and partly intensive type. In this system, there is a poultry house followed by a run. The run is a small land surrounded by wire mesh and is attached to the poultry house. Birds spend their day time in the run and take shelter in the house during night. Approximate floor space per bird is 3–4 sq ft for house and 150–200 sq ft for run area.

5.1.3 Folding Unit System

The general theme of this system of poultry rearing is same as that of semi-intensive system. Here also, there is a poultry house followed by a run. The whole area of the run is enclosed by wire nettings. But the space requirement is less and the total poultry unit can be shifted from one place to another. Hence the name of the system is folding unit. One can keep small number of birds in this system on the roof top of their house with sophistication. Approximate floor space per bird is 1 sq ft for house and 3 sq ft for run area, i.e. total 4 sq ft/bird. A folding house unit measuring 20 ft × 5 ft can accommodate 25 birds.

5.1.4 Intensive System

Commercial poultry farming is done only with this system. It is of 2 types, viz.

i. **Deep litter system:** This system is widely used for scientific and successful poultry farming. It is very popular for small as well as large units of commercial poultry farms. Birds are kept in large pen. The floor of the house is covered with dry litter materials like rice husk, sawdust, wood shavings, chopped straw, dried leaves, groundnut shells, *etc.* as per the cost and availability. Minimum floor space requirement under this system of management is 1 sq ft per broiler and 1.75–2.00 sq ft per layer chicken. (*See Fig. 10.1, Chapter 10*)

ii. **Cage system:** It is the latest system of poultry rearing. It is also called battery system. The birds are confined in a cage just large enough to permit limited movement and allow them to stand and sit comfortably. The cage is made up of strong galvanized wire and a tray is fixed underneath of the floor for collection of droppings. The feeder and waterer remain outside the cage. In case of cage rearing, minimum floor space requirement is 0.33 sq ft per chick, 0.42 sq ft per grower and 0.64 sq ft per layer chicken. Broiler birds are not generally reared in cages. (*See Fig. 10.2, Chapter 10*)

5.2 RAISING CHICKENS UNDER SCAVENGING SYSTEM OF MANAGEMENT

In rural India, number of chickens are reared under scavenging system of management. Though very small number of birds (say, maximum 10–20 birds) per farmer's family is reared in this system, but in totality a huge number of birds (approximately 45%) are raised under this system in our country. So, if it is possible to improve the productivity of these scavenging chickens, the total egg production of the country will be increased manifold. The following points may be considered for improving the productivity of these chickens raised under free range or scavenging system of management.

Scavenger feed base of village and feeding practices

The birds can manage their feed through scavenging in the nearby areas. The scavenger feed base is primarily composed of waste grains, grass seeds or shoots, insects, white ants, tender leaves, *etc.* The availability of such feed depends on the free area available in the backyards, intensity of vegetation, type of food grain cultivation, *etc.*

Only a few percentag of farmers used to provide supplementation to the birds in terms of broken rice, bajra, ragi, jowar, rice polish, rice bran and other grains as supplement as and when available. However, this is seasonal in most households, being practiced only during the harvesting season. It is observed that most of the farmers supplement and pour the feed on the ground, however, feed should be offered in flat type containers or at least in the containers similar to those used for providing water like earthen pot, plastic bowl, *etc.*

The birds under free range conditions can meet their protein requirements by taking insects, *etc.*, but the possibility of energy deficiency is common. So while supplementation is done, this point should be kept in mind and accordingly supplement should be rich in cereals along with equal parts of rice polish or rice bran. For more scientific feeding commercial poultry feed may be given to the bird (Table 5.1). For raising meat type chickens under this system commercial broiler starter feed may be used, and for raising egg type chickens grower ration may be used up to 6 weeks followed by layer ration. The weight of pullets should be regulated to maintain the egg production. At the age of sexual maturity (6–6½ months old), the weight of pullet should be about 2.2–2.5 kg. To minimise the laying of shell-less egg or broken egg, calcium supplementation is suggested. Besides commercial preparation, shell grit, stone grit, lime powder, chalk powder, *etc.* may be used as calcium source at 3–4 g/bird/day.

Supplement (either household grains or low density compounded feed) should be given preferably in the evening. The feed may be prepared for the free ranging poultry with the following composition.

Table 5.1: Formula of compounded feed for free ranging poultry

Sl no.	Ingredients	Parts
1.	Cereal by-product (rice bran/rice polish)	30
2.	Cereal (broken rice/broken wheat/jowar/bajra/ragi/maize or any cereal)	28
3.	Oil cake (mustard/sesame/linseed/groundnut)	40
4.	Vitamin and minerals (e.g. *Supplevite-M powder*)	2

Housing for night shelter

Night shelter should be provided to the birds (Fig. 5.1). Proper space should be given to the birds. The existing house, if any, should be modified. There should be window(s) in the house with protection from predators. Floor of the house should be kept dry as far as practicable. It should be cleaned daily and disinfected regularly.

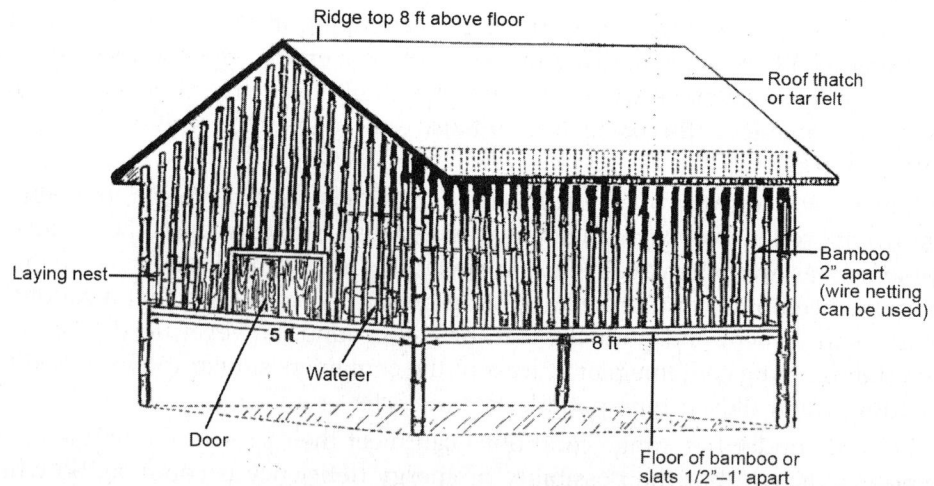

Fig. 5.1: Night shelter for scavenging poultry

Health management

i. **Regular vaccination against Ranikhet disease and fowl pox:** Generally, birds raised under scavenging system are frequently affected with Ranikhet disease and fowl pox. So these birds must be vaccinated against these 2 diseases. The schedule of vaccination of chickens under scavenging system is as follows:

For ranikhet disease—1st vaccine at the age of 4–7 days (RD F_1, nasal or ocular drop), booster dose at 5–6 weeks (RD F_1, nasal or ocular drop), then at the age of 10 weeks (RD R_2B, s/c injection), again at 18 weeks (RD R_2B killed type, s/c injection), then at 35 weeks of age (RD LaSota) and then at an interval of 8 weeks it may be repeated.

For fowl pox—single vaccine at the age of 8 weeks, if the disease is very predominant a booster dose may be given at the age of 13 weeks.

ii. **Regular deworming:** Internal parasitic infestation is very common in free range birds due to scavenging feeding habit. So regular deworming is essential. Piperazine hexahydrate (56.3% solution) may be used at monthly interval (1 dose every month) for this purpose. Dose is 2.5 mL per 10 birds aged 4–6 weeks, and 4–5 mL per 10 birds aged more than 6 weeks.

iii. **Prevent external parasitic infestation:** Precaution should be taken to prevent external parasitic infestation also. Sometimes birds are heavily infested with poultry lice. House should be kept clean to prevent parasitic infestation. If birds are already infested, Pestoban (an ayurvedic liquid preparation) can be used by spraying after mixing with water in the ratio of 1:10. Same medicine may be used in it also as it is a good hiding place for such external parasites. The alternative medicines are butox (Deltamethrin, 12.5% solution) or Clinar liquid (Cypermethrin, 100 g/L), *etc.* These medicines are dissolved with water in the ratio of 1 mL/L of water and is applied by spraying. One application is generally sufficient.

iv. **Use vitamin-mineral supplements:** One vitamin-mineral preparation may be used to curb the deficiency problems. Supplevite-M powder (vitamins A, B complex, D_3, E, K and minerals) may be used at the rate of 5 g/10 birds/day for at least 10 days consecutively on every month. It is very effective to use during laying period.

Other management pointers

- Before 6–7 weeks of age it is better not to let the birds in free range. At this age each bird should weigh 500 g. After this age they may be kept free in the free ranges during day time and given shelter in the night.
- Flock size should be restricted to 20 birds (maximum).
- Light management in poultry house kept for egg production is also very important. Provision may be created in the chicken house meant for night shelter so that light can enter at least 4 hours during the evening hours. It will certainly increase the egg production up to some extent.
- Introduction of new varieties of birds instead of existing deshi birds in the villages can improve the performanc of scavenging system of poultry keeping.

The genetic make up of these birds help them to lay more eggs than the existing ones. Nowadays new varieties of poultry were evolved by the Indian scientists for rural poultry farming, available at various institutes. These new varieties of poultry may be introduced to enhance the productivity of village poultry. One research study revealed that village chickens are an important source of income for household expenses, and the traditional free-range poultry production in the smallholder sector of developing countries can possibly be improved through the use of improved dual purpose birds (Kumaresan, 2008). (*See Chapter 2*)

5.3 BACKYARD AND SEMI-INTENSIVE UNITS OF VARIOUS SIZES

Poultry keeping has been practiced for centuries as a backyard operation among rural families in India. The practice of keeping *deshi* or indigenous chickens and their crosses under the scavenging system (backyard farming) is still popular in rural areas. Some farmers keep the chickens enclosed during the night under their houses and sometimes build an extension usually at the side of the dwelling house made up of wooden materials, wire netting and thatched roof for keeping the birds. Village fowls are generally kept to provide the family with income and protein diet.

The move towards semi-intensive system, whereby the birds are kept in enclosed areas with a shed for shelter and provided with feed, has become quite popular for medium-scale producers. Farmers in the rural areas can rear large number of chickens under the semi-intensive system. Normally, they have a ready market that pays a premium price for the birds. This scenario is also true to many South Asian countries as well as in Africa.

The free range system, sometimes also referred to as backyard production system, produces poultry at low-input, low-output levels and is the commonest type of family poultry production. This system is highly variable depending upon the local area resources and needs. This is also called extensive or scavenging management system. In this system of poultry production, different poultry species chickens, ducks, Guinea fowls, turkeys, *etc.* are kept. Chickens are dominant in terms of both numbers and economic contribution. Flock sizes in these production systems are highly variable, and larger flock sizes are associated with more intensification in housing, feeding, disease control and marketing.

The backyard and semi-intensive units of various sizes can be installed by the farmers as per the availability of land and resources. The unit cost of one such scheme under free range or scavenging **system of management** is depicted below. The total cost of the scheme will be ₹ 800.00, and about ₹ 5,000.00 earning is possible through implementation of this scheme. The birds are to be reared under confinement up to the period of about 28 days so the feed cost up to this period is considered in this scheme.

Capital investment

1. Cost of 20 numbers of RIR day-old chicks @ ₹ 12.00 per pc.   ₹ 240.00
2. Transportation charges   ₹ 40.00

3. Feed cost 1 kg per bird @ ₹ 11.00/kg up to 28 days of age	₹ 220.00
4. Medicine, *etc.*	₹ 100.00
5. Village type housing for night shelter (LS)	₹ 200.00
Total:	**₹ 800.00**

Note: A subsidy up to 75% may be available from the government department.

Recurring expenditure

Feed cost is nearly nil, as they manage their feed from surrounding areas. Other one time expenditures are included in the capital investment.

Income

1. At least 140 eggs will be available from each bird annually × 20 birds, i.e. total 2,800 eggs × ₹ 2.00	₹ 5,600.00
2. Poultry droppings as organic manure (LS)	₹ 100.00
Total annual income:	**₹ 5,700.00**

So a subsidiary income can be generated by the poor farmers through rearing of chickens under scavenging system of management.

EXERCISE

A. Objective Questions

i. **Indicate the correct answer by putting tick (√) mark (multiple choice).**

1. There is a poultry house followed by a run in which of the following systems of poultry rearing
   - (a) Intensive
   - (b) Semi-intensive
   - (c) Scavenging
   - (d) Deep litter

2. Which of the following is the oldest system of poultry keeping, but still popular in India
   - (a) Cage
   - (b) Semi-intensive
   - (c) Free range
   - (d) Deep litter

3. The common scavenger feed base for rural poultry farming is composed of
   - (a) Waste grains
   - (b) Grass seeds
   - (c) White ants
   - (d) All of these

4. Which of the following is an intensive system of rearing poultry?
   - (a) Scavenging system
   - (b) Folding unit system
   - (c) Battery system
   - (d) None of these

5. Which of the following new varieties of poultry may be introduced to enhance the productivity of village poultry?
   - (a) Kadaknath
   - (b) Cornish
   - (c) Punjab Brown
   - (d) Vanaraja

ii. Fill in the blanks.

1. To minimise the laying of shell-less egg or broken egg, _____ supplementation is suggested.
2. Under scavenging system of poultry keeping, the flock size should be restricted to _____ (no. of birds, maximum).
3. Free range system of poultry keeping is also known as _____.
4. Before _____ weeks of age, it is better not to let the birds in free range.
5. Generally, the birds raised under scavenging system are frequently affected with _____ and fowl pox.

iii. Write True (T) or False (F) against each statement.

1. Free range system of poultry keeping is not suitable for commercial purpose.
2. Scavenging poultry management, the commonest poultry production system in rural India, is a low-input, low-output production system.
3. Space requirement is less in deep litter system than cage system of poultry keeping.
4. Deep litter system of poultry housing is a semi-intensive system.
5. Deep litter system is the latest system of poultry rearing.

B. Subjective Questions

1. What are the systems of keeping poultry? Which system is generally used for commercial poultry farming in rural India and why?
2. What are range-fed chickens?
3. Describe in short about raising of chickens under scavenging system of management.
4. How egg production of *deshi* hens under free range system can be increased?
5. Write short notes on the following.
   (a) Scavenging system of management
   (b) Scavenger feed base of village for poultry
   (c) Semi-intensive system of poultry keeping

Answers of the Objective Questions

i. Multiple choice

1. (b) Semi-intensive
2. (c) Free range
3. (d) All of these
4. (c) Battery system
5. (d) Vanaraja

ii. Fill in the blanks

1. calcium
2. 20
3. extensive system/scavenging system
4. 6–7
5. Ranikhet disease/worm infestation

iii. True or False

1. T
2. T
3. F
4. F
5. F

6

Hatching, Brooding and Rearing Norms for Poultry

6.1 WHAT IS HATCHING?

Hatching means production of baby chicks from fertile eggs. The term 'hatching' is also known as incubation. The process of hatching seems nearly magical, because by means of this process within a period of 21 days (in case of chicken) a fertile egg is converted into a chick (Fig. 6.1), which is capable of walking, eating and expressing its needs by its voice and action. The average period required for hatching (incubation period) in case of duck, turkey, Guinea fowl and goose is 28 days and in Japanese quail 17–18 days.

Nowadays hatching of eggs is taken as a business, and it is known as hatchery enterprise. The whole venture of hatchery enterprise includes procurement of fertile eggs, their hatching and finally selling of chicks to the poultry farmers.

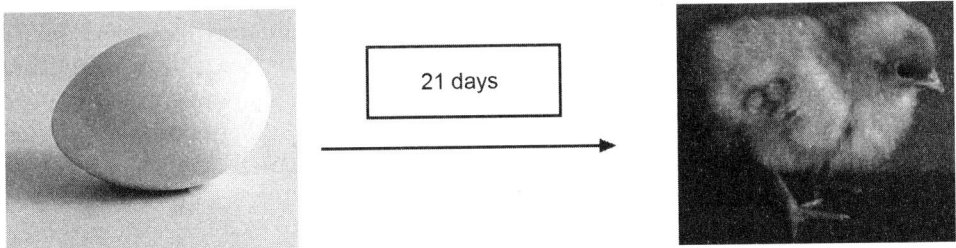

21 days

Fig. 6.1: Hatching of chicken egg

6.2 INCUBATION PERIOD OF VARIOUS POULTRY SPECIES

The period between setting of egg and hatching is known as incubation period. It varies from one species to other species as depicted in Table 6.1.

Table 6.1: Incubation period of various poultry species

Species of bird	Incubation period (days)
Chicken/fowl	21
Duck	28
Japanese quail	17–18
Turkey	28
Guinea fowl	28

Contd.

Table 6.1: Incubation period of various poultry species *(Contd.)*

Species of bird	Incubation period (days)
Goose	28
Muscovy duck	35
Emu	52
Ostrich	42
Pigeon	17–18
Swan	35
Pheasant	24

6.3 METHODS OF HATCHING—NATURAL AND ARTIFICIAL

The **methods of hatching** are of two types, viz.

1. Natural hatching (with the help of live bird/broody hen) and
2. Artificial hatching (with the help of machine/incubator).

Eggs can be hatched by placing them under broody hen. It is called natural hatching. It is a very primitive method, but still popular in rural areas in many parts of our country. As only 10–15 eggs can be hatched by one hen, it is not satisfactory for large scale production. In artificial hatching, thousands of eggs can be hatched at a time with the help of an egg incubator. It provides similar environment as that of broody hen for hatching of eggs. Generally, in commercial poultry production, hatching is done by the artificial method.

6.3.1 Natural Hatching

It is a very primitive method of hatching of eggs for production of chicks (Fig. 6.2). However, the percentage of hatching in this method is very high, sometimes 100 %. This method is still popular with the small poultry keepers in remote rural areas in many parts of our country. The following points should be taken into consideration for successful hatching of eggs by natural method.

- **Selection of broody hen**

Broody hen is used for natural hatching of eggs.

The hen should be thoroughly broody and broodiness may be tested with dummy eggs. She should be healthy, quiet and a good sitter, and have a good body size with all feathers on her body. She should be free from internal and external parasites. The ordinary *deshi* hen is ideal for this purpose.

- **Nest**

Nest should be roomy, fairly dark, cool and well ventilated, readily accessible and easy to clean. An earthen pot, about 15″ in diameter and 8″ deep may be used for this purpose. The nest may be made up of fine soft hay, straw or dry leaves and placed on the ground. The nest should be placed where hens will be safe from dogs, cats, rats and other vermin.

- **Best time to set hen**

The best time to set hen is at night because:

i. Broody hen is more likely to settle down on the eggs at night.

ii. Chicks are more likely to appear on the night of 21st day and will have the whole night to take rest and gain strength.

- **Number of eggs under a hen**

It depends on the size of hen. Maximum 10–15 eggs can be placed under one hen.

- **Care of sitting hen**

The sitting hen should be provided with water and feeds regularly. Cold clean water should be provided at least 2 times a day and whole grains are the desirable feed for sitting hen. Sloppy feeds of all description should be avoided as they tend to produce loose droppings and consequently soiling of eggs. The hen should be taken out from the nest at least for 2 times a day for about 30 minutes to be fed and watered. Exposure of hatching eggs to the fresh air during this time is also beneficial.

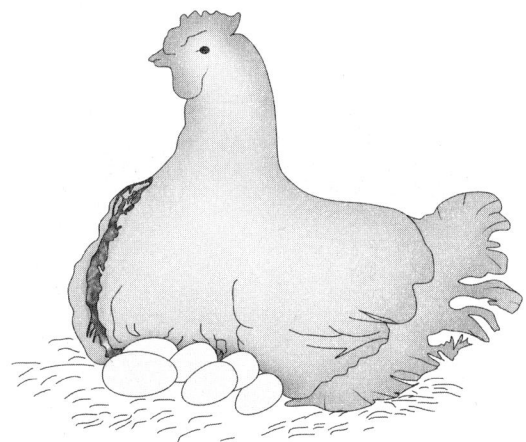

Fig. 6.2: Natural hatching by a broody hen

Advantages of natural hatching

1. It requires no capital investment for purchasing any machine (egg incubator), and it is profitable for small number of chicks production.
2. There is no need of skilled person. Broody hen itself provides all the necessary requirements for hatching of eggs.
3. No need of brooder/brooding management and broody hen will take care the new born chicks.

Disadvantages of natural hatching

1. It is not suitable for large scale production on commercial basis.
2. It is not always possible to get broody hen as and when required.
3. The broody hen, may sometimes, leave the eggs before completion of hatching. All the eggs will be spoiled in such case.
4. Some eggs may be broken due to faulty sitting of broody hen.
5. Hens do not lay eggs when they are engaged in hatching business and thereby total number of eggs production will be less.
6. Some diseases may get transmitted from broody hen to newborn chicks.

6.3.2 Artificial Hatching

Artificial hatching is done by means of a machine known as 'egg incubator' or 'setter and hatcher'. All the necessary microenvironment is created by this machine (Fig. 6.3). Time required for artificial hatching is same as that of natural hatching.

Egg incubator may be operated by kerosene or electricity. However, presently kerosene incubator is not in use.

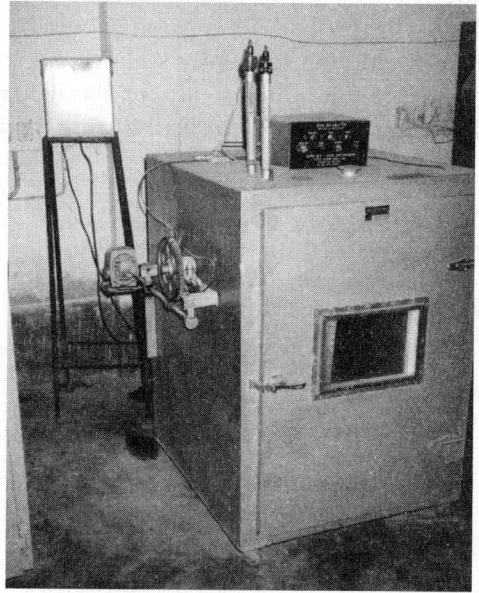

Fig. 6.3: An incubator—equipment used for artificial hatching

Advantages of artificial hatching

1. Large number of eggs can be hatched at a time.
2. Hatching may be done as and when required without broody hen.
3. Rate of hatching is very high and it is profitable from economic point of view.
4. Some diseases may be transmitted from broody hen to newborn chicks during natural hatching. There is no such possibility in case of artificial hatching, as brooding of newly hatched chicks are also done artificially.
5. It is most useful for the hatchery business.

Disadvantages of artificial hatching

1. Incubator and brooder are needed which involve large capital investment.
2. It requires skilful management otherwise whole programme will be upset.
3. The machinery defects at any time of incubation leads to heavy loss.
4. Disease may transmit through incubator, if cleaning and fumigation is not done properly.
5. The newly hatched chicks need special nourishment. The broody hen performs this function in case of natural hatching.

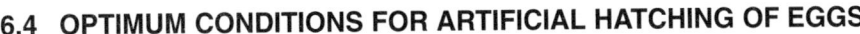

6.4 OPTIMUM CONDITIONS FOR ARTIFICIAL HATCHING OF EGGS

The most important conditions for successful hatching of eggs are maintenance of optimum temperature and humidity, proper ventilation and turning of eggs. These conditions vary from one species of poultry to other. In case of hatching of chicken eggs, the favourable conditions are (i) 37.5–37.7 °C temperature, (ii) 60–70% relative humidity, (iii) circulation of fresh air containing 21% oxygen, and (iv) turning of eggs during the first 18 days of incubation.

[For conditions for hatching of eggs of other poultry species, see Chapter 8. For details of hatchery practices, see Chapter 14]

6.5 BROODING AND REARING PRACTICES OF CHICKEN

6.5.1 Brooding of Chicks

The care and management of day-old birds during early part of their life, especially by providing heat, is called **brooding**. They require extra heat at this stage due to their ill-developed thermoregulatory mechanism. A heat source is required for the chicks until they are fully feathered, and generally up to 4–6 weeks of age in case of chicks. They should not be put out under direct sunlight to keep them warm.

Types of brooding: The brooding of chicks is of 2 types. These are natural brooding and artificial brooding. Natural brooding is done with the help of broody hen. Natural hatching is generally followed by natural brooding. This is very common for backyard poultry keeping for small number of birds. Artificial brooding is done with the help of artificial source of heat. Artificial hatching is followed by artificial brooding. Artificial brooding is done either on the floor or cage. Floor brooding is done under deep litter system of management, and cage brooding is done under cage system of rearing poultry. On the basis of heating arrangement, artificial brooding may be hot room brooding or cold room brooding. In cold room brooding, the house is kept at ambient temperature and limited area in the house is heated by artificial source of heat around the brooder. It is generally followed in tropical countries. In hot room brooding, the total area in the house is heated through central heating arrangement. It is generally followed in cold climate, mostly in Western countries. It is mostly suitable in environmentally controlled poultry houses.

The brooder unit consists of the following arrangements:

1. **A brooder with a heating source:** Usually it is a bamboo basket with electric bulbs as source of heat in case of floor housing with small number of birds. The height of the brooder should be about 6 inches in the first week. Some- times basket is not used and brooding is done on the floor of the deep litter house itself (See Fig. 6.5).

2. **Brooder guard:** A corrugated cardboard or a metal sheet or wire net may be used as brooder guard. In hot weather, hardware cloth or similar mesh material may be used instead of solid guard. Its height should be about 18–24 inches. It is to be placed around the heat source (hover), generally 2–3 feet away from the edge of the hover. In summer, the ring is to be enlarged to keep the chicks from getting too hot. After the first few days, the area is to be enlarged gradually to provide more floor space, and after 7–10 days, it can be removed completely.

A brooding unit with four 60 watt bulbs suspended with 6 inches above the floor and a brooder guard of 5 feet radius is sufficient for 250–300 chicks.

3. **Feeders and drinkers:** Four baby chick drinkers and 3 brand new egg trays (on which feed could be given) are sufficient for 250–300 chicks. Later, these would require to be increased gradually.

All the equipments should be in place in the brooder house, and brooder should kept on at least 24 hours before arrival of the chicks. For brooding, requirements are proper temperature, ventilation, floor space, appropriate feeders and drinkers. Optimum brooding temperature during the first week is 95 °F, and then temperature may be reduced at the rate of 5 °F on every successive weeks, until the room temperature of 60–70 °F (21 °C) is reached or the chicks are fully feathered (Table 6.2). At 5 weeks of age, chicks maintain their own body temperature, if the room temperature is kept near 70 °F.

However, chicks' behaviour is to be taken into consideration whether they are getting proper amount of heat or not. Since the temperature in our country varies a great deal, it is advisable to adjust the required comfortable temperature for the chicks as per their brooding behaviour. The comfort of the chicks is to be checked several times on each day, especially in the evening, and adjustments are to be made accordingly to maintain chick comfort. Contented peeping and even distribution of chicks around and under the brooder indicate comfortable conditions. If chicks chirp and huddle to one side of the brooder, there is a draft. When the temperature is too low/cold, the chicks chirp sharply and huddle together under the brooder. If chicks move away from the brooder, pant, and are drowsy, the temperature is too light warm (Fig. 6.4).

Table 6.2: Brooding temperature schedule for chicks

Age (days)	Brooder temperature (°F)	
	Summer	Winter
1–7	90	95
8–14	85	90
15–21	80	85
22–28	75	80
29–35	70	75
36 to market	70	70

Fresh air should be available continuously in the brooding house. But it is to be ensured that there should be no direct wind or draft that will chill the chicks.

The minimum floor space in the brooder house should be 3–4 inches/chick. However, not more than 500 chicks should be placed under one brooder.

During the first 3 days, feeds are offered on the newspaper or brand new egg tray. Regular chick feeders should be introduced after 3–4 days. Baby chick's drinks should be provided to the chicks.

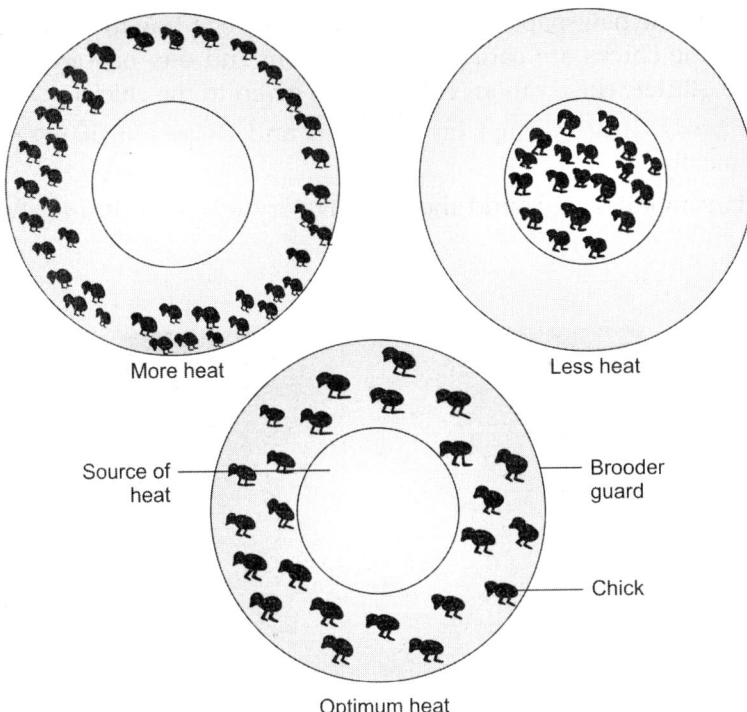

Fig. 6.4: Behaviour of chicks in the brooder

Few tips for brooding management

1. Chicks are to be placed in the brooder gently. Weak chicks should be separated from the others and should be placed in a separate brooder. They require more heat than other chicks.

2. They should receive fresh water only for several hours. Sugar may be added to this water. An 8% sugar solution containing 1% sodium chloride is usually given for first 15 hours after the chicks are placed in the brooder.

3. If the chicks are under stress due to long journey or inclement weather conditions, anti-stress medicine (vitamins + electrolytes) may also be added to the drinking water for the first 3–4 days. Zeetress (Indian herbs @ 0.5 g/100 birds/day), Stressban powder (Zeus @ 0.5 g/100 birds/day), Stresroak (Dabur @ 5 mL/100 birds/day) are some brand names of anti-stress medicine available in the market.

   Ensure that all the chicks are drinking water. Few chicks may be taught to drink water, by dipping their beaks.

4. Poultry must receive a diet containing adequate nutrients to meet their requirements for good health and vitality. Poultry must not be provided with feed that is deleterious to their health. To get a good start, newly-hatched chicks must be provided with feed within 24 hours of hatching. Generally, 3 hours after placing the chicks in the brooder, maize grits (chick maize) are

offered on the newspaper or on the brand new egg tray for them and ensure that all the chicks are eating. Usually, from 2nd day onwards, usual feed (broiler starter/chick ration/crumbles) is given to the chicks.

5. Dead birds, if any, must be removed and disposed of promptly and hygienically.

6. Constant monitoring round the clock is very essential during the first few days.

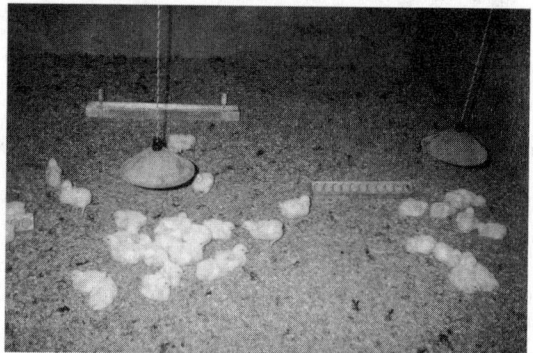

Fig. 6.5: Brooding of chicks with the help of electric bulb

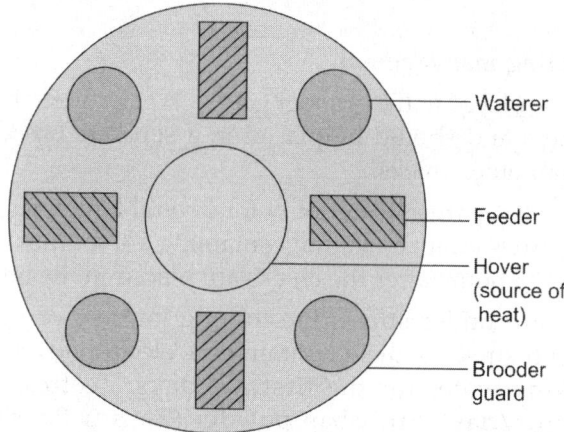

Fig. 6.6: Arrangement of feeders and waterers in a brooder

6.5.2 Feed Management for Chicks

- Generally, feed is offered to the chicks 3 hours after their arrival in the farm. Feed should be available all the time during first few days of life. During first 3–4 days feed is offered to the chicks on newspapers or brand new egg trays (Fig. 6.7). Generally, 1 egg tray (30 egg capacity) is sufficient for 100 chicks. After 3–4 days, newspapers or egg trays are to be replaced by chick feeders.

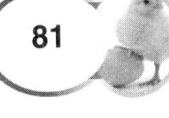

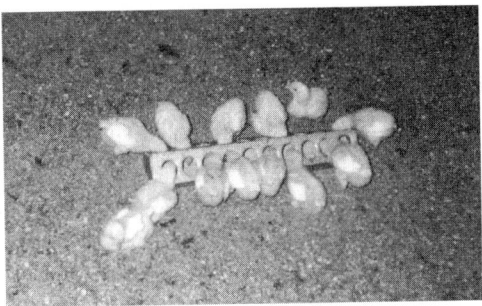

Fig. 6.7: Chicks taking feed

- Light and heat managements are important considerations for proper feeding. Insufficient light in the shed reduces the feed intake, as birds may not see the feed properly. If there is lack of proper brooding (less heat in the shed), birds may huddle together all the times without taking feed. (*See Chapter 11, Tables 11.7, 11.8 and 11.9*)

6.5.3 Water Management for Chicks

- Drinking water should be provided to the chicks within 24 hours of hatching (Fig. 6.8). Generally, water troughs are placed in the brooder before chick's arrival in the farm, so that they can get water just after entering in the farm. Four drinkers are sufficient for 250 birds. Waterers are to be placed properly on the litter materials to prevent leaking or splashing of water. During brooding, waterers are to be placed nearer to the hover (i.e. the source of heat). Height of the waterers should be increased as age of chick increases and should be at the bird's crop height.

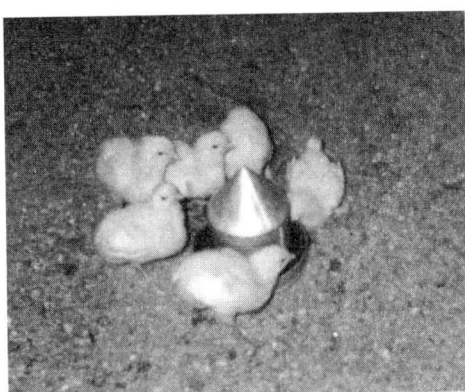

Fig. 6.8: Chicks taking water

- Waterers should be placed in such a way that birds need not walk more than 8 ft to drink water (Fig. 6.6). In general waterer space requirement is 1 inch/ bird up to the age of 4 weeks, then 2 inches/bird. In summer, waterer space should be increased by 2 times than normal.

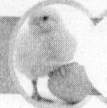
- Always clean and hygienic water should be provided to the birds. Waterers should be cleaned daily and it gives good result, if disinfectant is used during the cleaning process.

- Temperature of drinking water is important, especially in summer months. Fowls stop drinking water, if its temperature becomes 38 °C (110 °F). So, cold water is to be provided to the birds during hot summer.

- After arrival of chicks in the farm, first water is to be provided to the birds, then feed. Otherwise birds may take less water than required.

- Sometimes vaccine is provided through drinking water. In such cases, disinfectant should not be used for cleaning or disinfection of waterers, 24 hours before adding vaccine in it, otherwise the activity of vaccine may be reduced by the disinfectant.

- Water intake of birds depends on many factors like age, weather, *etc.* Water intake nearly doubles during summer than in winter. Sufficient quantity of drinking water should be provided to the birds. (*See Chapter 11, Tables 11.7, 11.8 and 11.9*)

6.5.4 Light Management

- Young birds reared away from the hen require a light intensity of about 20 lux on the feed and water, for the first 3 days after hatching, in order to learn to find feed and water. It may then be reduced to as low as 2 lux during rearing.

- Light is an important factor for growth and egg production of poultry. Bright light should be present in the poultry shed during first 3 weeks of their lives it attracts them towards feed and water.

- In broiler shed, 60 watt bulb may be used per 100 sq ft floor area during first 3 weeks (*See* Fig. 6.5). Then intensity of light is reduced to some extent for good result. After 3 weeks, one 60 watt bulb is sufficient for 200 sq ft. All time light (24 hours) may be present during chick stage, however, 1 hour darkness out of 24 hours gives better result. To avoid complete darkness a night bulb (25 watt) may be used. However, in layer type poultry, after 7 days, light may be reduced gradually during night hours till 9th week. (*See Chapter 12*)

6.6 BROODING AND REARING PRACTICES FOR OTHER SPECIES OF POULTRY

Brooding is an essential part for rearing other species of poultry also.

[*The brooding norms and other rearing practices for duck, quail, turkey, Guinea fowl and emu are described at the respective sections in Chapter 8.*]

EXERCISE

A. Objective Questions

i. **Indicate the correct answer by putting tick (√) mark (multiple choice).**

1. Production of chicks from fertile eggs is known as
    (a) Culling   (b) Hatching
    (c) Brooding   (d) Deworming
2. Maximum number of eggs that can be hatched by a broody hen is
    (a) 8   (b) 12
    (c) 22   (d) 25
3. Incubation period of chicken egg is
    (a) 17 days   (b) 21 days
    (c) 28 days   (d) 35 days
4. Incubation period of chicken egg by artificial hatching method (incubator) is
    (a) 7 days   (b) 14 days
    (c) 21 days   (d) 28 days
5. Incubation period of chicken egg by natural hatching method (broody hen) is
    (a) 7 days   (b) 14 days
    (c) 21 days   (d) 28 days
6. Temperature needed for artificial incubation of chicken eggs should be
    (a) 35.5 °C   (b) 37.5 °C
    (c) 39.5 °C   (d) 41.5 °C
7. Relative humidity needed for artificial incubation of chicken eggs should be
    (a) 50–60%   (b) 60–70%
    (c) 70–80%   (d) 80–90%
8. The incubation period of quail egg is
    (a) 15 days   (b) 17 days
    (c) 19 days   (d) 21 days
9. The incubation period of turkey egg is
    (a) 17 days   (b) 21 days
    (c) 28 days   (d) 35 days
10. The incubation period of duck egg is
    (a) 18 days   (b) 24 days
    (c) 28 days   (d) 32 days
11. Application of heat to the birds during their early part of lives is known as
    (a) Culling   (b) Brooding
    (c) Hatching   (d) Deworming
12. The incubation period of which of the following species of poultry is 28 days?
    (a) Chicken and turkey   (b) Turkey and Guinea fowl
    (c) Duck and quail   (d) Muscovy duck and Guinea fowl

13. Which of the following is true in relation to the artificial hatching of chicken eggs?
    (a) 60–70% relative humidity
    (b) 38.7 °C temperature inside the incubator
    (c) Turning of eggs during the total period of incubation
    (d) All of these
14. The favourable conditions for hatching of chicken eggs are:
    1. 65% relative humidity.
    2. 37.5 °C temperature inside the incubator.
    3. Circulation of fresh air containing 21% oxygen.
    4. Turning of eggs are must during the total period of incubation
    Select the correct answer from the code below:

Code (a) 1, 2 and 3 are correct   (b) 2, 3 and 4 are correct
     (c) 1, 2 and 4 are correct   (d) 1, 2, 3 and 4 are correct

15. Match List I with List II and select the correct answer using the code given below the lists.

List I (Species)	List II (Incubation period)
A. Duck	1. 35 days
B. Quail	2. 21 days
C. Muscovy duck	3. 28 days
D. Fowl	4. 17 days

Code (a) A B C D   (b) A B C D
        2 1 3 4   3 1 2 4
     (c) A B C D   (d) A B C D
        1 3 4 2   3 4 1 2

ii. Fill in the blanks.

1. Incubation period of chicken egg is _____.
2. Incubation period of duck egg is _____.
3. Incubation period of quail egg is _____.
4. Incubation period of turkey egg is _____.
5. Incubation period of Guinea fowl is _____.
6. Production of baby chicks from fertile egg is known as _____.
7. Day-old chicks should be kept under brooder at a temperature of _____ °F.
8. Birds require heat at their early part of lives as their _____ mechanism is ill-developed.
9. The hens engaged in natural hatching process are known as _____ hens.
10. Artificial hatching is done by means of a machine called _____.

iii. Write True (T) or False (F) against each statement.

1. Broodiness is negatively correlated with egg production.
2. *Deshi* hens are ideal sitter for hatching of eggs.

3. The minimum floor space in the brooder house should be 3–4 inches per chick.

4. Optimum brooding temperature during 2nd week of age of chicks, should be 90 °F.

5. Fowl may stop drinking water, if its temperature becomes 38 °C.

B. Subjective Questions

1. What do you mean by hatching and hatching egg? Mention the incubation period of any 3 poultry species. Discuss about natural and artificial hatchings with their advantages and disadvantages.

2. What is natural hatching? Describe this method of hatching along with its advantages and disadvantages.

3. What do you mean by artificial hatching? Indicate the optimum conditions for artificial hatching of chicken eggs.

4. What is brooding? Describe in short the rearing of chicks with special reference to brooding house requirement.

5. What is the recommended environmental temperature for a newly hatched chick?

6. Write short notes on the following.
   - (a) Natural hatching
   - (b) Artificial hatching
   - (c) Broody hen
   - (d) Incubator
   - (e) Incubation period

Answers of the Objective Questions

i. Multiple choice

1. (b) Hatching	2. (b) 12	3. (b) 21 days
4. (c) 21 days	5. (c) 21 days	6. (b) 37.5 °C
7. (b) 60–70%	8. (b) 17 days	9. (c) 28 days
10. (c) 28 days	11. (b) Brooding	

12. (b) Turkey and Guinea fowl

13. (a) 60–70% relative humidity

14. (a) 1, 2 and 3 are correct   15. (d)

ii. Fill in the blanks

1. 21 days	2. 28 days	3. 17–18 days
4. 28 days	5. 28 days	6. hatching/incubation
7. 90–95	8. thermoregulatory	9. broody

10. incubator

iii. True or False

1. T   2. T   3. T   4. T   5. T

7

Feeding Norms for Poultry

7.1 GENERAL FEEDING NORMS FOR CHICKEN

All the feed nutrients, viz. protein, fat, carbohydrate, vitamin, mineral and water should be fed to the poultry in balanced proportion. Feed nutrients are needed to support life, growth and production.

Out of the 6 classes of nutrients, carbohydrates and fats are required primarily as sources of energy. Fats are the most concentrated source of dietary energy providing essential fatty acids and is present in sufficient amount in oil cakes. Carbohydrates are mainly present in cereal grains. Energy is needed to maintain body temperature, their activity, growth and egg production.

Proteins are the complex organic compounds made up of amino acids. The critical amino acids for poultry are arginine, threonine, lysine, methionine, cystine and tryptophan, out of which the most critical amino acids are lysine, methionine and cystine in chick diets, and methionine and cystine in layer diets which should be considered while formulating these diets. Proteins are needed in the feed for tissue building and egg production. Fish meal and oil cakes primarily supply proteins to the birds.

Vitamins are organic compounds, usually not synthesized by the body and required through feed. They function as regulators of various metabolic processes. About 14 vitamins, required by poultry are classified into 2 groups, viz. fat-soluble vitamins (A, D, E and K) and water-soluble vitamins (B complex and C). Vitamins A, D and riboflavin are mostly critical in poultry. Sometimes choline, nicotinic acid and vitamin B_{12} are also needed. Grains may be fed to birds at the rate of 2 kg per 100 birds per day to provide vitamins. Synthetic vitamins are also available and generally incorporated in the commercial poultry feed.

Poultry requires 13 minerals which act as a part of certain proteins or enzymes. Poultry receives most of these minerals through feed. Special care should be taken to supplement at least 4 minerals in the feed, viz. calcium (Ca), phosphorus (P), manganese (Mn) and common salt (NaCl).

Clean and fresh water must be available all the times. Chickens must drink in every 15–20 minutes.

In general, the major sources of nutrients in poultry feed are cereal grains, oil cakes, fish meal and grain by-products. Distillery by-products, milk by-products, alfalfa meal and yeast are also used for poultry feed. If it is difficult to supply some nutrients through natural ingredients, synthetic materials available in the market are used. The major poultry ration ingredients in India are as follows.

Energy sources (60–65%): Corn, broken rice, pearl millet, wheat, sorghum and rice bran

Protein sources (30–35%): Soybean meal, fish meal, sunflower meal (decorticated), peanut meal and meat meal

Others (5%): Soy oil, sunflower oil and minerals

Poultry feed may be prepared at home by mixing various ingredients in proper ratio. However, in case of large farm, it is better to use compounded feed available in different brand names in the markets. Balanced feed should be given to the birds on the basis of their physiological needs (like chick, grower and layer stages of egg type birds, and starter and finisher stages of broiler type birds).

Feed is passed through the digestive tract of poultry, consisting of mouth, esophagus and crop, proventriculus (glandular stomach), gizzard (muscular stomach), small intestine and large intestine. Relatively speaking little digestion takes place until the feed reaches the small intestine. Feed passes through the digestive tract in 3½–4 hours when it is empty, while on continuous feeding it takes 12 hours.

Feeds should be offered 3–4 times a day during early part of life, and after that 2–3 times a day feeding is sufficient.

Feed should not be offered more than ⅓ to ½ level of the capacity of feeder, to avoid wastage. If hanging feeders are used, they must be shaken often. Feeders should be distributed in such a way that no bird has to move more than 8 ft for feed. Height of the feeder should be adjusted according to the height of the birds' back. Proper feeders should be used for different age groups and categories of birds. Required space of feeder should be given for proper feeding.

Feed should be essentially free from fungal and bacterial contaminations like *E coli*, *Salmonella*, Mycoplasma, *Aspergillus*, *etc*. Poultry feed should be free from toxic principles present in some feed ingredients like gossypol, aflatoxin, *etc*. It is better not to store the feed for more than 1–1½ months to avoid fungal infection and to restore vitamins properly. All feeds must be stored in cans or bins which have tight fitting lids to prevent contamination by insects or other vermin.

Feeder should be cleaned regularly to avoid any cake formation, which invites fungal growth. It is better to disinfect the feeders with potassium permanganate $(KMnO_4)$ at least once in a week.

Poultry are sensitive to abrupt diet changes. When necessary, changes should be done gradually. For changing diet in poultry, small amount of new feed should be mixed with larger portions of the existing feed and gradually, day by day, the portion of the new feed is to be increased while decreasing the portion of the old feed. As for example, for changing feed from chick mash to grower mash, initially 25% grower and 75% chick mash should be mixed and offered for first 4 days. Then, 50:50 in the next 4 days, then 75% grower mash and 25% chick mash for another 4 days, and finally 100% grower mash. Birds should be observed carefully as coccidiosis outbreak may take place during the changeover period.

Feeding should be encouraged during cooler part of the day as temperature higher than 30 °C reduces feed intake which may result into reduced intake of essential nutrients with adverse effects.

Poultry must have continuous access to clean and fresh drinking water. Waterer must be cleaned and disinfected daily. Height of the waterers should be equal to that of the birds' back. Birds generally stop drinking, if the temperature of water is more than room temperature. So cold water should be provided to the birds in summer season. Waterers should be placed in such a way that birds should not have to move more than 8 ft for water. Waterers should be checked frequently to avoid overflow or shortage. *(For detailed information see Chapter 11)*

7.2 FEEDING NORMS FOR OTHER SPECIES OF POULTRY

The feed ingredients used for chicken are also used for other species of poultry.

(For other detail of species see Chapter 8)

EXERCISE

A. Objective Questions

i. **Indicate the correct answer by putting tick (√) mark (multiple choice).**

1. The most critical vitamin(s) in poultry diet is/are
   (a) Vitamin A   (b) Vitamin D
   (c) Riboflavin   (d) All of these

2. The most critical amino acid(s) in layer diets is/are
   (a) Methionine   (b) Lysine
   (c) Cystine   (d) Both a and c

3. Special care should be taken to supplement which of the following minerals in poultry diet?
   (a) Calcium   (b) Phosphorus
   (c) Manganese   (d) All of these

4. Greens may be fed to poultry birds to provide vitamins @
   (a) 0.5 kg/100 birds per day
   (b) 2 kg/100 birds per day
   (c) 6 kg/100 birds per day
   (d) Greens should not be fed to the poultry birds.

5. Poultry needs energy to maintain
   (a) Body temperature   (b) Growth
   (c) Egg production   (d) All of these

ii. **Fill in the blanks.**

1. Relatively speaking in case of poultry, little digestion takes place until the feed reaches the _____.

2. Feed should not be offered more than _____ level of the capacity of feeder to avoid wastage.

3. The most critical amino acids in layer diets are _____ and
_____.

iii. Write True (T) or False (F) against each statement.

1. The most critical amino acids are lysine, methionine and cystine in chick diets.
2. Chickens must drink every 15–20 minutes.
3. Feed passes through the digestive tract in 8 hours when it is empty.
4. Feed should not be offered more than $\frac{1}{3}$ to $\frac{1}{2}$ level of the capacity of feeder to avoid wastage.
5. Height of the waterers should be equal to that of the birds' back.

B. Subjective Questions

1. Describe in detail the feeding norms for chicken.
2. Why is it not desirable to store the feed for more than 1–1½ months for feeding poultry?
3. What is the method of changing diets in poultry?

Answers of the Objective Questions

i. Multiple choice

1. (d) All of these   2. (d) Both a and c   3. (d) All of these
4. (b) 2 kg per 100 birds per day   5. (d) All of these

ii. Fill in the blanks

1. small intestine   2. $\frac{1}{3}$ to $\frac{1}{2}$ 3. methionine, cystine

iii. True or False

1. T   2. T   3. F   4. T   5. T

8

Other Poultry Species: Duck, Quail, Turkey, Guinea Fowl, Emu and Goose

Chicken or fowl is the primary poultry species. Other important poultry species are duck, quail, turkey, Guinea fowl, emu, *etc*. Many aspects of these species of poultry were described in various chapters of this book. Some special features of these poultry species are presented in this chapter.

8.1 GENERAL IDEA ABOUT DUCK

8.1.1 Introduction

Duck is an important species of poultry in India (Fig. 8.1) and it enjoys the next position just after chicken so far the total poultry population is concerned. Duck population in India is estimated to be 27.64 million constituting approximately 4.26% of the total poultry (18th All India Livestock Census, 2007). Duck egg and meat have become an important source of nutrients in human diet. In Europe and the USA, ducks are reared for meat, whereas in Asia they are primarily reared for eggs. In India, coastal states of India and some parts of Assam and Bihar constitute the major breeding tracts of ducks. Important duck producing states of our country are West Bengal (12.16 million), Assam (8.44 million), Tamil Nadu (1.04 million) and Kerala (0.99 million). Out of the total ducks available in the country, more than 90% comprises of indigenous type. Majority of duck keepers belong to small and marginal farmers and landless labourers. Duck production in India remains neglected due to lack of attention from research workers, planners, developmental agencies and private sectors. However, after introduction of Khaki Campbell duck, in India duck farming, particularly for egg production, is gaining popularity.

Top 10 duck meat producing countries in the world are China (67.23%), France (5.95%), Malaysia (3.00%), Vietnam (2.52%), USA (2.43%), Thailand (2.43%), Taiwan (2.00%), Hungary (1.95%), India (1.86%) and Republic of Korea (1.37%).

Top 10 egg producing countries (excluding hen eggs) in the world are China (84.58%), Thailand (6.06%), Indonesia (3.52%), Philippines (1.41%), Brazil (1.163%), Taiwan (0.62%), Republic of Korea (0.55%), Bangladesh (0.51%), Myanmar (0.28%) and Romania (0.20%). (The figures within parentheses are world figures, FAOSTAT, 2007.)

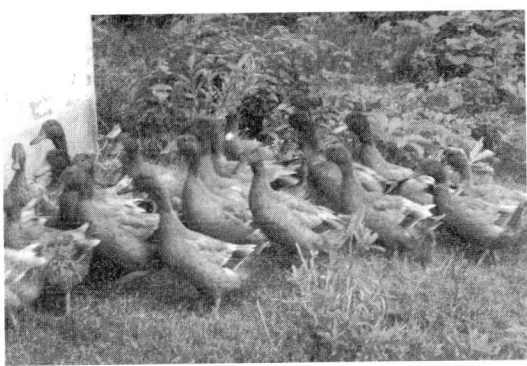

Fig. 8.1: A flock of Khaki Campbell ducks

8.1.2 Salient Characteristics of Duck in Comparison to Chicken

- The scientific name of duck is *Anas platyrhynchos* (Family: Anatidae).
- Ducks lay more number of eggs than chicken (Khaki Campbell duck can lay about 300 eggs/year).
- Duck egg (65–70 g) is larger in size than chicken egg (55–60 g). So more nutrients are present in duck egg than chicken egg.
- Ducks have a more profitable life span than chicken from commercial egg laying point of view. Ducks are kept in the farm for 36 months whereas chickens are kept in the farm for 18 months for economic laying. So replacement cost in duck farming is less than chicken farming.
- Ducks do not require elaborate houses like chicken. They are quite hard and more resistant to common avian diseases. Marsh, wetland and barren moors, upon which chicken or no other type of livestock will flourish, are excellent quarters for duck farming.
- Ducks generally completes their egg laying within morning hours. They lay 95–98% of their eggs in the morning before 9.00 am. So collection of eggs in duck farm is easier, and from research point of view data can be accurately collected in less time and labour.

8.1.3 Reproduction and Hatching

For fertile egg production the ratio of male and female duck is 1:5. Generally at the age of 18 weeks ducks start laying eggs. The incubation period is 28 days. For commercial purpose, the duck eggs can be artificially hatched with the help of incubator just like chicken eggs. The optimum temperature and relative humidity for hatching of duck eggs are 37.0–37.5 °C and 70–75% respectively.

Apart from these, there should be proper air circulation inside the incubator. Eggs are sprinkled with lukewarm water having sanitiser, once a day from 2nd day to 25th day and cooled for a maximum period of half an hour. Candling is done on 7th day. The eggs are turned hourly and are transferred to hatcher on 25th day.

Duck can also hatch eggs naturally just like chicken. Normally Khaki Campbell ducks do not like to hatch. Hence, the process of hatching is carried out with the help of broody hen or *deshi* ducks. A single broody hen can hatch 8–10 duck eggs.

8.1.4 Feeds and Feeding of Duck

A duck requires less feed, if reared under semi-intensive system with facility of water bodies. They can manage their feed requirements up to 60% from the range land and pond in terms of insects, food grains, grasses, *etc*. In such cases 50–60 g feed per head per day may be offered to them. However, feed requirement increases when the ducks are reared under complete confinement. A layer type duck requires 4–5 kg feed up to 8 weeks of age and 12–13 kg up to 20 weeks of age. Every layer duck takes about 120–130 g feed per day depending on the rate of egg laying. Total feed requirement for a layer duck (e.g. Khaki Campbell) from day-old stage up to 1 year laying period is about 60 kg (maximum).

Readymade duck feeds are not popular in the market. The feed ingredients, which are commonly used for preparing chicken feeds, can also be used for preparation of duck feed. Nutritional requirements and feed formulae of ducks at different ages are given in Tables 8.1 and 8.2 respectively. Further, feed consumption of Khaki Campbell duck for egg production is given in Table 8.3.

Table 8.1: Nutrient requirements for ducks

Characteristic	Starter duck	Grower duck	Layer duck	Broiler starter duck	Broiler finisher duck
Moisture (max %)	11	11	11	11	11
Metabolisable energy (min Kcal/kg)	2,600	2,500	2,600	2,800	2,900
Crude protein (max %)	20	16	18	23	20
Crude fibre (max %)	7	8	8	6	6
Acid-insoluble ash (max %)	4	4	4	3	3
Salt (NaCl max %)	0.6	0.6	0.6	0.6	0.6
Calcium (min %)	1	1	3	1.2	1.2
Available phosphorus (min %)	0.5	0.5	0.5	0.5	0.5
Linoleic Acid (min %)	1	1	1	1	1
Lysine (min %)	0.9	0.6	0.65	1.2	1
Methionine (min %)	0.3	0.25	0.3	0.5	0.35

NB: BIS 1992 requirements for poultry feeds are taken as a guide.

Table 8.2: Feed formulae for Khaki Campbell ducks

Ingredients (%)	Starter duck	Grower duck	Layer duck
Wheat	45	48	42
Yellow maize	—	—	10
Deoiled rice bran	14	25.5	6.5
Soybean meal	25	15	20
Fish meal	10	6	10
Lucern leaf meal	2	2	2

Contd.

Table 8.2: Feed formulae for Khaki Campbell ducks *(Contd.)*

Ingredients (%)	Starter duck	Grower duck	Layer duck
Mineral mixture	2.5	2.5	2.5
Shell grit	—	—	5.5
Dicalcium phosphate	1	0.5	1
Vitamin mixture	0.5	0.5	0.5
Total	100	100	100

Source: This formula is used at Central Poultry Development Organisation (CPDO), southern region, Bengaluru.

Table 8.3: Feed consumption of Khaki Campbell ducks

Age (weeks)	Weekly feed consumption (kg/bird)	Progressive total (kg)
1	0.115	
2	0.255	
3	0.425	
4	0.620	
Total	1.415	1.415
5	0.720	
6	0.770	
7	0.785	
8	0.790	
Total	3.065	4.480
9	0.690	
10	0.730	
11	0.755	
12	0.755	
Total	2.930	7.410
13	0.595	
14	0.605	
15	0.630	
16	0.705	
Total	2.535	9.945
17	0.615	
18	0.655	
19	0.665	
20	0.745	
Total	2.680	12.625

NB: From 20 weeks onwards feed consumption varies from 125–150 g/bird/day, depending upon the rate of production.

Source: Central Poultry Development Organisation (CPDO), southern region, Bengaluru.

8.1.5 Systems of Rearing Duck

Duck may be reared in intensive, semi-intensive or range system. Ducks by nature prefer to graze on fields and swim in ponds. They can be reared conveniently, if there are water bodies and garden. But attention should be paid to cleanliness. The pond water should be clean and hygienic. Rearing ducks in dirty water may lead to diseases.

In absence of pond or other water body, duck rearing is still possible in close confinement. Khaki Campbell ducks are suitable in such cases. Ducks should be supplied with adequate water in big tubs made up of plastic or cement. It is not essential for ducks to swim, but water is needed for drinking and cleaning of beaks and eyes. Neck deep water source will serve their purpose. Balance feed should be supplied to the ducks as per their requirements.

Duck rearing is also popular in integrated farming system. Ducks can be reared in ponds profitably along with fish culture. In this system of farming, cost of fish production is low as droppings (faeces) of ducks are used as fish feed and no other feed or manuring in the pond is required for fishes (200–300 ducks per hectare of water area). Under integrated duck farming with rice cultivation, the ducks perform 4 essential functions, viz. intertillage (as they search for food, their bills loosen up the soil around the rice plants), weeding, insect control and manuring.

8.1.6 Care and Management of Duck

8.1.6.1 Care and Management of Duckling

- Ducklings need special care during first 3 weeks of age. The mortality rate among ducklings during this stage is more due to lack of proper care.
- At this stage the ducklings are reared on wire floor. Mud floor or cemented floor with saw dust may also be used for this purpose. Depending on the health status, ducklings can be set free in pond or other water body, after 21–30 days of age.
- The care of ducklings at their early part of lives is called brooding. Brooding temperature during 1st week should be 30 °C. In the following weeks 3 °C per week is reduced till it reaches 24 °C. In summer the atmospheric temperature remains high, but in winter season, if the required temperature is not provided, the ducklings may die due to chilling effect. Heat may be provided by electric bulbs. Those villages which do not have electricity, can provide heat to the ducklings by kerosene lamps.
- The new born ducklings do not need any feed in the first 24 hours. Sometimes the new born ducklings are fed upon glucose water or electrolyte water. They should be served liquid or semi-liquid diet after mixing with water on 1st and 2nd days. Afterwards general feed should be mixed with little water and served. The quantity of feed required at various stages of life is depicted in Table 8.3.
- While serving feed to the ducks, it should be mixed well with water. But it should not be soaked in water overnight to avoid possibility of fungal growth, if any.

- **The following points have also to be kept in mind while taking care of ducklings.**
    i. The brooding temperature should be kept optimum to protect them from cold.
    ii. The ducklings should be protected from rats. Duck house must be rat proof.
    iii. Each duckling should have proper space according to its age (Table 8.4). They should not be kept in congested condition.
    iv. The water level in their drinking pots should be 5.0–7.5 cm. They may be drown, if the water level is high.

8.1.6.2 Care and Management of Grower Ducks

The grower ducks do not need extra heat. They do not need any artificial light also. The normal day light of 12 hours is sufficient for them. The level of water in the waterers is to be increased to 12.5–15.0 cm, so that they can dip their heads as well. Proper floor space (Table 8.4) and space for feeder and waterer should be provided (Table 8.5). Sufficient feed of proper quality should be given for proper growth.

8.1.6.3 Care and Management of Layer Ducks

The ducks, if reared in a proper way, start laying eggs at the age of 4½ months or even few days earlier. Each duck should be provided with specific floor space. The duck shed should be kept clean. They should be served sufficient feed and water as per their requirements. Duck house should have proper light for 16–17 hours. This is very important because laying eggs have a direct or indirect connection with the provision of light. Apart from natural day light of 12 hours, artificial light should be given for 4–5 hours. The house should have egg laying boxes for production of clean eggs. The ducks will lay eggs in the boxes. The size of each box is 30 cm × 30 cm × 45 cm. One such box for 3 ducks should be kept in the duck house. Soft and dry grasses, leaves, hay, *etc.* should be sprayed in the boxes and needs to be changed after every 2–3 days. Ducks are generally timid birds. They should be caught/hold by their necks and not the sides of their bodies.

Table 8.4: Floor space requirements for ducks (for rearing on floor)

Age of duck (week)	Floor space (m²/duck)*
0–4	0.093
5–16	0.279
17 and above	0.371–0.465

* 1 m² = 10.77 sq ft

Table 8.5: Feeder and waterer space requirements for ducks

Age of duck (week)	Feeder space (cm /duck)	Waterer space (cm /duck)
0–3	1.4	1.2
3–6	2.0	1.8
6–9	3.5–4.0	2.0
10 and above	10.0	5.0

8.1.7 Maintenance of Duck Health

Just like any other birds ducks too fall ill. But in comparison to chicken the rate of sickness in ducks is less. A few infectious diseases like duck plague, duck cholera, duck viral hepatitis and fungal diseases may be fatal for ducks. Proper preventive measures should be taken to fight against these diseases as depicted below.

- Ducklings should be purchased from renowned and dependable institutions.
- Allowing proper floor space per duck is important for intensive rearing of ducks. Overcrowding must be avoided.
- There should be better air circulation in each and every shed. Otherwise the suffocation may occur due to the formation of ammonia and other pollutants. This leads to the difficulty in breathing of the ducks which may fell upon the health and productivity of the ducks.
- The floor should be kept dry as far as possible. The damp and wet floor may lead to incidence of some diseases like coccidiosis and worm infestation.
- Surroundings of the duck farms should be kept clean. The utensils utilised in the farms, viz. feeders, waterers, etc. should be cleaned daily and disinfected regularly. They may be washed with potassium permanganate ($KMnO_4$) solution at least once in a week.
- Proper feed should be given to the ducks at their various stages, viz. duckling stage, growing stage and egg laying stage. Sufficient clean drinking water should be given to the ducks.
- To avoid fungal diseases, ducks should not be given previously soaked feed. Their feeds should be stored in a dry place. Fungal infection is commonly seen in GNC, wheat, soybean, rice bran, etc.
- Antibiotics against bacterial diseases and anticoccidials against coccidiosis should be mixed with drinking water and/or feed, routinely. Some commonly used antibiotics are vendox-vet, tetracycline hydrochloride powder, neodox forte, etc. These antibiotics, if started, should be continued for at least 4–5 days. Codrinal (hoechst), amprolium soluble powder (merind), Esb_3 (cadila) are some of the brand names of medicines which prevent coccidiosis. Anyone of these anticoccidial medicines, if given in proper dose in the 3rd and 5th weeks and a few days before the laying of eggs, then the chance of the disease occurrence is less.
- Deworming medicines should be given in proper dose to prevent worm infestation. Levamisole HCl, piperazine hexahydrate, fenbendazole are some of the anthelmintic medicines commonly used against worm infestation.
- Various infectious diseases like duck plague, duck cholera, etc. can be prevented, if they are properly vaccinated (Table 8.6).
- Inspite of the above measures, if any disease appears in the duck farm then the sick bird should be isolated apparently from the healthy birds. Local veterinary doctor should be consulted immediately and urgent measures should be taken as per his advice.

Table 8.6: Vaccination schedule of the ducks

Name of disease	Name of vaccine	Age at which vaccination should be done	Dose and route of administration*
Duck plague	Duck plague vaccine	1st at 4 weeks of age; 2nd at 8–10 weeks of age; 3rd at 16–18 weeks of age; after that twice a year	0.5 mL; subcutaneous injection
Duck cholera	Duck cholera vaccine	1st at 3–4 weeks of age; 2nd at 1 month after the 1st injection; after that twice a year	1 mL; subcutaneous injection

* manufacturer's instruction should be followed.

8.1.8 Duck at a Glance (as per CPDO, Govt. of India)

Performance indicators of Khaki Campbell (egg type)

- Age at first laying — 120 days
- Age at 50% production — 146 days
- Annual egg production — 300 eggs
- Egg weight at 40 weeks — 66 g
- Body weight at 40 weeks — 1.80 kg
- Daily feed consumption per bird — 120–130 g
- Ducklings mortality (0–8 weeks) — 2–3%
- Grower mortality (8–20 weeks) — 0.2–0.5%
- Adult mortality (20–72 weeks) — 5–7%

Performance indicators of Vigova Super-M (meat type)

- Day-old body weight — 47–48 g
- Body weight at 4 weeks — 1.3–1.5 kg
- Feed consumption up to 4 weeks — 3.0–3.2 kg
- Body weight at 6 weeks — 2.3–2.5 kg
- Feed consumption up to 6 weeks — 5.8–6.2 kg
- Mortality (0–6 weeks) — 2–3%

8.2 GENERAL IDEA ABOUT QUAIL

8.2.1 Introduction

Quail meat and quail eggs are sometimes featured on the menu of fancy hotels to satisfy the demand of wild bird taste. Quail is not only popular as a producer of meat and eggs, but is also a research animal (Fig. 8.2). This bird is an ideal laboratory animal for testing especially in the field of embryology as well as for endocrinological, nutritional, onchological and genetic studies. Many researchers prefer working with this bird because of its hardiness, ease of handling, great laying ability, low generation interval, producing 3–4 generations per year and easy accessibility of the embryo. These features make this small avian not only suitable as pilot animal for biological research but also for commercial exploitation.

Quails have been reared through centuries in many countries of the world like China, Taiwan, UK, *etc*. During late 50, its commercial production started in Italy. It has also been very popular in Japan, France, Hong Kong, Singapore, Korea, Germany, *etc*. from long time. In Hong Kong, thousands of farmers have taken up quail farming of various sizes ranging from thousands to lakhs per year.

As far as India is concerned, Japanese quail was introduced by Indian Veterinary Research Institute (IVRI) in 1974 by importing hatching eggs from University of California, USA. Since then researches were done in many central institutes and agricultural universities. Nowadays commercial production of quail is also being initiated in many states of our country. However, its marketing has been limited to some of the urban pockets which requires to be developed further.

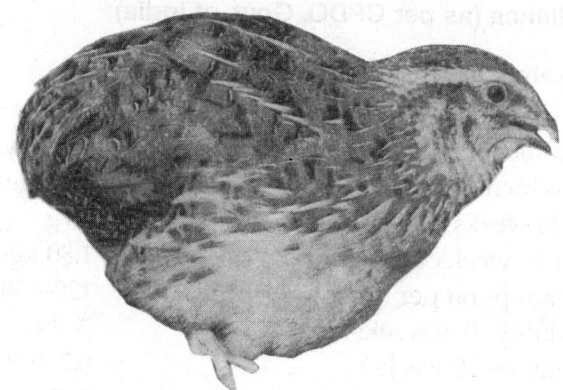

Fig. 8.2: A Japanese quail

8.2.2 Salient Characteristics of Quail

- Scientific name of Japanese quail is *Coturnix japonica* (Family: Phasianidae).
- Average body weight of quail:

Age	Average body weight (g)
Day-old	6 g
Adult	150–170 g
Adult females	140–160 g
Adult males	120–140 g
Quail egg	10 g

- Males and females are easily recognisable at about 3 weeks of age. The females have long and pointed feathers with grey and black speckles on the throat and upper breast, whereas males have an even coloured rusty brown breast with only very few speckles.
- They start laying egg at the age of 6 weeks and annual egg production is about 260–280. Most of the quails lay eggs in the afternoon during 3 to 5 pm.

- Broiler quails can be marketed at the age of 6 weeks with an average body weight of 150 g. The FCR is 3.3 and dressing percentage is 70.
- Quail meat is nutritive and palatable. It is considered as a delicacy having low fat (6.8%), low cholesterol (25–30 mg/100 g) and high protein (25%). From nutritional quality point of view, quail egg is comparable to chicken egg; however, 5 quail eggs are considered equivalent to 1 chicken egg. Quail eggs are multicoloured (Fig. 8.3).

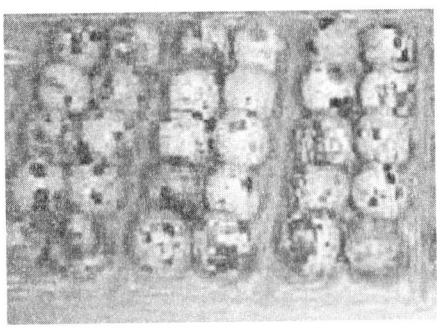

Fig. 8.3: Multicoloured quail eggs

8.2.3 Reproduction and Hatching

The male:female ratio in breeding stock, to be maintained is 1:3 for production of hatching eggs. Eggs can be collected before hatching, 4 days after keeping male with female breeder birds. Eggs collected from the parents aged between 10–24 weeks are highly fertile. The hatching eggs can be stored at 13 °C with 80% relative humidity for 7–10 days. The optimum temperature for hatching quail eggs is 37–37.5 °C with 60–70% relative humidity. The turning of eggs should be done for at least 4–5 times a day for first 14 days, with adequate ventilation. Eggs are transferred to hatching tray on 14th day of incubation. The incubation period of quail egg is short (17–18 days). The hatchability is about 60–70% under artificial incubation.

8.2.4 Systems of Rearing Quail

Quails can be reared under deep litter or cage system of management, however, for their commercial rearing, cage system or battery system is better. The method of rearing quail is similar to that of chicken, but quails need much less space. The space requirement for quails under cage system of rearing is given in Table 8.7.

Table 8.7: Floor space, feeder space and waterer space for a quail in cage system

Age (week)	Floor space (sq cm)	Feeder space (linear, cm)	Waterer space (linear, cm)
0–3	75*	2–2.5	1
4–6	150–175	2.5–3	1.5

* During this age group (0–3 weeks), in addition to brooder/hover space, 75 sq cm run space to be provided to each bird.

The space requirement is to be increased with the increase of age of quails. Roughly a commercial colony cage with the specification of 60 cm × 60 cm × 25 cm can accommodate 25 quails, and 120 cm × 60 cm × 25 cm colony cage can accommodate 50 quails. A pair of breeding quails can be kept in an individual cage measuring 12.5 cm × 20 cm × 25 cm.

8.2.5 Brooding of Quail

Rearing of quail during the first 3 weeks, called brooding, is very vital. Battery system of brooding is the best for quails. Brooding temperature during the 1st week of life should be 37 °C which is to be reduced to 3 °C on every 5th day till it reaches to 22 °C by the end of 3rd week. It is better to cover the floor with corrugated paper or clean gunny bag to provide them foothold. Besides brooding (i.e. giving artificial heat to the birds), light management is also important. Continuous light may be provided during the first 2 weeks, and then it is to be gradually reduced from 3rd week of age to 12 hours during the growing period. Layer quails require 15 to 18 hours of light per day during laying period.

8.2.6 Feeds and Feeding of Quail

Types of quail feed

For layer quails, 3 types of feed are used, viz. **starter mash** (0–3 weeks), **grower mash** (4–5 weeks) and **layer mash** (6 weeks onwards) (Tables 8.8 and 8.9).

For broiler quails, 2 types of feed are used, viz. **starter mash** (0–3 weeks) and **grower mash** (4–6 weeks). Details regarding types of feed and feeding are shown in Tables 8.8, 8.9 and 8.10.

Feed requirement for quail

Total feed requirement for a broiler quail up to 6 weeks of age is about 500 g with feed conversion ratio (FCR) 3.3.

Total feed requirement for a layer quail from day-old stage to up to one year laying is about 9.6 kg.

Chick mash (0–3 weeks) @ 4 g/day/bird	—	85 g
Grower mash (4–5 weeks) @ 18 g/day/bird	—	250 g
Layer mash (6 weeks to 1 laying year) @ 25 g/day/bird	—	9300 g

(*See* Table 8.10)

Table 8.8: Nutrient requirements for quail

Nutrients	Starter mash (0–3 weeks)	Grower mash (4–5 weeks)	Layer/Breeder mash (6 weeks and above)
ME (Kcal/kg)	2,850	2,750–2,800	2,700
Crude protein (%)	27.5	24.0	22.5

Table 8.9: Feed formulae for quail

Ingredients (kg / 100 kg feed)	Starter mash (0–3 weeks)		Grower mash (4–5 weeks)		Layer / Breeder mash (6 weeks and above)	
	1	2	1	2	1	2
Maize crushed (yellow)	33.5	45.5	30.5	40.5	36.5	46.5
Rice polish / Jowar	10	–	10	–	10	–
Wheat bran / Rice bran (deoiled)	–	–	7	7	6	8
GNC (43% protein)	12	5	10	12	10	7
Soybean meal (45% protein)	15	20	12	10	12	14
Sunflower cake (37.5% protein)	12	15	14	15	10	10
Fish meal (44% protein)	8	12	7	7	7	6
Meat meal	7	–	7	6	6	6
Mineral mixture	2.5	2.5	2.5	2.5	2.5	2.5

Table 8.10: Feeding schedule of quail

Age (week)	Average weight (g)	Daily feed intake per bird (g)	Weekly feed intake per bird (g)
1	25	5	35
2	50	10	70
3	85	15	105
4	105	17	119
5	135	20	140
6	150	22	154
Total	–	69	623

NB: From 6 weeks onwards feed consumption varies from 22–25 g per bird per day, depending upon the rate of production.

8.2.7 Maintenance of Quail Health

Quails do not seem to be susceptible to any of the common diseases of poultry and thus do not demand routine vaccination and deworming. It is seen that quails are refractory to Ranikhet disease virus and *Ascaridia galli* infestation.

They are also resistant to 8 species of *Eimeria* which are pathogenic to chicken. Other strain may produce disease. To prevent this, an anticoccidial (viz. *Codrinal* @ 1 g/L of drinking water) may be used routinely for first 14–15 days of life.

Quails are very sensitive to environmental changes. They may be affected by brooder pneumonia caused by *Aspergillus fumigatus*. To check this, calcium propionate may be added at 2 kg/tonne of feed. Besides this, an antibiotic (viz.

Tetracycline powder @ 500 mg/L of drinking water) may be used during first 3–4 days of life, and again during 4th week of life to prevent any bacterial infection.

8.3 GENERAL IDEA ABOUT TURKEY

8.3.1 Introduction

Turkeys are mainly reared for meat and are well-known for their delicacy (Fig. 8.4). The native land of turkey is North America. They are being mainly domesticated in European countries and America for meat, since long time. They have a great demand during Christmas, New Year and other special occasions.

As far as India is concerned, turkey has not gained much popularity and it is still in infant stage. However, West Bengal, Kerala, Tamil Nadu and eastern parts of Uttar Pradesh are some of the states where a considerable number of turkeys are being reared for meat.

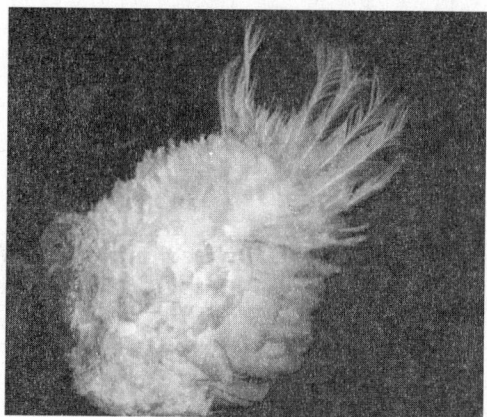

Fig. 8.4: A turkey

8.3.2 Salient Characteristics of Turkey

- The scientific name of turkey is *Meleagris gallopavo* (Family: Phasianidae).
- The turkey eggs are tasty and have almost the same nutrients as that of chicken eggs. The average weight of a turkey egg is 80–85 g. The average weight of new born poult is 50 g.
- Turkey meat is palatable and nutritious. It is rich in protein (24%), but has low fat content (6.6%) and low cholesterol. The meat is also rich in minerals, particularly calcium, potassium, magnesium, iron, zinc, *etc*. It is rich in vitamins like niacin, vitamin B_6 and B_{12}. Essential amino acids and fatty acids are also present in turkey meat.
- Turkeys start to lay eggs from the age of 30 weeks, i.e. approximately 7½ months. Proper care and feeding management can help them to lay about 80–100 eggs per year. The eggs are pointed at one end and have thick shell. The eggshell is tinted in nature.
- The marketing age of turkeys for meat is about 16 weeks. At this time a hen turkey weighs about 5.5 kg and a tom turkey weighs about 7.5 kg. The FCR of

broiler turkey is 2.7–2.8, i.e. marketing for every 1 kg body weight 2.7–2.8 kg feed is required. The dressing percentage is 80–87, which is quite high in respect to other meat animals.

- Turkeys cannot be classified into breeds. However, according to American Standards for Poultry, there are 8 varieties of turkeys, viz. Bronze, Bourbon Red, White Holland, Narragansett, Black, Slate, Royal Palm and Beltsville Small White. Apart from these, there are about 12 non-standard varieties, which are not very significant. At present only 3 varieties are used for commercial breeding and best suited in Indian conditions. These are Bronze, White Holland and Beltsville Small White.

- Turkeys are likely to panic when any type of sudden change occurs in their environment (e.g. loud noise, light turns on or a wild bird flies through their house, *etc*). When panicked, turkeys may trample one another and often pile up against the wall or in corners, with some birds smothering and killing other birds. So sudden changes or movements should be avoided. If possible, young poults should be allowed to be exposed to any noise, light, movement or other environmental variables that they will face as adults. The young poults are more able to learn and habituated to these variables.

8.3.3 Reproduction and Hatching

For fertile egg production the ratio of male and female turkeys is 1:5. Generally, at the age of 30 weeks hen turkeys start laying eggs and tom turkeys become biologically ready for reproduction.

The incubation period is 28 days. For commercial purpose the turkey eggs can be artificially hatched with the help of incubators just like chicken and duck eggs (Table 8.11).

Table 8.11: Optimum temperature and relative humidity for hatching of turkey eggs

Incubator	Temperature (°C)	Relative humidity (%)
Setter	37.5	60–65
Hatcher	37.5	85–90

Apart from these, there should be proper air circulation inside the incubator.

Turkey can also hatch eggs naturally just like chicken. A good broody turkey can hatch about 10–15 number of eggs. Hatchability is generally 60–80%.

8.3.4 Systems of Rearing Turkey

Turkeys can be reared under 2 systems, viz. free range system and deep litter system.

Under free range system each turkey requires 3–4 sq ft area for resting at night. About 200–250 adult turkeys can be reared in 1 acre land. Turkeys can be ideally reared along with agroforestry models.

The deep litter system of rearing turkeys is similar to that of chicken. But in this system turkeys need more floor space and feeder and waterer spaces (Table 8.12).

Table 8.12: Floor space, feeder space and waterer space for a turkey under deep litter system

Age (week)	Floor space (sq ft)	Feeder space (linear, cm)	Waterer space (linear, cm)
0–4	1.25	2.5	1.5
4–16	2.5	5.0	2.5
16–29	4.0	6.5	2.5
Breeder turkey	5.0	7.5	2.5

Turkey house should be in long axis preferably in east-west direction. Its width should be maximum of 9 m and its height may vary from 2.6–3.3 m. The shelter should be constructed in such a way so as to avoid rain water. The depth of the deep litter in turkey's house should be initially 2 inches and gradually it should be increased to 3–4 inches.

8.3.5 Brooding of Turkey

The brooding period in turkey management is up to 4 weeks. But in winter this period may extend up to 5–6 weeks.

The method of brooding is similar to that of chicken, only difference is that the turkeys need more brooding space in comparison to the chicken. Brooding temperature is initially 95 °F, which should be reduced by 5 °F per week. Maintaining proper brooding temperature is very important.

The poults are generally timid and panick in nature. Sometimes they refuse to eat and drink water properly. So special care should be taken for feeding baby turkeys. Initially they may be fed milk and boiled eggs up to 15 days (100 mL milk mixed with 1 L water and 1 boiled egg). Turkeys are slow feeding learner. So they may get attracted to the feeders, if some coloured marbles or catchy items are kept in their feeders. Higher intensity of light (3 watts/poult) may be preferred to prevent 'starve outs'.

Paper and other smooth surfaced materials should not be used on the floor during brooding. Gunny bags or thick corrugated paper boards are preferred for this purpose.

8.3.6 Feeds and Feeding of Turkey

Readymade turkey feeds are not available in the market. The feed ingredients, which are commonly used for preparing chicken feeds, can also be used for preparation of turkey feed. Nutritional requirements and feed formulae of turkeys at different ages are given in Tables 8.13 and 8.14 respectively. Further, the feeding schedule of the turkeys reared for meat production is given in Table 8.15.

Turkeys like to eat fresh green grasses. Lucerne, berseem, stylo may be chopped and fed to them. About 50% of the total diet of turkey may be constituted with greens which should be fed on dry matter basis. Introduction of green fodder or vegetable wastes, along with compounded feed after 8 weeks of age, helps in reducing the feed cost.

Hanging type feeders and waterers are preferred for growing turkeys. Young poults should be carefully observed for feeding for first 3–5 days of life.

Table 8.13: Nutrient requirements of turkey

Age (weeks)	ME (Kcal/kg)	Crude protein (%)
0–4	2,800	28
4–8	2,900	26
8–12	3,000	22
12–16	3,200	16
16–20	3,300	14
> 20	2,900	14

Table 8.14: Feed formulae of turkey

Ingredients (kg / 100 kg feed)	Poult	Grower
Maize	42	49
Soybean meal	40	26
Sunflower meal	8	8
Fish meal	5	13
Dicalcium phosphate	2	2
Soaked lime	1	1
Mineral mixture	2	1

Apart from this, for every 100 kg of feed 10 g vitamins A, B_2 and D_3, 150 g choline chloride, 20 g vitamin B complex and 100 g microminerals may be mixed.

Table 8.15: Feeding schedule of turkey

Age (weeks)	Average body weight (kg)		Total feed intake (kg)		FCR	
	Male	Female	Male	Female	Male	Female
Up to 4	0.72	0.63	0.95	0.81	1.3	1.3
Up to 8	2.36	1.90	3.99	3.49	1.8	1.7
Up to 12	4.72	3.85	11.34	9.25	2.4	2.4
Up to 16	7.26	5.53	19.86	15.69	2.8	2.7
Up to 20	9.62	6.75	28.26	23.13	3.4	2.9

Source: Central Poultry Development Organisation (CPDO), southern region, Bengaluru.

It may be mentioned that on an average an adult turkey consumes 200–250 g feed daily.

8.3.7 Maintenance of Turkey Health

Vaccination against infectious diseases

Turkeys need to be vaccinated regularly especially against Ranikhet disease and fowl pox. If situation demands, vaccine against fowl cholera may also be given (Table 8.16).

Table 8.16: Vaccination schedule for turkey

Sl no.	Disease/ Type of vaccine	Age at which vaccine is to be given
1.	Ranikhet disease vaccine (F_1)	7 days
2.	Ranikhet disease vaccine (LaSota)	28 days
3.	Fowl pox vaccine	42 days
4.	Ranikhet disease vaccine (R_2B)	56 days
5.	Ranikhet disease vaccine (R_2B)	25 weeks
6.	Fowl cholera	8–10 weeks

Regular deworming

The turkeys should be given anthelmintic (dewormer) medicines, if they are being reared under free range system. Deworming should be done at the age of 16 weeks and then at an interval of 3 months. Turkeys reared under free range system, get easily infested by round worms. Piperazine citrate is an effective medicine against this type of worm infestation.

Measures against Ectoparasites

Fowl mite is commonly found in the turkeys. It affects feathers on tail and around the abdomen portion, *etc.* This can be avoided by keeping the turkey houses clean and, if necessary *Pestoban* (an ayurvedic medicine) may be used by mixing with water in 1:10 proportion.

Proper care and management

Turkey keepers should take special care of their feeds. Balanced feed should be provided to the birds. Their houses should be kept dry, neat and clean. Every care should be taken for proper brooding at their initial stages.

With good management, sound sanitation and vaccination program, overall turkey mortality can be reduced to less than 5%.

8.4 GENERAL IDEA ABOUT GUINEA FOWL

8.4.1 Introduction

Guinea fowl can be reared for their eggs and meat. Guinea fowl have good adaptation and high resistance against many diseases, and perform better even under stress conditions. Guinea fowl production seems to be one of the most simple and effective ways to support poor families to raise their incomes. Guinea fowl have the potentiality to become an alternative source of chicken in our country. Moreover, it is the natural germplasm for the subcontinent.

Guinea fowl are referred by various local names as *Chittra* in Western region, *Titri* in northern plains, and *China Murgi* (*Cheena Murgi*) in southern peninsular and eastern parts (Fig. 8.5). Scientific name of Guinea fowl is *Numida meleagris*.

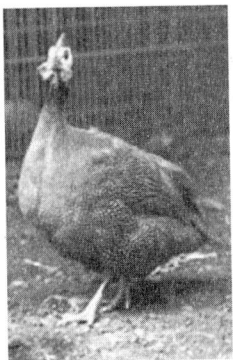

Fig. 8.5: A Guinea fowl

8.4.2 Characteristics of Guinea Fowl

- Guinea fowl are hardy birds and have better resistance against common avian diseases in comparison to chicken.
- Guinea fowl have gregarious habits, which in turn reduces the feed cost and long neck and legs, suitable for grazing. They can eat insects, earthworms, and variety of green leaves, vegetables and fruits and variety of feeds in harvested land also. In this way, it is helpful in development of low-input grain saving aviculture system. It has got better tolerance of aflatoxin in comparison to chicken and hence, eat somewhat bad ration to produce good quality of meat.
- Guinea fowl eggs are smaller in size (30–40 g), but hardy and hence have better storage capability.
- Guinea fowl egg and meat have less cholesterol.
- They can be raised under a range of climatic conditions and needs of special type of housing, *etc.*
- They don't cause any loss to the field, but increases the productivity.
- Its gregarious habits, flocking instinct, long neck, and strong and sufficiently long legs are some of the special advantageous points in favour of the species.
- Growth in Guinea fowl is low in comparison to domestic fowl.

8.4.3 Brooding Management

The baby chicks of guinea fowl are called as keets. These keets are very sensitive during their early life and hence, need more attention than chicken. Guinea fowl are brooded in the same way as chicks with slight reduction in brooding space. However, temperature should be maintained at 95 °F for first 2 weeks and then reduced by 5 °F on every week, by lowering it down to 70 to 75 °F. During summer season, there is no need of additional temperature after 2nd week.

8.4.4 Feed and Feeding of Guinea Fowl

Guinea fowl are mostly raised in small flock. They are not profitable on full feeding under intensive system. They are provided feed only in the morning and evening. After 10 days of brooding, they are allowed to forage and amount of feed which is provided to them is reduced by 25%. Thereafter, the reduction may be up to 75% gradually as the grazing hours increase. The Guinea fowl have flocking tendency and they eat insects, grasses, *etc.* in the grazing fields and household waste. The timings of grazing can be decided as per convenience. The average feed consumption of Guinea fowl is given in Table 8.17.

Table 8.17: Average feed consumption of Guinea fowl

Age (week)	Feed required on full feeding/day/bird (g)	Feed required on grazing + feeding/day/bird (g)
1	5	5
2–4	10	10
4–6	25	15
6–8	40	20
8–10	45	22
10–12	55	25
12–14	60	30
14–16	65	32

8.4.5 Reproduction and Egg Production

Guinea fowl is a seasonal breeder. The ratio of male to female should be 1:5 for optimum fertility. The males mature 15 days later than females. Female birds start laying from March–April and ends in August–September. Preferential mating, observed in Guinea fowl, is one of the important causes of reduction in fertility. Average fertility is 60–65%. The summer season is good for better fertility. Artificial insemination is not practiced in Guinea fowl because of difficulty in training of males to donate the semen and lesser number of good quality sperms. One male can give 0.03–0.1 mL semen in a single ejaculation. Guinea fowl attain sexual maturity at 270–330 days and lay well for 2–3 years. The annual egg production ranges from 60–80 eggs under free range conditions, however, it can lay about 100–150 eggs, depending upon genetic quality and management conditions.

8.4.6 Disease Resistance

General disease resistance is comparable or higher than indigenous fowl (like Kadaknath) and commercial broilers. Guinea fowl show lower susceptibility to poultry lice (*Menopon gallinae* and *Lipeurus tropicalis*) and ticks (*Argas persicus*) infestation. Guinea fowl also seemed to possess high innate tolerance to aflatoxin as compared to chicken and other poultry species.

8.4.7 Egg and Meat Quality Traits

The egg quality parameters of Guinea fowl are presented in Table 8.18. Guinea fowl eggs are relatively smaller in size than those of the chicken. Shell weight and thickness of Guinea fowl eggs are more than the chicken and hence, eggs can be stored for many days and make the transportation easier. The shell colour is light pink, which is due to the porphyrin pigments and does not have any adverse effect, so far as nutritive value of the egg is concerned. Thicker shell with lower porosity makes Guinea fowl eggs relatively stronger against shocks, better resistance against contamination and thus more wholesome.

Table 8.18: Egg quality parameters of Guinea fowl

Parameters	Average	
	Pearl	Lavender
Egg weight (g)	34.69	35.92
Yolk weight (g)	11.88 (34.25%)	12.45 (34.69%)
Albumin weight (g)	17.56 (50.62%)	17.82 (49.62)
Shell weight (g)	5.25 (15.13%)	5.62 (15.65%)
Shell thickness (mm)	0.39	0.41
Shape index	78.29	77.19
Albumin height (mm)	4.82	4.98
Yolk height (mm)	14.66	14.73
Albumin index	0.08	0.08
Yolk index	0.38	0.37
Haugh unit score	77.88	78.43

Source: Singh B, Singh B and Barwal RS (2009). Prospects of Guinea fowl rearing in India, Lead paper presented in ISAPM National Symposium at Kolkata.

Eggs are used traditionally for popular preparations like omelettes, poached egg, scrambled egg, hard boiled egg, egg curry, *etc.* A comparable sensory evaluation study for different egg preparations of Guinea fowl and chicken was conducted by Mahapatra *et al.* (1986) and observed non-significant difference in colour, texture and chewability of the preparations. However, overall acceptability for most of the preparations was comparatively higher for Guinea fowl egg preparations because of its taste, flavour, *etc.* The low total lipids and cholesterol in Guinea fowl eggs were reported against the chicken eggs (Mahapatra *et al.*, 1986). The lesser fat and cholesterol content in comparison to chicken eggs make it preferable for people having cardiac problems.

Guinea fowl are basically reared for meat purpose. Guinea fowl are better than chicken in respect of dressing percentage (Table 8.19). Guinea fowl seem to have about 77% dressing yield which is higher than those for commercial broilers. Guinea fowl meat has lesser cholesterol and fat contents in comparison to broiler chicken. In this era of ban on hunting of wild birds, Guinea fowl is the only species having gamy flavour because of its feeding habits.

Table 8.19: Live weight and different cut-up parts of Guinea fowl at 16 weeks of age

Parameters	Pearl Guinea fowl	Lavender Guinea fowl	Broiler chicken
Live weight (g)	1002.00	1175.50	2925.00
Dressed weight (g)	739.10	842.20	2020.00
Eviscerated weight (g)	936.00	790.30	1836.00
Giblet weight (g)	43.10	46.90	84.00

Contd.

Table 8.19: Live weight and different cut-up parts of Guinea fowl at 16 weeks of age *(Contd.)*

Parameters	Pearl Guinea fowl	Lavender Guinea fowl	Broiler chicken
Breast weight (g)	217.00	230.00	495.00
Drumstick weight (g)	89.90	103.10	435.00
Thigh weight (g)	99.25	118.45	330.00
Back and neck weight (g)	174.25	206.65	352.00
Wings weight (g)	110.50	135.50	199.00

Source: Singh B, Singh B and Barwal RS (2009). Prospects of guinea fowl rearing in India, Lead paper presented in ISAPM National Symposium at Kolkata.

8.4.8 Marketing of Guinea Fowl

Guinea fowl become ready for marketing at about 12 weeks of age. They attain about 1 kg live weight with dressing yield of 75%. Guinea fowl has tremendous potential as organic meat because of the existence of traditional backyard system in the country. These birds are mainly kept as foragers and insectivorous under semi-range and range conditions and produce organic products that fetch high price in the market.

8.5 GENERAL IDEA ABOUT EMU

8.5.1 Introduction

Emu (*Dromaius novaehollandiae*), a flightless bird belongs to Ratite group, was originated in Australia. **It happens to be the second largest bird of the world by height, after its relative Ostrich.** They are very hardy and adaptable to diversified climatic conditions ranging from hot deserts (56 °C) to very cold regions (0 °C). Long emu is very popular due to its oil having medicinal value. Emu oil has been used for thousands of years by Australian Aborigines. They apply emu oil or fat on cuts, muscle injuries and sunburns. Emu farming is currently the fastest growing livestock industry in the world and it is very popular in America, Australia and China. However, it is slowly gaining popularity in India. Emu breeding is in operation in many states of our country like Tamil Nadu, Andhra Pradesh, Maharashtra, Karnataka, Pondicherry, Goa, Odisha, parts of Kerala, Uttar Pradesh and Uttarakhand.

Nowadays emu is considered as an alternative livestock (Fig. 8.6). The high quality emu oil, meat, hide feather, empty eggshell and toenails are available from emu farm. At market age (15–18 months), an emu can yield approximately 5 L of oil. This oil is unsaturated fat devoid of any colour, odour and taste and it contains both omega 3 and omega 6 fatty acids. Emu oil is currently used in skin care products, hair oils, soaps, massage oils and topical analgesic creams. Emu meat is low in fat and cholesterol, but is rich in protein, and tastes like red meat. A 100 g ready-to-eat emu meat contains 23.3 g protein, 1.7 g fat, 57.5 mg cholesterol and 109 kilocalories energy. Emu leather, a fine grained hide, is being used in fashion industry. The eggshells are used for painting and decorative items due to its special colour. Toe nails are strong and decorative, and used in ornaments and craft goods.

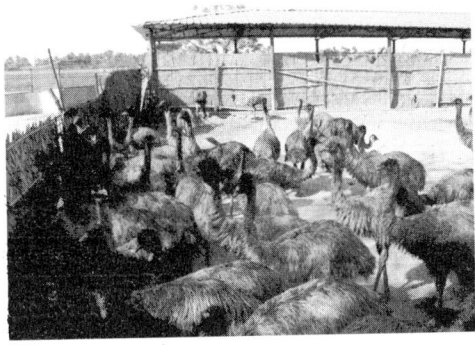

Fig. 8.6: A group of Emus

8.5.2 Characteristics of Emu

Emu chicks are about 10 inches tall at birth, with silky feathers having longitudinal black and white stripes. After 3 months of age they turn nearly solid black and change into tan, brown and black mixture at the age of 12 months. Adult birds have bluish neck and mottled feathers. The feathers are downy, with no stiff vein running through the centre. Emu feathers are unique because both the primary and secondary feathers are of the same length. Female birds are heavier and taller than males. Body temperature of female is more (101 °F) than male (100 °F). Under captive condition, birds sit on their haunch and run frequently along the fence. They spent many times in standing (25–30%). There is no visible difference between male and female birds, however, adult female usually makes a deep booming/drumming sound, especially in breeding season, and males grunt. Emu chicks make a whistling/chirping sound usually up to a period of 1 year. Identification of male and female can be done by fibre optic proctoscope and by 2-primer cleaved amplified polymorphism sequence assay.

An Emu hen may lay as early as at 18 months, but normally laying begins after 2 years age. The Emu hen can be productive for 25 years or more. They lay 10–20 eggs during the first laying year and subsequently up to 50 eggs in a year. They generally lay eggs during November to March, which is considered as breeding season.

8.5.3 Housing and Space Requirement

Emu birds are usually reared in large paddocks. The paddock should have a fence of 6 ft height with 2 × 4 sq inch wire mesh. The floor space requirement for different categories of emu is given in Table 8.20.

Table 8.20: Floor space requirement for emu

Category	Floor space requirement
Chicks (0–3 weeks)	4 sq ft/bird
Chicks (4–14 weeks)	30 sq ft/bird with run space
Growers (15–34 weeks)	100 sq ft/bird with run space
Above 34 weeks and layers	125 sq ft/bird with run space
Mating (from 18–24 months and above)	2,500 sq ft/pair in paddock

8.5.4 Brooding

Dry litter materials (especially rice husk) should be spread on clean and disinfected brooding shed, and is covered with new gunny bags. It is better to accommodate 25–40 chicks in one brooder. One feeder and one waterer should be provided for 5–8 chicks. A chick guard of 2.5 ft height must be provided to avoid jumping and staying of chicks, which may be removed after 7 weeks. Optimum brooding temperature is 90 °F up to 10 days and then 85 °F till 28 days of age. Brooding comfort can be assessed by noting the distribution of faecal matter on the gunny bags spread over the litter. Starter feed (mash type) should be provided to the chicks during brooding period. Occasionally a piece of cucumber or carrot or papaya per chick may be offered in the brooder.

8.5.5 Feeding and Management

Emu can be maintained on variety of plants and insects and readily manufacture feed. Like broiler or layer chicken, the quality of feed is different for different categories of emu (Table 8.21). During growing stage, the size of waterer and feeder is to be increased. The thickness of litter material is also to be increased. It is better to rear male and female separately during growing stage. They should be adapted to feed fibrous diet during growing stage and hence, 10% greens may be added to the grower ration. During breeding season (November–March) feed intake is reduced (550–750 g/bird) and so breeder diet should be offered during this period, preferably 3–4 weeks before breeding. Some vitamins and minerals may be added to the breeder ration for getting better result. Layer ration should have sufficient calcium (2.7%). Provision of trees and shrubs in the paddock for privacy during breeding season helps in inducing mating.

Table 8.21: Nutrient requirements for emu

Nutrients	Starter (0–9 weeks)	Grower (10–42 weeks)	Finisher (43 weeks to slaughter)	Breeder (43 weeks and above)	Maintenance (non-breeding)
ME (Kcal/kg)	2 700	2 600	2 600	2 600	2 400
CP (%)	20	18	16	20	15
Lysine (%)	1.00	0.80	0.70	0.90	0.63
Methionine (%)	0.45	0.40	0.35	0.40	–

8.5.6 Healthcare

The birds are very hard and adaptable to extreme climatic conditions. They can play in water or mud. Chick survival rate is excellent. Eighty percent survivability rate is common up to the age of maturity. No diseases have yet been diagnosed as common to the species. Initial chick mortality is seen generally due to starvation, malnutrition, leg abnormality, intestinal obstruction, and *aspergillus*, clostridial and *E. coli* infections. However, Ranikhet disease on the basis of gross lesion is reported in emu farms in India. Emu birds can maintain themselves on a simple diet and requires lot of water, drinking 7.5 to 15 L daily. Health problem in emu farm can be controlled by improving the farm management conditions.

8.5.7 Important Facts About Emu

Scientific name	*Dromaius novaehollandiae*
Life span	30–40 years
Purpose of rearing	Oil, meat, skin, feather
Weight of day-old chick	400–450 g
Adult body weight (1–1.5 years)	40–50 kg
Height	5–6 ft
No. of toenails/leg	3
Age at sexual maturity	18–24 months
Slaughter age	15–18 months
Sex ratio for breeding	1:1
Space requirement in paddock for breeding	2,500 sq ft/pair
Egg weight	475–650 g
Eggshell colour	Emerald green (ranging from light medium to dark green, look like tough marble)
Incubation period	52 days
Hatchability	70% on total eggs set
No. of eggs produced per year	40–50 eggs
Dressing percentage (meat yield)	50–60%
Oil production per bird	5–6 L
Leather produced per bird	8–10 sq ft
Feather yield per bird	400–600 g
Feeding habit	Omnivores
Laying pattern	Lay an egg on every 3rd day
Laying time	Late evening (5.00 to 7.00 pm)
Running speed	50 km/hour

8.6 IMPORTANT FACTS ABOUT GOOSE (Fig. 8.7)

Scientific name	*Anser anser*
Male goose	Gander
Female goose	Goose
Young goose	Gosling (Broiler is known as green gosling.)
Important breeds	African, Embden, Toulouse, Canada, Chinese, Egyptian, Tufted Roman, American Buff, Pilgrim, Saddleback Pomeranian, Sebastopol, *etc.*
Life span	20–60 years
Purpose of rearing	Meat. Goose meat is palatable and has high energy value.
Body weight at 10 weeks	5 kg
Age at sexual maturity	270–300 days

Contd.

(Contd.)

Scientific name	Anser anser
Egg weight	140–220 g
Incubation period	30 days
Laying characteristics	Seasonal layer
Feeding habit	Excellent foragers, commonly raised on green pasture. They can manage their most of the feed requirements, if kept on pasture with succulent grass.
Feed efficiency	1:3 in case of geese broilers
Growth	Fastest growing bird generally up to 10 weeks of age with 5 kg body weight at this stage.

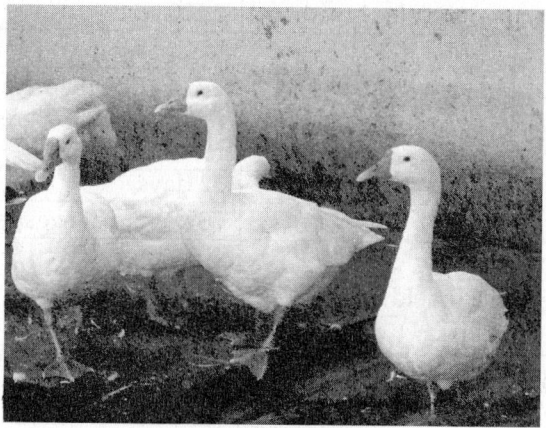

Fig. 8.7: A flock of geese

EXERCISE

A. Objective Questions

   i. **Indicate the correct answer by putting tick (√) mark (multiple choice).**

   1. The average weight of a duck egg should be
      - (a) 10 g
      - (b) 60 g
      - (c) 70 g
      - (d) 95 g

   2. A standard chicken egg weighs about
      - (a) 40 g
      - (b) 55 g
      - (c) 65 g
      - (d) 70 g

   3. The average weight of a quail egg is
      - (a) 10 g
      - (b) 18 g
      - (c) 70 g
      - (d) 150 g

   4. A quail starts to lay egg at the age of
      - (a) 6 weeks
      - (b) 8 weeks
      - (c) 10 weeks
      - (d) 12 weeks

5. Average weight of broiler quail at the time of marketing is
   - (a) 150 g
   - (b) 260 g
   - (c) 300 g
   - (d) 500 g
6. A cage measuring 60 cm L × 60 cm W × 25 cm H can accommodate
   - (a) 10 quails
   - (b) 25 quails
   - (c) 50 quails
   - (d) 150 quails
7. A broiler quail requires the following quantity of feed up to 6 weeks of age:
   - (a) 0.5 kg
   - (b) 1.6 kg
   - (c) 1.9 kg
   - (d) 3.8 kg
8. Average weight of a newborn quail chick is
   - (a) 10 g
   - (b) 6 g
   - (c) 16 g
   - (d) 58 g
9. Which of the following diseases must be prevented by means of vaccination in duck?
   - (a) Ranikhet disease and Gumboro disease
   - (b) Duck cholera and Gumboro disease
   - (c) Duck cholera and duck plague
   - (d) Duck plague and duck pox
10. Turkeys are generally vaccinated against
   - (a) Ranikhet disease
   - (b) Fowl pox
   - (c) Both of these
   - (d) None of these
11. Quails are commonly vaccinated against
   - (a) Ranikhet disease
   - (b) Fowl pox
   - (c) Both of these
   - (d) None of these
12. Quails are resistant to
   - (a) Ranikhet disease
   - (b) *Ascaridia galli* infestation
   - (c) Both of these
   - (d) None of these
13. Age of sexual maturity in turkey is
   - (a) 18–24 weeks
   - (b) 24–28 weeks
   - (c) 28–32 weeks
   - (d) 32–40 weeks
14. Young one of turkey is known as
   - (a) Chick
   - (b) Gosling
   - (c) Poult
   - (d) Capon
15. Male duck is known as
   - (a) Gander
   - (b) Gosling
   - (c) Drake
   - (d) Cock

ii. **Fill in the blanks.**
1. The average weight of chicken egg is _____.
2. The average weight of duck egg is _____.
3. The average weight of quail egg is _____.

4. After introduction of _____ in India, duck farm-ing, particularly for egg production, is lately gaining popularity.

5. The weight of day-old chick of emu is _____ g.

6. Turkeys start to lay eggs from the age of _____ weeks.

iii. Write True (T) or False (F) against each statement.

1. Duck enjoys the second position just after chicken in India.

2. Ducks lay more than 95% of their eggs in the morning before 9.00 am.

3. Guinea fowl become ready for marketing at about 12 weeks of age.

4. The annual egg production in Guinea fowl ranges from 60–80 eggs under free range conditions.

5. Weight of an emu egg may be 650 g.

B. Subjective Questions

1. Why duck farming is becoming popular in India?

2. What is the present position of duck in poultry industry in India? Discuss in brief why duck rearing is preferred to bring better rural economy. Describe in brief the breeds, management and disease control programme in ducks.

3. What is the future of turkey production in the poultry business in India?

4. What are the factors which limit the quail production in India?

5. Describe the important characteristics of Guinea fowl.

6. Write short notes on the following.
   (a) Brooding of duckling
   (b) Characteristics of quail as poultry
   (c) Importance of turkey as an alternative species of poultry

Answers of the Objective Questions

i. Multiple choice

1. (c) 70 g	2. (b) 55 g	3. (a) 10 g
4. (a) 6 weeks	5. (a) 150 g	6. (b) 25 quails
7. (a) 0.5 kg	8. (b) 6 g	

9. (c) Duck cholera and Duck plague

10. (c) Both of these	11. (d) None of these	12. (c) Both of these
13. (c) 28–32 weeks	14. (c) Poult	15. (c) Drake

ii. Fill in the blanks

1. 55–60 g	2. 65–70 g	3. 10 g
4. Khaki Campbell duck	5. 400–450	6. 30

iii. True or False

1. T	2. T	3. T	4. T	5. T

9
Economic Production and Marketing of Poultry

9.1 ECONOMIC PRODUCTION OF POULTRY

Economic production of poultry requires sound planning, considerable amount of capital, scientific technological knowhow and business understanding. Other important factors that affect the profitability of poultry farm are location of the farm, size of operation, genetic quality of the stock, feed and labour efficiency, and finally marketing. These are discussed in short in the following section.

Location of the farm: Location of poultry farm is an important consideration for economic poultry production. Urban or peri-urban farms are better than rural farms for better facilities of procurement of inputs of the farm and easy marketing of poultry and poultry products. However, the land cost and labour would be higher in urban or peri-urban areas than rural areas. Electricity in rural areas is another constraint. *(See Chapter 10, Section 10.1)*

Size of operation: It is always true that larger the size of poultry farm, greater is the margin of profit. This is primarily due to bulk purchase of inputs of the farm and better labour utilisation.

Genetic make up of the stock: Nowadays high yielding hybrid stock is available both for broiler and layer farms. One should select the renowned stock as per the cost and availability. The quality of chicks should not be compromised for economic production. *(See Chapter 14, Section 14.11.1)*

Feed: Feed alone accounts for about 70% of the total cost of poultry production. So good feed and efficient feeding management are the keys to success for economic poultry production. Quality of feed should be judged periodically and it should not be compromised at any situation.

Labour efficiency: Efficient use of labour is very important for economic poultry production. Usually labour efficiency is better in large farms than small farms. Skilled labour should be employed for carrying out different activities of poultry farms.

Timely marketing: Marketing of poultry and poultry products is the ultimate goal of commercial poultry farming. Timely marketing is very much essential as both egg and meat are perishable items. Moreover, in broiler farming the feed conversion efficiency will be reduced, if birds are kept in the farm for longer duration. Recently, they are marketed at the age of 42 days or below. *(See Section 9.4)*

Capital investment: Capital is the most important item of any business. In poultry farming, it is required for purchase and development of land, development of infrastructural facilities including shed, equipment, *etc.*, meeting day to day expenses including purchase of birds, purchase of feed, medicines, insurance coverage, payment of electric and water bills, *etc.* and transportation cost. If this capital is borrowed, the rate of interest and credit terms add further dimension to the production cost.

9.2 SETTING OF FARMS FOR DIFFERENT CLASSES OF POULTRY

The objective of setting poultry farm is mainly to produce egg and/or meat. For commercial production of eggs, chickens and ducks are preferred. For commercial production of meat, all the poultry species may be reared as per the demands of the specific products. The meat type poultry may be chicken, quail, turkey, Guinea fowl and even emu. Emu is also economically important for its fats and oil. For setting up of farms and economic production of poultry, a project report is to be prepared before starting the enterprise, and then it is to be implemented by following the technical norms. *Project reports for commercial production of various categories of poultry are presented in Chapter 15 of this book, viz.* **broiler, layer, duck** *(free range system),* **duck** *(intensive system),* **Japanese quail** *(broiler type),* **turkey** *(free range system) and* **cockerel** *(all in all out system).*

9.3 MIXED FARMING AND POULTRY RAISING

The mixed farming system is generally composed of crop production combined with livestock production. Such type of mixed farm unit is more relevant to Indian conditions, where livestock component is complimentary to crop production and *vice versa*. Mixed farm unit provides more returns from a unit of land holding. It also results in balanced labour utilisation in the farmers' family. In a mixed farm units avian farms (fowl, duck, quail, turkey, *etc.*) can play an important role. The grains and grain by-products from agriculture component (like maize, jowar, bajra, damaged grains, rice-kani, rice polish, oil cakes, pulse chuni, *etc.*) can be used efficiently as poultry feed ingredients. The cost of poultry feed can be reduced by using these farm-produced. On the other hand, large quantity of poultry manure, rich in fertiliser value, are available from the avian farms which can be used to increase the fertility of soil. This high quality biofertiliser also prevents bleaching of soil, a major problem due to chemical fertilisers.

However, in India poultry farming is very well-organised. Large poultry farm (layer for egg production or broiler for meat production) can be established as a specialised farm for sole income generation. So large specialised and sophisticated poultry farms can not be operated under mixed farming pattern. Only small and medium sized poultry farm units can be operated under mixed farming system.

9.4 MARKETING OF POULTRY AND POULTRY PRODUCTS

The marketing of poultry and poultry products (eggs and meat) is not organised in India rather this is the weakest side of poultry industry in this subcontinent. We have high standards of production technology, and many large poultry farms are being operated in various parts of our country. But the market is not stabilised rather price is fluctuating very frequently.

Existing strategies of poultry marketing

Most of the broiler chickens are sold in live form either at the producer's farm or at the local vegetable markets. In India, less than 2% of the total broilers are sold as processed and packed form. Consumers prefer broilers processed before them due to assurance of fresh chicken, lack of awareness about the quality of processed chicken, and unable to realise hidden costs of feathers and offal discarded during processing. However, selling of processed or ready-to-cook chicken is becoming popular in big cities because of convenience. Eggs are also sold at local markets, however, a good number of eggs are moved to the distant markets, though eggs are moved from one state to others. There is middlemen involvement in poultry marketing systems for transacting both eggs and live birds. It cuts the profit margin of the actual producers.

NECC (National Egg Coordination Committee) is a cooperative for promotion of egg industry in India involving poultry farmers, poultry businessmen and hatcheries. This organisation, established in 1982, has many regional centres in various parts of our country. It has been actively involved in stabilising the prices of eggs. Another agency Bromark is trying to stabilise the broiler or live poultry market by declaring the price, based on market dynamics. However, these are purely voluntary organisations without any statutory power. The National Agricultural Cooperative Marketing Federation of India Ltd (NAFED) handles marketing of eggs at national and regional levels, giving due consideration of recommendations of NECC. After receiving the prestigious International Egg Commission 1991 award for national egg campaign, the NECC aims to achieve a per capita consumption of 180 eggs, by the year 2015. This was based on minimum nutritional requirements per person laid down by the Indian Council of Medical Research (ICMR).

Recently Poultry Development Corporations in different states have set up retail booths to sell eggs and related products at reasonable rates. West Bengal Dairy and Poultry Development Corporation, Tamil Nadu Poultry Development Corporation, Andhra Pradesh Meat and Poultry development Corporation, etc. are few examples of such type of corporation.

Common marketing channels of eggs and meat

In India, 5 channels are commonly seen through which eggs are moved from the producer (farmer) to the ultimate consumers as follows:

Channel I　Producer–Trader–Wholesaler (consumption centre)–Retailer–Consumer.

Channel II　Producer–Trader–Retailer (consumption centre)–Consumer.

Channel III　Producer–Wholesaler–Secondary Wholesaler (consumption centre)– Retailer–Consumer.

Channel IV　Producer–Wholesaler–Retailer (consumption centre)–Consumer.

Channel V　Producer–Consumer.

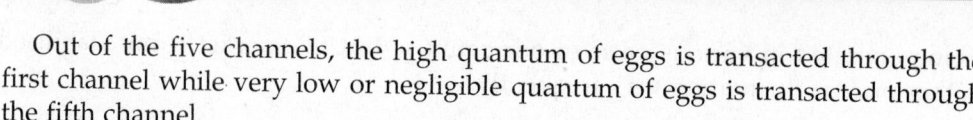

Out of the five channels, the high quantum of eggs is transacted through the first channel while very low or negligible quantum of eggs is transacted through the fifth channel.

On the other hand, 3 channels are commonly seen in marketing of meat. They are as follows:

Channel I   Producer–Wholesaler–Retailer–Consumer

Channel II   Producer–Retailer–Consumer

Channel III   Producer–Consumer

Out of the 3 channels, channel I handles large quantum of meat, while channel III handles a negligible quantity of meat.

Suggestions for improving poultry marketing system

i. There is a need of an APEX body to monitor the growth of the poultry industry including rural poultry farming. A National Poultry Development Board may be constituted on the line similar to NDDB (National Dairy Development Board) to look after the poultry development in India. It is necessary to set up a poultry marketing cell under the Directorate of Animal Husbandry to collect and compile information on marketing of poultry, poultry products and by-products for designing developmental activities. On the other hand, the activities of NAFED and NECC need to be strengthened/encouraged.

ii. To avoid the exploitation by middlemen, poultry farmers should be encouraged to sell their products directly to the consumers by forming functional cooperative society, exclusively for this purpose.

iii. Poultry products are perishable items. Government may set up cold storage plants and hire them for farmers at nominal rent, so as to store their products prior to marketing. This will avoid spoilage of this perishable commodity, thereby increasing the profit margin. Precaution should be taken during packaging and transportation of eggs.

iv. Brand development may be encouraged to be taken up by private commercial firms. Selling of ready-to-cook chicken may be encouraged, however, scientific and hygienic processing, packing, maintaining cold chain, *etc.* should be given due to importance.

v. The consumers should be properly educated through mass media like radio and television, by giving importance of nutritive value of poultry eggs/meat, for creating more demand of the products. Wide publicity should be given to the poultry products of rural poultry farming under scavenging system for its near-organic and non-synthetic nature. Indian market can be broadly divided into urban and rural sections. The key requirement is to develop marketing channels in rural areas. Increasing the egg consumption can be brought about by getting the non-egg eaters to start eating eggs and turning occasional egg eaters to regular egg eaters.

9.5 ORGANIC POULTRY FARMING

Organic poultry farming, comparatively a new approach in India, is discussed in the following sections.

9.5.1 What is Organic Farming?

'Organic agriculture is a holistic production management system which promotes and enhances agroecosystem health, including biodiversity, biological cycles and soil biological activity. It emphasises the use of management practices in preference to use of off-farm inputs, taking into account that regional conditions require locally adopted systems. This is accomplished by using, where possible, agronomic, biological and mechanical methods, as opposed to using synthetic materials, to fulfill any specific function with the system' (FAO/WHO Codex Alimentarious Commission, 1999).

Organic livestock farming is an integrated system of farming based on ecological principles. It uses environment-friendly methods of crop and livestock productions without use of synthetic fertilisers, growth hormones, growth-enhancing antibiotics, synthetic pesticides or gene manipulation. The aim of organic livestock farming is to increase the production of livestock with minimum reliance on chemicals while at the same time conserving resources. Above all, organic livestock farming is a 'sustainable, ecologically sound, economically viable, socially humane' production system. The use of synthetic growth-promoters, synthetic appetisers, preservatives, artificial colouring agents, synthetic amino acids, emulsifiers, solvent-extracted oil cakes, urea, genetically engineered organisms or products are prohibited. However, seaweed powder, rock salt and natural sources of vitamins, such as cod liver oil and yeast are the most preferred supplements, if any, are needed.

9.5.2 Global Market Opportunity for Organic Food Items

- Market share of organic farming is presently about 2 per cent of world market, with annual growth of 20 to 30 %, which is very impressive.
- Total estimated market for organic foods is around US $ 30 billion. The USA is leading followed by Germany, the UK and other European countries. Worldwide about 130 countries produce certified organic products in commercial quantities, which include 30 countries in Africa, 30 countries in Asia, 20 countries in Central America and the Caribbean, 10 countries in South America, 5 countries in Australia and the Pacific and most countries in Europe as well as the USA and Canada.
- In the USA and EU markets, the fastest growing categories between 1999 and 2000 included meat and eggs (64% growth), and dairy (40% growth) along with other foods.
- In global market, the most popular organic products are fruits and vegetables followed by poultry and livestock products.
- In the USA, organic meat and meat products including poultry are the 6th fastest growing organic commodity group.
- Among global organic industry's top producers, organic poultry and dairy productions have shown stronger growth rates than organic beef and pork production.
- As per reports, the chief motivations for purchase of organic food are increasing consumers' awareness about personal health, food safety, enhanced taste of organic products, environmental issues and animal welfare, *etc.*

- Various studies in abroad indicate that organic foods are generally priced higher than conventional foods, and organic consumers generally have higher average income, a good education, awareness about health and environmental issues, and are of young age or young families. Consumers with high meat consumption are more likely to purchase the labeled ('Organic' or 'Bio' or 'Green') meat.

9.5.3 What is Organic Poultry Farming?

The key principles for organic poultry production are:

- Management of poultry as land-based systems (excluding intensively housed poultry units).
- Reliance on feed resources produced organically.
- Maintenance of health through preventive management and good husbandry in preference to preventive treatment.
- Housing systems to allow natural behaviour patterns with high priority to animals' welfare, along with emphasis on free-range system for poultry.
- Breeds and rearing systems suited to the production systems employed in terms of disease resistance, productivity, hardiness, suitability for foraging and eco-friendliness.

9.5.4 Advantages of Organic Poultry Farming

The advantages of poultry products (egg and chicken) as reported by some workers are mentioned here.

- Organic poultry products reduce the risk of potential public health problems by prohibiting the use of antibiotics, hormones and pesticides, which are suspected to have endocrine disrupting, carcinogenic, teratogenic, immuno-suppressive and ill-effects on nervous system.
- In India, organic poultry farming has enormous potentiality for export as the demand of organic poultry products are increasing rapidly in the developed countries.
- There is a growing demand of organic poultry products in domestic markets also as urban consumers are paying remarkably more for free-range poultry meat and eggs.
- As per reports, organic poultry products taste equal or better than conventional animal products. It is important from consumers' point of view as taste plays an important role while purchasing of any product. Hence, many consumers (middle and upper middle classes) are willing to pay more for unique taste of organic poultry products.
- Cost of veterinary treatment is significantly lower in organic poultry farms than conventional one.
- It is better for environment as there is lower stocking rate of poultry and products are free from chemicals. Besides, synthetic fertilisers and pesticides are prohibited in poultry feed and thus ensures eco-friendly agriculture which protects soil, water and air from pollution caused by conventional agriculture.

- Organic poultry framing ensures strict animal welfare measures and recognises animal comfort and animal behaviour.
- It ensures better sustainability of poultry production over long term including boost to indigenous technologies.

9.5.5 Standards for Organic Poultry Production in India and Abroad

Most of the countries including India have national certifying body for certification of organic agricultural products including livestock and poultry. Without their certification, agricultural products cannot reach to the consumers as certified organic products. A lot of organic standards exist at present at international and national levels which are subject to continual amendment. These standards are described below:

- At the international level, FAO/WHO Codex Alimentarious Commission (the intergovernmental body that sets standards for all foods) has produced international guidelines for production, processing, labeling and marketing of organically produced foods. It does not certify, but provides guidelines for developing organic standards to certifying bodies.
- The private sectors equivalent to the Codex Alimentarious guidelines is the International Basic Standards for Organic Production and Processing, created by the International Federation of Organic Agriculture Movements (IFOAM). This is a worldwide standard, which guides others and have a strong impact on national standards.
- In India, the National Standards for Organic Production (NSOP) developed by Ministry of Commerce and Industry, Govt of India provides general guidelines for organic crop production and animal husbandry including poultry. Henceforth, no certified organic products could be exported from India as such from 1st October, 2001 unless they are certified by an inspection and certification agency duly accredited by one of the accreditation agencies designated by Govt of India. The Indian Standards on Organic Poultry and Livestock Husbandry is largely based on the IFOAM basic standards.
- Besides Indian standards, some of the important standards of other countries include EU Regulation, Organic Food Products Act (OFPA) of the USA, the UK Register of Organic Food Standards (UKROFS) of the UK and Japan Agricultural Standard (JAS) of Japan.

9.5.6 Salient Features of Indian Organic Poultry Production

Management

Management of organic poultry farm is the key to success. Management should be directed for good health and welfare of birds so that they can exhibit their basic behavioural habits through following measures:

- Sufficient free movement, fresh air, natural day light, protection against excessive sunlight, temperature, rain and wind
- Enough lying and/or resting area with ample access to feed and fresh water
- Poultry should not be kept in cages.

- No compounds used for construction materials or production equipment shall be used which might detrimentally affect animal or human health.
- Adequate facilities for expressing behaviour

Origin of Stock

- All the organic birds should be born and raised on organic holding.
- In case of non-availability of organic birds, the accredited certification programme shall allow to brought in conventional birds of the age of 2-day-old chicks for meat production, 18-week-old hens for egg production and 2-week-old for any other poultry.
- Breeding stock may be brought in from conventional farms, but maximum replacement will be 10% of adult birds per year of the same species on the farm.

Breeds and Breeding

- Breeds should be chosen which are adapted to local condition.
- Reproduction techniques should be normal.
- Use of genetically modified organisms (GMO) is not allowed.

Feeding

- Poultry should be fed 100% organically grown feed to provide balanced ration. If certain feed ingredients are not available from organic farming sources, then 15–20% conventional feeds may be allowed.
- All feed ingredients should be produced on the farm or procured from organic farms in the region.
- Some products such as synthetic growth promoter or stimulants, synthetic appetisers, preservatives (except when used as processing aid), artificial colouring agents, droppings or other manure (all types of excreta) even if technologically processed, solvent extracted oil cakes, pure amino acids, genetically engineered organisms or products thereof should not be included or added in organic and conventional feeds.
- Vitamins, trace elements and supplements should be used from natural origin.

Healthcare

- Management practices should be directed to achieve maximum resistance against disease and preventing infections.
- When illness does occur, the aim should be to find the cause and prevent future outbreaks by changing management practices.
- Natural medicines and methods, including homeopathy, ayurvedic medicine and acupuncture, shall be emphasised.
- The use of conventional veterinary medicines are allowed when no other justifiable alternative is available. If veterinary medicines are used, the withholding period shall be twice the legal period.
- Vaccinations shall be used when diseases are known or expected to be a problem in the region.

Conversion Period

- The establishment of organic poultry husbandry requires an interim period, termed as the conversion period. Conversion may be accomplished over a period of time.

- Replacement poultry should be brought to the holding at the start of the production enterprise.

Apart from the aforesaid standards, there are several other standards concerning transport, slaughter, *etc.*

9.5.7 Opportunities for Farmers Producing Organic Poultry

Indian poultry farmers have definitely an edge over others in respect of organic poultry farming. The existing extensive poultry farming system in India is mostly traditional in nature where animal confinement is very limited. These traditional small poultry farmers (about 70% of farming community) of India are mostly using organic methods, but are not aware of it. External inputs like growth hormones, antibiotics and other drugs, *etc.* are generally not used. Indigenous poultry breeds are well-adapted to Indian climate and feed resource situations. They possess natural resistance against many diseases whereas the exotic and crossbreds/strain birds are susceptible to many diseases. India has vast reservoir of Indigenous Technical Knowledge (ITK) which can effectively be used in organic poultry production system as well as can be exported to developed countries to earn foreign exchange. For implementation of organic poultry, organic agriculture is a must. The production of non-toxic organic food is a tough task for the developed world because of rampant use of chemical fertilisers, pesticides and herbicides. India has an edge because it is still rainfed and use of chemicals are much low compared to developed countries. Traditional Indian Agrarian Society has an inbuilt culture and systems which are closer to organic production system. Thus the traditional Indian farming system should be well-utilised to promote domestic and export markets of organic foods.

In this context it may be mentioned that as organic farming especially poultry and livestock sectors, is in the stage of infancy, though there are many information gaps and lack of knowledge and data in India. Besides, too many unrealistic environmental and animals' welfare related legislation may hinder the growth of animal industry. So there is an urgent need for research and development in organic farming sector in order to apply the modern knowledge and improve its performance. Research institutes and universities should start research programmes together with farmers. Government assistance in matter of policy support, incentives, training and market development are urgently required to boost this frontline technology.

EXERCISE

A. Objective Questins

i. Indicate the correct answer by putting tick (√) mark (multiple choice).

1. Which of the following organisations received the prestigious International Egg Commission 1991 award for national egg campaign?
   - (a) NAFED
   - (b) NECC
   - (c) ICMR
   - (d) None of these

2. Which of the following is/are commonly seen channel(s) for marketing poultry meat in India?
   - (a) Producer–Wholesaler–Retailer–Consumer
   - (b) Producer–Retailer–Consumer
   - (c) Producer–Consumer
   - (d) All of these

3. The weakest link in broiler production system in India is
   - (a) Cost of feed
   - (b) Lack of marketing facility
   - (c) Availability of medicine not assured timely
   - (d) None of these

4. The following are the major constraints for growth of poultry industry.
   1. Shortage of quality feed
   2. Delayed return of profit
   3. Disorganised marketing
   4. Inadequate health coverage

   Select the correct answer from the code below:
   - Code (a) 1, 2, 3 and 4 are correct
   - (b) 1, 2 and 3 are correct
   - (c) 1, 3 and 4 are correct
   - (d) 1, 2 and 4 are correct

ii. Fill in the blanks.

1. The full form of NECC is _____.
2. The full form of NAFED is _____.
3. In case of organic poultry farming, if certain feed ingredients are not available from organic farming sources, then _____% conventional feeds may be allowed.

iii. Write True (T) or False (F) against each statement.

1. In India less than 2% of the total broilers are sold as processed and packed form.
2. In the USA, organic meat and meat products including poultry are the 6th fastest growing organic commodity group.
3. Cost of veterinary treatment is significantly lower in organic poultry farms than conventional one.
4. Feed alone accounts for about 70% of the total cost of poultry production.

B. Subjective Questions

1. Describe the existing strategies of poultry marketing in India. Do you have any suggestion for improving the poultry marketing system?
2. Write a note on 'mixed farming and poultry raising'.
3. What do you mean by organic farming? How is the term 'organic' used on poultry products?

Answers of the Objective Questions

i. Multiple choice

1. (b) NECC
2. (d) All of these
3. (b) Lack of marketing facility
4. (c) 1, 3 and 4 are correct

ii. Fill in the blanks

1. National Egg Coordination Committee
2. National Agricultural Cooperative Marketing Federation of India Ltd
3. 15–20

iii. True or False

1. T   2. T   3. T   4. T

PART II

Commercial Poultry Production and Hatchery Management

10

Housing of Poultry

10.1 LOCATION OF POULTRY FARM

Location is a very important consideration to establish a large poultry farm, because a considerable amount is needed to construct the poultry houses and other farm buildings, which are somewhat permanent structures and cannot be changed/shifted frequently. It is necessary to choose the most suitable location from technical as well as marketing point of view. The following points should be duly considered for choosing the site for poultry farm.

i.   **Transport facility:** The site should be accessible to all types of transport, i.e. the place should be well-connected with road. It will minimise the cost of transport, and facilitate transportation of input and output items of the farm. However, there should not be any unauthorised vehicles and visitors for maintaining biosecurity. The farm should be away from public habitation, busy roads and industries to avoid pollution and other sources of suffocations.

ii. **Market:** Better marketing facility shall be available, if the place is nearer to peri-urban area. It may be located at a place where more non-vegetarian people are residing so that market is available for the poultry products (as eggs and meat being primarily non-vegetarian food items). The poultry farm should not be located near religious areas where there is no demand of egg and meat. Nearby market is essential for ready and easy availability of raw materials (like feed, equipment, etc.) easy disposal of eggs and meat and to stabilise price also. On the other hand, it reduces the cost of storage/refrigeration of eggs and meat.

iii. **Availability of water and electricity:** The farm should be located at a place where adequate quality of water and electricity are available at reasonable cost. Enough and continuous supply of electricity is needed for better efficiency of labours and speedy work. It is needed for maintaining brooders, as a source of light inside the poultry sheds, running of machines noiselessly without much pollution, etc.

iv. **Topography and soil:** The highland with leveled surface and loamy soil is good for poultry farm as it provides good drainage to prevent wet floors/dampness. At least the site should have higher elevation than the surroundings for effective drainage. It should be ensured that the area is not flooded during rainy season and there is no water logging due to poor drainage facility. If it is intended to establish the poultry farm in hilly areas, it is better to locate the farm on a sloping hillside rather than on a hilltop or in the bottom of a valley. Sloping hillside provides good drainage and some protection from wind.

v. **Extra space:** Sufficient extra space should be available for possible future expansion.

vi. **Open area:** The farm should be located in open space so that it will provide good ventilation and exposure of floor to sunlight. Such condition removes dampness of the area, checks germs and keeps floor dry.

vii. **Shade and protection:** Surrounding of the farm may have tall shady trees which provide shade in the summer months and serve as windbreak in the winter. However, shrubs are not desirable in the nearby place as such type of plants may prevent sunlight to enter the farm. The area should not have prolonged cloudy weather, cyclonic weather, storm, dust, *etc.* as these may induce physiological stress to the birds. The birds also have to be protected from heavy rains, snow and intense heat. The poultry house needs to be properly oriented to protect against wind, but permits some air movement for proper ventilation.

viii. **Cheap labourer:** Cheap, reliable and honest labourers are the assets of any establishment. It reduces the cost of production and increases efficiency of the farm.

ix. **Social condition:** The surrounding areas adjacent to the proposed site of poultry farm should be clean and safe. Otherwise, thieves and unsocial people may cause difficulties in smooth running of poultry farm business. There should have a control over visitors of the farm also to maintain the biosecurity of the farm.

x. **Miscellaneous points:** It is better to have facilities like banking, postal communication, shopping complex, *etc.* nearby for welfare of farm workers/ employees in case of very large establishment.

10.2 TYPES OF POULTRY HOUSES

Various types of poultry houses are outlined below:

i. **On the basis of system of intensive management**, poultry houses may be of 2 types, viz.

a. **Deep litter house**

In this, house birds are reared on floor which is commonly made up of various bedding materials like cinder, sawdust, wood shavings, chopped straw, hay, *etc.* (Fig. 10.1).

b. **Cage house**

Birds are kept totally confined on wire netting floor. Cages may be arranged in poultry house in many ways, like flat deck cages or single-tier system, battery cages or multi-tier cages, Californian cages or reverse cages, *etc.* (Fig. 10.2).

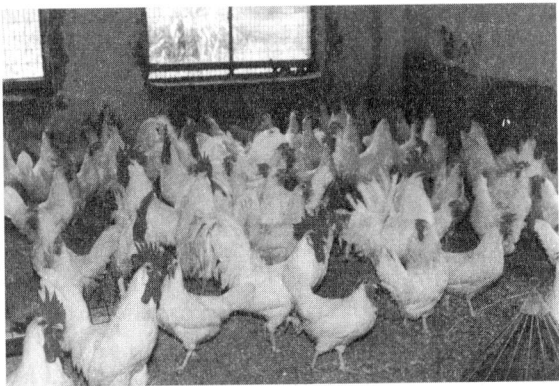

Fig. 10.1: Rearing of poultry in deep litter system

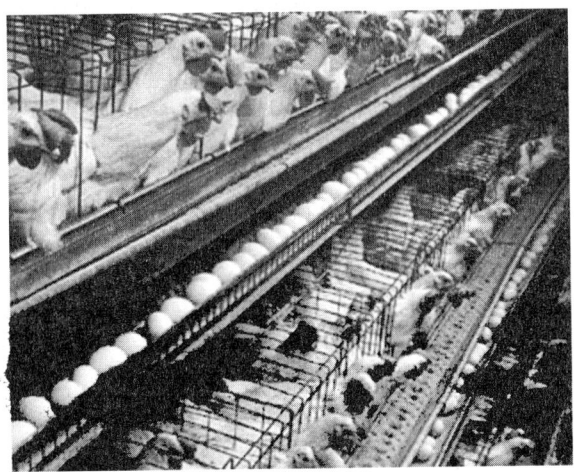

Fig. 10.2: Rearing of poultry in cage system

ii. **On the basis of purpose of rearing,** the poultry houses may be:

a. **Brooder house**

In this house chicks are kept generally up to 3–4 weeks of age in broiler and 6–8 weeks in layer type birds. It provides heat to the birds at their early part of lives.

b. **Grower house**

Growing birds of egg type chickens are kept from 9–20 weeks of age or up to the point of lay.

c. **Layer house**

Birds are kept during laying period, from 20–72 weeks of age in chickens and the 1st laying year is considered as economic egg laying period.

d. **Broiler house**

Broiler chickens from day-old stage to 42 days of age are kept in this house and 42 days of age is considered as marketing age in broiler chicken.

e. **Breeder house**

Breeder birds are kept in this house for production of hatching eggs.

f. **Hatchery**

This house is used for artificial incubation of eggs for production of chicks.

iii. **On the basis of style of roof**, poultry houses may be:

a. **Shed type**

It is very simple type of house and can be used in different climatic conditions. The slope of roof is usually less in plain areas, but it is to some extent steep in hilly areas or high rainfall areas. The shed type houses may be portable or permanent. In case of free range system or semi-intensive system of poultry keeping, a small portable house is generally constructed for accommodating less number of birds, but in case of commercial poultry farm, permanent type of house is constructed.

b. **Gable type**

The gable type house has sloppy roof so it is popular in high rainfall areas. More roof materials and labourers are needed for construction of this type of house. Sometimes a false ceiling is made below the gable roof, and the space between roof and ceiling is used as a storage space. Gable type house may be portable or permanent as per the need of the farmers.

c. **Combination type**

This type of house has double pitch roof in which the ridge is not at the middle from the front to back. Most of the houses have the long slope at the rear. This type of house also needs more roof materials and labourers than shed type house.

d. **Monitor type**

Ridge ventilation is provided at the middle of monitor type roof, other conditions are like the shed type house. In hot-humid areas, monitor type roof having ridge ventilation is preferred for escape of heat, gases and moisture produced in the house.

iv. **On the basis of microenvironment**, poultry houses may be of 2 types, viz.

a. **Open-sided poultry house**

Open-sided poultry houses are common in tropical regions having warm-humid conditions. The open-sided houses are generally oriented from east to west and the long sides are left open to maximise air movement. Actually a low wall of 25–30 cm height (60–80 cm in severe climatic condition) is made to prevent water penetration inside the house and the remaining portion is covered with wire netting or bamboo slats as a protection against predators or theft.

b. **Environmentally controlled poultry house**

The house in which microenvironment is controlled in such a way that it satisfies the optimum requirements of birds is called environmentally controlled house. Such houses are completely closed, even without any window. These are artificially lighted instead of sunlight and are artificially ventilated. The expired air is removed from the house by exhaust fans and fresh air is taken in through intake opening. Usually air inlets are made in the front wall and exhaust fans are installed in the back wall. The quantity of air exchange depends on type and age of birds, outside temperature and humidity. The insulation of the house is very important. The roof may consist of a double aluminium sheet with an insulating material in between the 2 layers. The walls can be insulated by fixing 4 cm mineral wool sheets against the inner side of the wall. The insulating materials should be resistant to water, dust, insects and fungi. The most important tools to maintain optimum environmental conditions, i.e. ambient temperature, humidity and quality air in closed houses, are ventilation and cooling.

The controlled environment houses are more appropriate in hot and dry regions. The controlled environment houses also help to reduce the stress due to greater bird density, rapid growth rate, increased metabolic rate and higher body weight, *etc.* The cost involvement in such type of houses is more. However, the space requirement is less in controlled house than open-sided poultry house. Till date controlled environment poultry houses are popular in western countries, but not so in India.

10.3 DIFFERENT SYSTEMS OF REARING COMMERCIAL POULTRY

Generally four systems are found for rearing poultry. These are:

  i. Free range or extensive system
 ii. Semi-intensive system
iii. Folding unit system
 iv. Intensive system

Out of these only the intensive system of housing is followed for commercial poultry production. It is of 2 types, viz.

  a. Deep litter system
  b. Cage system or battery system

The details of deep litter and cage housing for commercial rearing of poultry are discussed in the following sections. (*See Chapter 5*)

10.3.1 Deep Litter System

This system is widely used for scientific and successful poultry farming. It is very popular for small as well as large units of commercial poultry farms (both for broiler and layer). Birds are kept in large pen. The floor of the house is covered with dry litter materials up to the depth of 3 inches in broiler and 6 inches in layer houses. Feed and water are provided in respective containers.

Litter materials

The common litter materials are rice husk, sawdust, wood shavings, chopped straw, dried leaves, groundnut hulls, sugarcane bagasse, *etc.* These litter materials are used on the floor just like bedding as per the cost and availability.

Floor space requirements

Minimum floor space requirement under deep litter system of management is 1–1.2 sq ft per broiler and 1.75–2.00 sq ft per layer chickens (Tables 10.1 and 10.2). However, the floor space may be increased to some extent in summer months.

Litter management

Success of deep litter system depends on proper management of litter materials. So management of deep litter is very important. The following points should be considered for scientific care and management of deep litter.

- The floor of the poultry shed should be cleaned and disinfected with phenyl or bleaching powder, *etc.* before placing the deep litter materials. It should be ensured that the litter materials are sufficiently dry. The depth of the deep litter is to be maintained as 3–4 inches, however, it may be increased or decreased as per the requirement on the basis of environmental conditions. In no case, the depth should not be less than 2 inches. The best time to start deep litter is the dry period of the year.
- The deep litter should be kept dry always. If any part of litter becomes wet, that part should be replaced by new litter materials. If waterers are placed on the deep litter, the place of waterers should be changed frequently to avoid the dampness of litter below the waterers. In spite of all precautions, in some areas particularly in coastal humid areas in rainy season, litters become wet due to environmental reason. In such cases to keep the litter dry, 0.5 kg hydrated lime or super phosphate may be thoroughly mixed with litter for every 10–15 sq ft floor area.
- Proper ventilation is to be maintained to keep the litter dry.
- Litter should be stirred at regular interval. It is better to stir the litter daily to prevent cake formation. But precaution should be taken to avoid dusting of the litter materials which may cause respiratory problems among the birds.
- Same litter may be used for 6 weeks in broiler house, 18–20 weeks in case of brooder-cum-grower house and 1 year in case of layer house. New litter should be used for every batch of broilers and layers; that means old litters should be disposed off along with broilers and layers at the end of production.

Advantages of deep litter system

i. Safety and comfort of poultry

The birds are kept totally confined within the deep litter house. So they are safe from predator animals like dogs, cats, wolves, *etc.* The deep litter house also protects the birds from inclement weather. The litter materials on the floor act as bedding which provides comfort to the birds. This litter also acts as an insulating agent due to bad conductor of heat. In hot weather, it provides coolness and in winter it provides warmth to the birds.

ii. Providing scientific management is easy

There is full control over the birds, as they are confined in sheds under deep litter system of management. So scientific care and management especially in terms of feeding, vaccination and medication, culling, *etc.* can be applied easily. The sick birds can be detected, isolated and treated promptly.

iii. Labour saving

It needs no daily cleaning of floor as needed in other animal farms. Feeding and watering management is also easy and, if automation in feeding and watering is practiced, it will be easier. As the day to day management in deep litter system is easier, it saves labour.

iv. **Less land requirement**

Land requirement is less in deep litter system than free range or semi-intensive system. So farms can be established nearer to market to reduce the transportation cost and better marketability of products.

v. **Maintenance of heath**

Well-managed deep litter house can control many poultry diseases. The heat generated in deep litter due to fermentative action can kill some bacteria like *Salmonella* and also some parasites. If the deep litter is kept dry the coccidiosis and worm load will be very less, which is a major problem in free range poultry.

vi. **Poultry litter—a source of feed supplements**

Built up deep litter supplies some feed supplements to the birds. Built up deep litter generates animal protein factor (APF, vitamin B_{12} or cyano-cobalamin) and riboflavin (vitamin B_2). Birds can take these valuable supplements through deep litter.

vii. **Poultry litter—a valuable by-product**

a. **Poultry litter is a high quality manure.** It can be utilised directly as a fertiliser on agricultural land to increase soil fertility. It can also be processed into more stable products such as dried manure in pellet form, which is preferred to use as fertiliser in horticulture land. One study indicates that approximately 40 birds, kept on deep litter for about a year produce 1 tonne of manure, which will provide the full fertiliser needs of 1 hectare of paddy or maize or two hectares of sorghum or half a hectare of intensive vegetable cultivation (*Ghatnekar and Ghatnekar, 1999*). Poultry manure is rich in fertiliser value, containing 1.0–1.8% nitrogen, 1.4–1.8% phosphorus (P_2O_5) and 0.8–0.9% potassium (K_2O). (*See Table 1.1, Chapter 1*)

b. **Poultry litter can be recycled through ruminant animals** by using the treated manure as a feed ingredient. As the undigested remainder of ingested feed, the poultry manure contains high amount of fibre. It is also rich in uric acid, a non-protein nitrogen constituent, which is excreted as a part of poultry droppings. These fibres and uric acid can be efficiently utilised by ruminant animals through microbial fermentation process in their rumens. Besides, a part of energy of the ingested feed is left with droppings which can be recycled through animals. One study indicates that broiler litter contains 31.3% crude protein, 23.3% digestible protein, 16.8% crude fibre, 2.4% calcium and 1.8% phosphorus (*Saxena and Ketelaars, 1993*).

c. **The poultry litter may be used in fish ponds.** Some poultry droppings may be eaten by the fish (carp and other cultivated fish) directly. However, most of the poultry litter is utilised through fertilisation of fish ponds to improve the aquatic food resources consisting microalgae and bacteria.

d. **The poultry litter can be utilised for power generation** by producing biogas through anaerobic digestion. The other available materials are biogas slurry. Biogas mainly consists of methane (50–80%) and carbon dioxide (CO_2). This methane can be used for heating process as well as for generating electricity. The slurry can be used as a fertiliser on agricultural land or in fish ponds.

Disadvantages of deep litter system

There is no demerit of deep litter system for commercial production of broiler as well as layer, if management is done on scientific line. However, in certain conditions the following problems may be associated with this system of poultry keeping.

i. It may act as a source of some diseases called **litter-borne diseases**, if litter is not managed properly. The most important litter-borne diseases are respiratory diseases, coccidiosis, worm infestation and fungal disease. If the moisture of deep litter is not maintained properly, the litter becomes damp leading to generation of ammonia gas. It causes irritation of respiratory system, coughing and related diseases. It also causes irritation of eyes leading to less feed intake and less production. Damp litter is also the predisposing factor of coccidiosis, worm infestation and fungal growth. On the other hand, if the litter is too dry, it will be dusty leading to again respiratory problem. So the moisture level of deep litter (20–25%) should be maintained properly. Besides disease problem, wet litter may be responsible for foul smell, soiled egg and soiled feathers of broiler which reduce the market demand. However, good litter management can overcome these problems.

ii. As the birds are totally confined in this system, special care should be taken to supply feed and water timely and as per their requirements. Otherwise deficiency of nutrients may occur.

iii. Feed and water may be soiled by the birds, if the feeding and watering devices are placed on the deep litter. So precaution should be taken, by using specially designed feeders and waterers to prevent soiling.

10.3.2 Cage System

It is the latest system of poultry rearing. The birds are confined in a cage just large enough to permit limited movement and allow them to stand and sit comfortably. The cage is made up of strong galvanised wire with variable dimensions. The droppings are heaped up underneath the cages, or conveyer belt or a tray is fixed underneath of the floor for collection of droppings, at frequent interval, manually or by mechanical means. The feeders and waterers are attached outside the cage, mostly at the front side. The cage floor slopes to one side to let the eggs roll away to the egg collection area, which remains outside the cage. Initial investment in this system is very high, so this system is not suitable for small units of poultry. However, this system of poultry rearing is very efficient and is being used in case of large commercial egg production. However, cage rearing is not preferred for broilers as it may cause skin lesions and other quality defects.

Floor space requirement

Floor space requirement for birds is least in cage system (*See* Table 10.3). However, in hot-humid area the cage density should not be too high.

Types of cages

Different types of poultry cages are outlined below.

i. **On the basis of arrangement and design,** the poultry cages may be of three types as follows:

a. **Californian cages or reverse type cages:** The other name is stair-stepped cages. The name Californian is given to these cages as they were first invented in California. The compartments of cages are arranged stepwise in 2 or 3 tiers on stands in 2 or 3 rows. The droppings are accumulated on the ground or in deep pit under the cages. These droppings can be removed at a long interval, say 6 months or even 12 months interval depending upon the capacity of pit.

b. **Battery cages or multi-tier cages:** The other name is vertical cages. The compartments of cages are arranged one above the other on stands in two or three rows. A tray or sheet belt is provided under each cage for collection of droppings, and the droppings are preferably removed every day or an alternate day.

c. **Flat deck cages or single-tier cages:** The cages are arranged on stands in single-tier in 3–4 rows. These cages are generally used for rearing of chicks up to 8 weeks of age. The droppings may be collected in a tray or on the ground below the cages, which may be removed after 8 weeks at the time of shifting of chicks to grower house. Quantity of droppings is less due to smaller size of birds at this stage.

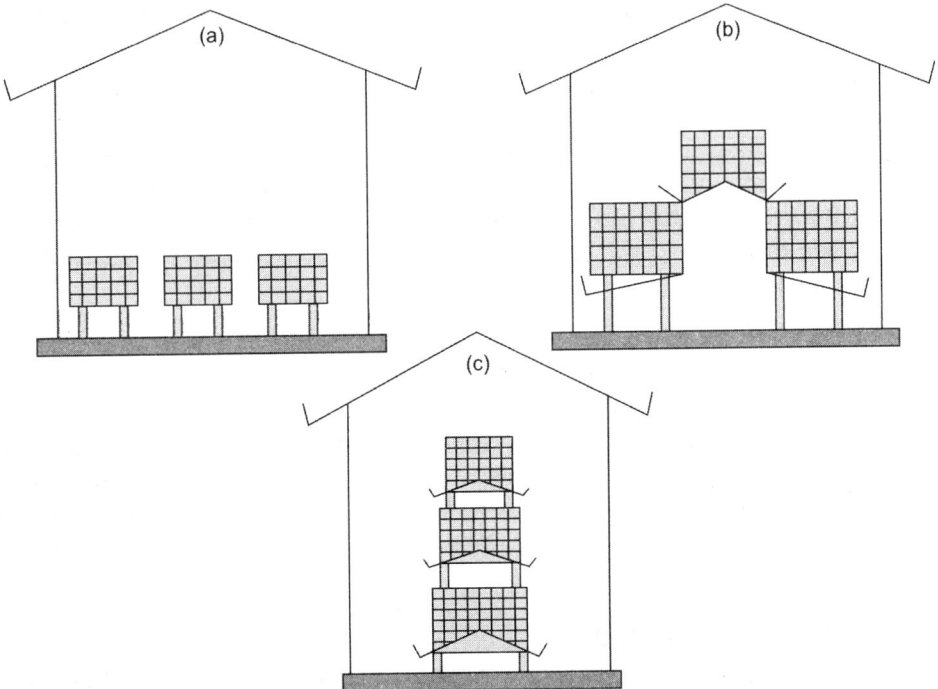

Fig. 10.3: Different types of cages. (a) Flat deck cages or single-tier cages, (b) Californian cages, (c) Battery cages or multi-tier cages

ii. **On the basis of categories of birds to be kept,** the cages may be of various types, viz.

    a. Brooder cage (for keeping chicks up to 8 weeks of age)

    b. Grower cage (for keeping growing chickens from 9–20 weeks of age or up to the point of lay)

    c. Layer cage (for keeping laying birds)

Advantages of cage system

The cage system of rearing poultry is the latest invention. It has many advantages as follows:

i. **Less space and land requirements:** The space requirement of birds and land requirement for operating poultry farm in this system of management is the least in comparison to other systems of poultry rearing. About 20–25 thousand birds can be reared in 1 hectare of land. So this system reduces the overall cost of housing to a great extent.

ii. **Better supervision and maintenance of birds:** The birds are under complete control so flock supervision is better in this system. Scientific management practices in terms of feeding, watering, healthcare, culling, debeaking, *etc.* can be carried out easily with minimum stress on birds.

iii. **Less disease incidence:** Birds are kept on wire floor. There is no scope of occurring many litter-borne diseases particularly coccidiosis and worm infestation. This system does not need the recurring cost of litter materials, and there is no litter management problem. Dust and ammonia problems are usually less prevalent in this system.

iv. **Clean egg production:** In cage system, just after laying eggs are rolled out and accumulated in the extended egg tray outside of the wall. So there is no scope of soiling of eggs by the birds. Egg eating habit is also prevented for this arrangement. The breakage of egg is very minimum (about 0.5–1.0%) which increases the profit margin. On the other hand, there is minimal contact between the egg and the hen in this system. This decreases the possibility of bacterial contamination of the egg.

v. **Better record keeping:** Record keeping is easier, even individual records can be kept in this system; which helps the poultry breeders to carry out efficient breeding programme.

vi. **Efficiency of production:** In this system, feed consumption is reduced due to less movement of birds. Labour requirement is also less depending on the level of automation followed. Ultimately the cage system of poultry rearing offers economy in space, feed, labour and medication, and increases the efficiency of production.

Disadvantages of cage system

i. The initial cost of involvement is high for manufacturing welded iron wire cages. Though it is very efficient system of poultry keeping, it is not suitable for small scale operation.

ii. Sometimes layer birds develop a problem called 'cage layer fatigue' or cage paralysis. They show weakness or leg paralysis along with reduction in egg production. If it is continued, birds may die. Calcium and phosphorus levels of birds should be higher in cage rearing than deep litter system.

iii. As the birds are fully confined in this system, special care should be taken to supply feed and water timely and as per their requirements. Otherwise birds may go for starvation.

10.4 SPACE REQUIREMENTS FOR POULTRY

Space requirement depends on systems of housing, category of birds to be kept, breeds, seasons, *etc.* A space requirement is generally increased to some extent during summer months and in case of heavy breeds.

Space requirement for floor rearing under deep litter system

Space requirement for layer and broiler chickens under deep litter system of management is presented in Tables 10.1 and 10.2.

Table 10.1: Space requirements for commercial layer chicken under deep litter system

Category of space	Chick (0–8 weeks)	Grower (9–20 weeks)	Layer (21–72 weeks)
Floor space	0.75 sq ft	1 sq ft	1.75–2 sq ft
Feeder space	2 inches	2.5 inches	3.5 inches
Waterer space	0.6 inch	0.75 inch	1 inch

Table 10.2: Space requirements for commercial broiler chicken under deep litter system

Category of space	Broiler starter (0–4 weeks)	Broiler finisher (5–6 weeks)
Floor space	0.35 sq ft	1–1.2 sq ft
Feeder space	1.5 inches	3 inches
Waterer space	0.75 inch	1 inch

Note: Generally up to 1 kg body weight, 1 sq ft floor space per broiler chicken is sufficient. If it is planned to keep the birds for a longer period of time after 1 kg of body weight, floor space must be increased especially in hot-humid areas. In case of heavy birds it is better to provide about 2 sq ft floor space per bird.

Space requirement for rearing of chickens in cages

In case of cage rearing, the minimum floor space requirement is 0.33 sq ft per chick, 0.42 sq ft per grower and 0.64 sq ft per layer chicken. Broiler birds are not generally reared in cages. Depth (breadth) and height of the cage are 1 ft and 1½ ft respectively; and the length depends on the number of birds to be kept in the cage. It is better not to keep more than 10–12 birds per cage, provided they are debeaked. The dimension of various cages for accommodating commercial layers, growers and chicks are given below.

Dimension of layer cages: It may be Californian or reverse type cage having 3 tiers with stair-step arrangement. The floor wires (GI weld) are of 10 gauge with 3 inches × 1 inch mesh size (wirenetting). The floor is extended up to 9 inches which is moulded upwards by 2 inches at the edge to form an egg tray. The floor should slant downward of 3 inches back to front so that eggs will roll through a 2 inches gap in the front wall. The cage roof, front and back mesh size may be of 2 inches × 3 inches with 8 gauge wires and cage partition mesh size may be of 3 inches × 1 inch with 12 gauge wires. The specification of layer cages is as follows (Table 10.3):

Table 10.3: Dimension of various commercial layer cages

Width / Depth (inches)	Length (inches)	Height (inches)	No. of birds to be accommodated
12	15	18	3
12	20	18	4
15	20	18	5
18	20	18	6

The dimension of grower cages: It may be Californian or reverse type cage having 2–3 tiers with stair-step arrangement. The floor wires (GI weld) are of 12 gauge with 2 inches × 1 inch mesh size (wirenetting). The specification of grower cage is as follows:

Length	—	24 inches
Depth (Width)	—	12 inches
Height	—	14 inches
Capacity	—	6 growers

The dimension of brooder cages: It may be flat deck or single-tier type cage. The floor wires (GI weld) are of 14 gauge with 1 inch × ½ inch mesh size (wire-netting). The specification of brooder cage is as follows:

Length	—	40 inches
Depth (Width)	—	40 inches
Lengthwise partition	—	At the middle, 20 inches + 20 inches
Height	—	12 inches
Capacity	—	40 chicks (20 chicks in each compartment)

10.5 CONSTRUCTIONAL DETAILS OF POULTRY HOUSES

Poultry house should not be very expensive. However, its durability, comfort and safety of birds should not be overlooked. The architecture of an ideal poultry house should be such that it provides a regular and efficient exchange of air, thus removing excessive moisture, ammonia gas and heat from sheds. The comfortable temperature zone for poultry is 18.3–21.5 °C, however, temperature range of 11–17 °C (minimum) to 22–28 °C (maximum) are also comfortably tolerated by them. The body temperature of poultry is 40–41°C. The optimum relative humidity inside the poultry house should be 38–42%. There is no restriction to the length, but the width should not exceed more than 26–28 ft as wider house may cause improper ventilation. The high environmental temperature may exhibit various adverse effects on poultry production through low feed intake, alkalosis and low level of blood calcium, increased body temperature, *etc.* Poultry houses may be constructed with concrete pillars with brick and cement walls. The 2 sides are to be made up of solid brick wall. The house is to be provided with 3-phase power supply. There should be provision of sufficient space for any expansion, if needed in future.

Floor: The floor should be moistureproof, easily cleaned, ratproof and durable. Various types of floors are litter floor, wire floor, slat floor, slat and litter floor, wire and litter floor, *etc.* The floor may be plastered with cement and elevated 1 ft above the ground level. All litter floors in case of deep litter system and all wire floors in case of cage rearing are commonly practiced in our country.

Roof: The roof must be moistureproof and draftproof. Insulation of roof is advantageous both in summer and winter seasons. There should be 2½–3 ft overhang of roofs to offer full protection from direct solar radiation and rains. Roof structure is to be built by seasoned wood and tiles. Roof materials may be thatch, asbestos sheet, corrugated iron and zinc sheet and cement concrete. Asbestos cement sheets are commonly used as they have more insulation capacity. The gable type roof, i.e. roof with 1 in 50 slope is commonly used for poultry houses. In warm-humid areas the roof should have ridge ventilation to escape gases, heat and moisture.

Wall: The inside height at eaves should be at least 7 ft, while at ridge height should be around 12 ft. The side walls may be kept open from half to two-third area in open-sided house and is fitted with wire mesh. Generally out of 7 ft high wall, 2 ft is constructed as solid brick wall and then remaining portion is covered with wirenetting for open air ventilation. The open-side of the shed may be covered with 1 inch GI 12 gauge chain link mesh throughout except at the doors.

Door: The doors are to be made up of MS angle frame and 1 inch × 3 inches mesh of 10 gauge thickness, with provision to lock from both sides. The size of the door may be 4 ft wide × 7 ft high, so that a man can conveniently get through.

Other buildings: The feed room, office, store and workers' quarters will have brick side walls to the full height.

10.6 LAYOUT PLANS FOR POULTRY FARMS

Type of house: Poultry houses may be of 2 types, viz. open-sided house (conventional type) and environmentally controlled closed house (non-conventional type). Open-sided poultry houses are very popular in almost all parts of India except temperate climatic conditions where ambient temperature is exceptionally low. This is the conventional poultry house followed in our country. Initial cost involvement in this type of house is comparatively less. Closed house with controlled environment needs high cost involvement so it is not generally followed for commercial purpose in India.

Orientation: Efforts should be made to build the house in such a direction that maximum availability of sunshine from early morning to late evening can be achieved. Houses with east-west direction having long axis facing north and south, and short axis on east and west is better. Shape of the building should be preferably L, E, C or Y in order to facilitate good sunshine.

Gap between various buildings: At least 10–15 m gap should be there in between 2 layered houses. The layer houses may be constructed in single row or double rows. In big poultry farms having separate brooder, grower and layer houses, 50–60 m gap should be there between layer house and brooder or grower house. The distance between brooder house and grower house should be about 30 m.

Location of various sheds in the farm: The brooder house and grower house should be located away from the entrance of the farm, preferably at the western side.

Number of sheds: Number of sheds in the poultry farm depends on the rearing/selling schedule of birds.

In case of broiler chicken farm, if there is 1 shed, 6 batches of broilers can be sold. One batch requires 1½ months and 15 days gap is necessary before bringing the next batch, i.e. at an interval of 2 months each batch of birds can be sold. However, one extra shed should be kept to accommodate the unsold birds, if any. In this way, for selling the birds at monthly interval 3 sheds (2 + 1) are necessary, at fortnight interval 5 sheds (4 + 1) are necessary and at weekly interval 9 sheds (8 + 1) are necessary.

In case of layer chicken farm, various rearing schedules are found to be followed by the farmers. In case of small farm, one brooder cum grower cum layer house is used for rearing layer chickens and is very common in small farms under deep litter system of management. In case of medium farms, (1 + 3) system, i.e. one brooder-cum-grower house and 3 layer house is followed and is very common under cage system of rearing poultry. In case of large farms, (1 + 1 + 4) or 5 housing system is followed, where there are one brooder house, one grower house and 4 or 5 layered houses.

10.7 COST OF CONSTRUCTION OF POULTRY HOUSE

An economical poultry shed should be built with locally available materials. However, the comfort of the birds should not be compromised because it will have positive influence on the productivity of birds.

The cost of construction may vary from time to time. To get an idea the cost for construction of various items in poultry farm is given in Table 10.4. It may be recast on the basis of current price of various items in the locality where the poultry farm is to be established.

Table 10.4: Cost of poultry house and equipment

Sl no.	Types of poultry house	Cost/sq ft (₹)
1.	Thatched roof with wooden structure and mud floor	30.00
2.	Tile roof with country wood support and stone pillars	45.00
3.	Asphalt/light roofing with country wood support and stone or brick pillars	40.00
4.	Asbestos roof with country wood support and stone or brick pillars	50.00
5.	Asbestos roof with iron truss and iron or concrete pillars	80.00
6.	Aluminium roof with iron truss and concrete pillars	100.00
7.	Elevated raised platform cage house with iron and concrete structures and asbestos roof	100.00
8.	Environmental control house with foggers and tunnel ventilation	110.00
9.	Cost of equipment per bird (cost/bird in ₹) i. Under deep litter system • For a layer bird up to point of lay • For a layer bird during laying period • For a broiler ii. Under cage system • For a bird (excluding cage cost)	6.00/bird 8.00/bird 8.00/bird 2.00/bird
10.	Barbed wire fence with 5 ft height and stone pillars	₹ 15.00/ running ft
11.	Compound wall with 5 ft height and 5 inches thickness	₹ 120.00/ running ft
12.	Borewell 150 ft depth with pipe	₹ 120.00/ft
13.	Overhead tank	₹ 6.00/L
14.	Pipeline with pump having 3 HP motor and compressor	₹ 20,000.00
15.	Pipeline with pump having 1 HP jet motor	₹ 15,000.00

10.8 POULTRY FARM EQUIPMENT

Common poultry farm equipments are feeder, waterer, nest, catching appliance, weighing balance, debeaker, brooder, *etc.*

1. Feeder

Two types of poultry feeders are in use, viz. **hopper type** (tube or circular feeder, Fig. 10.4 (a)) and **trough type** (linear or longitudinal feeder, Fig. 10.4 (b)). Sometimes egg trays are used as chick feeder. Four feeders (trays) are usually provided for about 250–300 chicks up to 7 days of age, and then additional feeders (3–4 per 100 birds) are provided.

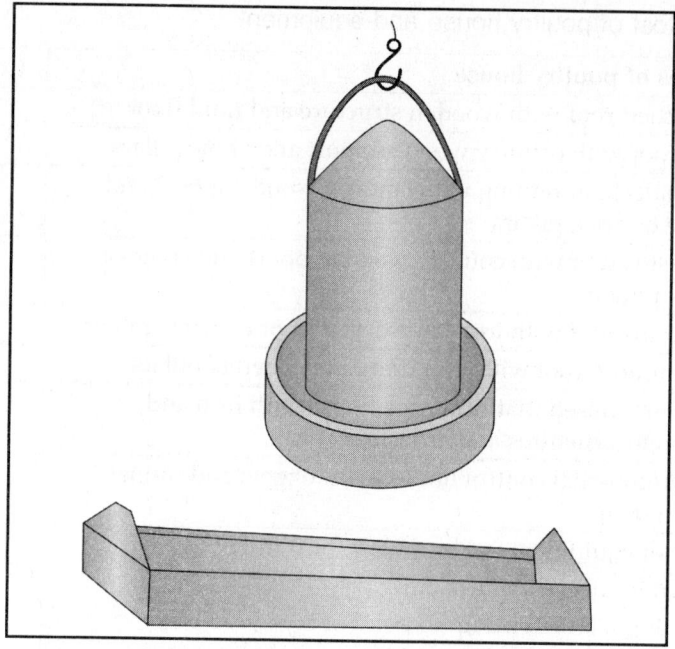

Fig. 10.4: Types of feeder for poultry (a) Hopper type feeder,
(b) Trough type feeder

Feeder space requirement is as follows:
In case of broiler farm under deep litter system—
0–2 weeks: 1 inch/bird
3–6 weeks: 2–2.5 inches/bird

2. Waterer (Drinker)

Different types of waterers are in use, viz. plate and jar, water bowl, water trough (linear or channel type), pipeline with nipples, deep water pan with guard grill, *etc* (Fig. 10.5).

Four waterers (drinkers) are usually provided for about 250–300 chicks up to 7 days of age, and then additional waterers (3–4 per 100 birds) are provided.

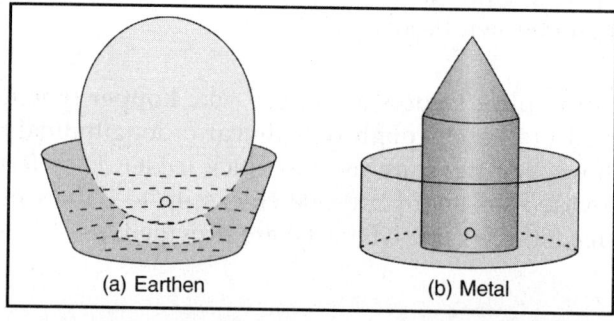

(a) Earthen   (b) Metal

Fig. 10.5: Waterer for poultry (a) Earthen, (b) Metal

Waterer space requirement is as follows:

In case of broiler farm under deep litter system—

0–4 weeks:	1 inch/bird
5 weeks onwards:	2 inches/bird

One automatic round waterer is sufficient for 50 birds. No birds should have walk more than 8 ft for a waterer. Water intake generally increases by 2–3 times during summer months. So adequate number of waterers is to be provided by introducing more numbers as per needs so that fresh clean drinking water will be available always. Generally, water space is increased by about 50% in hot weather. Under normal conditions, chicken of all age groups consume about two times as much water by weight as they eat feed.

3. Nest

The nest is provided in the layer house only, generally under deep litter system of management. It helps in proper collection of eggs as well as production of clean eggs. Nest may be of several types, viz. individual nest, community nest, community roll away nest, trap nest, *etc.* They are made up of wooden or steel with sufficient space for birds.

Individual nest: One individual nest box measuring 35.5 cm × 35.5 cm × 30.5 cm is sufficient for 4–5 laying hens of commercial flock.

Community nest: One community nest measuring 1.5 m × 0.6 m × 0.6 m is sufficient for 50 layers. It is commonly used at commercial layer farm under deep litter system of management.

Community roll away nest: It is generally used in case of breeding flock under cage system of management. It helps in clean egg production, but if wrongly installed, it may increase breakage of eggs.

Trap nest: It is used for breeding poultry farm. After entering in the nest box the door is automatically closed and the bird cannot come out. After completion of laying the bird is to be left out manually, and egg is collected and marked for the research purpose.

4. Catching appliance

Catching appliances are used to catch the birds with minimum possible stress for various operations like vaccination, weighing, debeaking, culling, *etc.* The important catching appliances are catching hook and catching crate/wire panel.

5. Debeaker

Cutting of about ⅓ to ½ of upper mandible and trimming of lower mandible for just making it blunt is known as debeaking. This is done to reduce the wastage of feeds and to minimise the chance of cannibalism. This is generally done for egg type chicken and usually not required for broiler chicken. Debeaker is used for this purpose. Both manual and electric debeakers are available in the market; however, in commercial layer farm electric debeaker is commonly used.

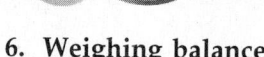

6. **Weighing balance**

   Weighing balances of various capacities are needed in the poultry farm for weighing chicks and adult birds, feeds, eggs, *etc*. Special egg weighing balance is also available.

7. **Brooder**

   It is a device which provides heat to the birds at their early part of lives, generally up to 4–6 weeks of age, or until they are well-feathered. There are various types of brooders. In case of deep litter system, various types of brooders that may be bamboo basket, hover or canopy (round, conical or angular-shaped structure usually made up of galvanised iron sheets fitted with bulbs), infrared lamps (electricity), infrared brooder (gas), and radiant brooder (gas).

   Cage brooders are used in case of cage system of rearing.

   Choice of brooder depends on the system of keeping poultry, economy, number of chicks to be reared, and source of fuel, *etc*. Under deep litter system usually bamboo basket with electric bulbs is used as a source of heat in small farms. The height of the brooder should be about 6 inches in the first week. Sometimes basket is not used and brooding is done on the floor of the deep litter house itself. Under cage system of rearing poultry, use of cage brooder is common (Fig. 10.6).

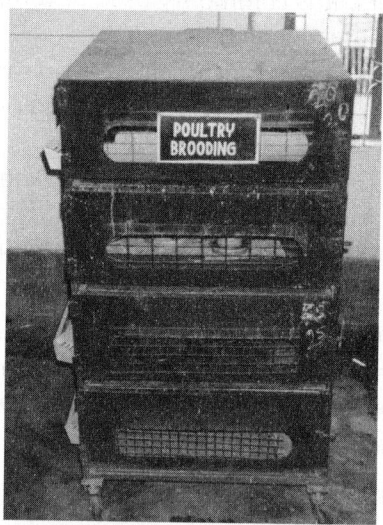

POULTRY BROODING

Fig. 10.6: Cage brooder of poultry

8. **Electric bulb**

   Electric bulbs are used for light management as well as brooding management under conventional system. Four 60 watt bulbs suspended 6 inches above the floor are generally provided for 250–300 chicks for brooding management at the initial period.

EXERCISE

A. Objective Questions

i. **Indicate the correct answer by putting tick ($\sqrt{}$) mark (multiple choice).**

1. Which system is the best for commercial poultry keeping at rural India?
   - (a) Free range system
   - (b) Semi-intensive system
   - (c) Deep litter system
   - (d) Cage system

2. The minimum floor space requirement for a broiler (chicken) under deep litter system is
   - (a) 1.00 sq ft
   - (b) 1.75 sq ft
   - (c) 2.00 sq ft
   - (d) 2.50 sq ft

3. The minimum floor space requirement for a layer (chicken) under deep litter system is
   - (a) 1.00 sq ft
   - (b) 1.75 sq ft
   - (c) 3.50 sq ft
   - (d) 3.75 sq ft

4. A broiler poultry shed of 25 ft × 10 ft under deep litter system can accommodate
   - (a) 125 birds
   - (b) 250 birds
   - (c) 325 birds
   - (d) 375 birds

5. Poor ventilation in poultry house may cause
   - (a) Accumulation of carbon monoxide
   - (b) Accumulation of ammonia
   - (c) Wet litter condition
   - (d) All of these

6. For harvesting broiler crops per week, the number of poultry sheds needed is
   - (a) 3 sheds
   - (b) 5 sheds
   - (c) 7 sheds
   - (d) 9 sheds

7. Cage layer fatigue is a problem associated with
   - (a) Deep litter system
   - (b) Battery system
   - (c) Semi-intensive system
   - (d) Folding unit system

8. What type of roof of poultry house is preferred in hilly areas?
   - (a) Monitor type roof having ridge ventilation
   - (b) Sloppy roof
   - (c) Straight roof
   - (d) None of these

9. High environmental temperature may exhibit adverse effects on poultry production through
   - (a) Low feed consumption
   - (b) Increased body temperature
   - (c) Alkalosis and low blood calcium level
   - (d) All of these

10. Animal protein factor available from built-up of deep litter is nothing, but
    (a) Vitamin B$_6$
    (b) Vitamin B$_{12}$
    (c) Biotin
    (d) None of these

11. The optimum temperature of poultry house should be
    (a) 11–17 °C
    (b) 18–21 °C
    (c) 22–28 °C
    (d) 40–41 °C

12. Poultry birds are housed for
    (a) Better care and management
    (b) Efficient production
    (c) Comfort
    (d) All of these

13. Consider the following statements in relation to the location of large establishment of commercial poultry farm.
    1. The place should be well-connected with road.
    2. It should be located at the place where more vegetarian people are residing.
    3. The highland with leveled surface and loamy soil is good.
    4. It is better to have facilities like banking, postal communication, shopping complex, *etc.*, nearby.
    Select the correct answer from the code below:
    Code (a) 1, 2, 3 and 4 are correct
    (b) 1, 2 and 3 are correct
    (c) 1, 2 and 4 are correct
    (d) 1, 3 and 4 are correct

14. Poultry house should be properly ventilated for the following reasons.
    1. It keeps the house dry.
    2. It removes the gases like CO_2, CO, NH_3, CH_4, *etc.*
    3. It reduces the chance of occurrence of worm infestation.
    4. It cools the house in summer months.
    Select the correct answer from the code below:
    Code (a) 1, 2, 3 and 4 are correct
    (b) 1, 2 and 3 are correct
    (c) 1, 2 and 4 are correct
    (d) 2, 3 and 4 are correct

15. Consider the following statements in relation to the space requirement in poultry farm.
    1. The space requirement is the least in battery cage system of poultry housing.
    2. Space requirement is generally increased to some extent during summer months.
    3. Generally up to 1 kg body weight, 1 sq ft floor space per broiler chicken is sufficient.
    4. A layer cage having the specification of 15″ × 12″ × 18″ can accommodate 6 laying chickens.
    Select the correct answer from the code below:
    Code (a) 1, 2, 3 and 4 are correct
    (b) 1, 2 and 3 are correct
    (c) 1, 2 and 4 are correct
    (d) 2, 3 and 4 are correct

ii. Fill in the blanks.

1. Floor space requirement per broiler chicken on deep litter is _____.
2. Floor space requirement per layer chicken on deep litter is _____ (minimum).
3. Poultry deep litter is a source of _____ (vitamin).
4. Air used for ventilation in incubator should have _____% oxygen.
5. Four 60 watt bulbs suspended 6 inches above the floor are generally provided for _____ chicks for brooding management at the initial period.
6. Flat deck cages for poultry are _____ -tier cages.
7. Californian cages for poultry are also known as _____ cages.
8. Battery cages for poultry are _____ -tier cages.
9. The optimum moisture level of deep litter should be _____ %.
10. The gable type house of poultry has _____ roof.

iii. Write True (T) or False (F) against each statement.

1. Damp litter is a predisposing factor for coccidiosis and fungal disease in poultry.
2. The gable type house has sloppy roof, so it is popular in high rainfall areas.
3. Californian cages are also known as single-tier cages.
4. Flat deck cages are multi-tier cages for rearing of poultry.
5. Approximately 40 layer type birds kept on deep litter for about a year, can produce 1 tonne of manure.
6. The distance between brooder house and grower house should be about 30 m to prevent cross infection.
7. Monitor type roof having ridge ventilation is preferred to escape heat and moisture, produced in the poultry house.
8. The moisture level of deep litter materials should be near about 40%.
9. The minimum floor space requirement in cage system is 0.33 sq m per chick.
10. The floor of layer cages is extended up to 9 inches which is moulded upwards by 2 inches at the edge to collect droppings and leftover feeds.

B. Subjective Questions

1. Mention the points to be considered for selection of site for poultry housing. What are the different types of poultry houses?
2. What are the different systems of housing poultry? Describe the deep litter system with its merits and demerits.
3. What is deep litter system? Indicate the advantages of this system. What are the space requirements for broiler and layer chickens under this system of housing?
4. Describe the cage system of rearing poultry. What are its advantages over deep litter system?

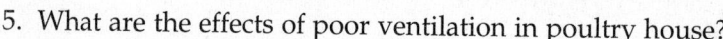

5. What are the effects of poor ventilation in poultry house?
6. Write short notes on the following.
   (a) Environmentally controlled housing
   (b) Deep litter system
   (c) Different types of cages for poultry

Answers of the Objective Questions

i. Multiple choice

1. (c) Deep litter system
2. (a) 1.00 sq ft
3. (b) 1.75 sq ft
4. (b) 250 birds
5. (d) All of these
6. (d) 9 sheds
7. (b) Battery system
8. (b) Sloppy roof
9. (d) All of these
10. (b) Vitamin B_{12}
11. (b) 18–21 °C
12. (d) All of these
13. (d) 1, 3 and 4 are correct
14. (a) 1, 2, 3 and 4 are correct
15. (b) 1, 2 and 3 are correct

ii. Fill in the blanks

1. 1 sq ft
2. 1.75–2 sq ft
3. vitamin B_{12}/cyanocobalamin/APF
4. 21
5. 250–300
6. single
7. stair-stepped/reverse type
8. multi
9. 20–25%
10. sloppy

iii. True or False

1. T
2. T
3. F
4. F
5. T
6. T
7. T
8. F
9. F
10. F

11

Feed and Water Management of Poultry

11.1 DIGESTIVE SYSTEM AND DIGESTION IN CHICKEN

The conversion of complex feed into simple form so that it easily gets absorbed in the blood is described as digestion. The digestive tract (alimentary tract/gastro-intestinal tract) with the help of accessory glands of digestion performs this function. The digestive system of birds is somewhat different from mammals.

11.1.1 Digestive System of Chicken

The digestive system of chicken includes the digestive tract and some digestive glands (Fig. 11.1). The digestive tract is a long tube through which feed passes. It begins at the mouth and terminates at the vent. The parts of digestive tract of chicken are mouth (beak, tongue and mouth cavity), oesophagus, crop, proventriculus, gizzard, small intestine, large intestine, cloaca and vent. The primary accessory glands are salivary glands, liver and pancreas. All these organs and glands are physiologically as well as anatomically linked. Digestion and absorption occur in different stages, each of which being dependent on the previous stage or stages. The various organs of the digestive system and their respective functions are described in the following section.

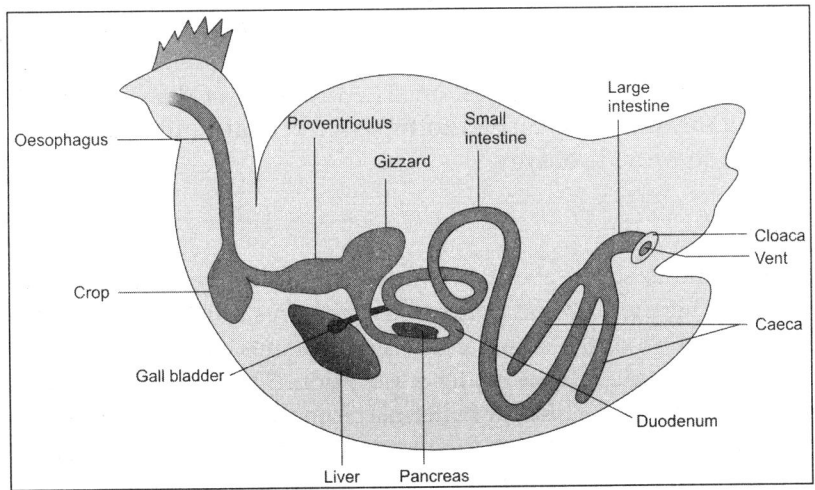

Fig. 11.1: Digestive system of chicken

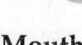

Mouth

The mouth of bird lacks teeth and lips. Instead, the horny beak serves to bite off feed. The shape of the **tongue** is just like barbed head of an arrow, which helps feed to be moved backward, so that it can be easily swallowed.

Esophagus and crop

The esophagus is a flexible tube which carries feed from the mouth to the crop. The **crop** is the bulging portion of the esophagus, where feed is stored for brief period and softened. The feed materials are gradually moved to the stomach by contraction of the wall of the crop.

Stomach

Poultry stomach is divided into 2 parts, viz. proventriculus and gizzard. The proventriculus is called the glandular stomach or true stomach as enzymatic digestion takes place here and gizzard is called ventriculus or muscular stomach, where mechanical digestion takes place. Gizzard is the largest single organ of the body. It is reddish-green in colour, oval-shaped and thick-walled with powerful muscles. Proventriculus receives feed from the crop, where hydrochloric acid and pepsin start the process of digestion. Then feed moves into the gizzard. The main function of the gizzard is to grind or crush feed particles into smaller sizes. The birds eat small amount of fine gravels or grits which help this process of grinding in the gizzard.

Small intestine

The small intestine is more or less similar to mammals. It is about 1.5 m long in adult fowl. The small intestine consists of duodenum, jejunum and ileum. The upper part of small intestine is called duodenum and its U-shaped portion having 2 limbs. The other parts of small intestine (jejunum and ileum) are not well-demarcated in poultry. From gizzard, the feed moves into the **duodenum**. Intestinal digestion together with pancreatic digestion takes place here. Bile is also added in the duodenum which helps in fat digestion. The products of digestion are absorbed from the small intestine and carried to the liver primarily to remanufacture into body tissues or to provide energy.

Large intestine

The large intestine is short, about 10 cm in length, but twice as the diameter of small intestine. There are 2 blind pouch-like structures called **caeca**, about 15 cm in length, at the junction of the small and large intestines. Some microbial digestion takes place here, besides minor water absorption. They also appear to serve as temporary storage organs of faecal materials. Sometimes large intestine is referred as **colon** and **rectum,** rectum being the terminal part. But in large animals, caecum is considered as the first part of large intestine followed by colon and rectum. Large intestine serves as a further absorption site especially for water.

Cloaca

It is the common passage for digestive, urinary and reproductive systems. Large intestine empties into the **cloaca**. It is responsible for the elimination of faeces and urine. Here faeces of birds mixed with urine and are excreted through the **vent**.

Digestive glands

Liver is the largest gland of the body and is divided into several lobes. The right lobe is the largest. The liver is dark brown or chocolate in colour except for the first 10–14 days when it may be quite pale due to the absorption of lipids from the yolk as an embryo. It weighs approximately 50 g. The gall bladder lies on the right lobe of the liver and beneath the spleen. The liver produces bile, metabolises carbohydrate, lipid and protein, and stores glycogen, fat and fat-soluble vitamins (e.g. vitamin A). It is also a major detoxification organ. **Pancreas** is the yellow organ present in between 2 limbs of duodenum. The functions of pancreas are production of pancreatic juice, a mixture of digestive enzymes, and production of the hormones like insulin and glucagon, that are involved in the metabolism of carbohydrate.

11.1.2 Digestion in Chicken

The chicken digestive system breaks down ingested feed into basic components by mechanical and chemical means. These basic components are then absorbed and used by the body. The digestion and absorption of feed takes place primarily in the small intestine of chicken. The secretion of digestive system and steps of digestion in chicken are described here.

- The **salivary glands** secrete mucous in the mouth cavity, which lubricates and softens feed. The enzyme amylase is also seen in **saliva** of poultry, but little or no digestion can occur as the feed quickly passes down from mouth to the esophagus. Saliva secretion varies from 7–30 ml per day and is somewhat acidic, with a pH range of 6.7–6.9.
- **Crop** secretes mucous which is acidic in nature and has a pH of 4.7–4.9. In crop, softening of feed takes place along with the digestion of a little amount of starch. The mucous secreted from crop helps to soften the feed and the enzyme amylase coming from mouth cavity helps in carbohydrate digestion in crop. Then the feed goes to the stomach.
- **Proventriculus** has 2 types of glands, viz. (i) simple mucosal glands that secrete mucous, and (ii) compound mucosal glands that secrete **mucous** and **gastric juices** (containing HCl and pepsin). About 8 mL of gastric juice is secreted per kg body weight per hour which is considerably higher than dogs, monkeys and human beings. The gastric juice is highly acidic with a pH range of 0.5 to 2.5. The acid proteolysis takes place in proventriculus. Protein is converted into proteoses and peptones. The acid proteolysis also takes place in **gizzard** with the help of gastric juices, secreted from proventriculus along with mechanical digestion of coarser feed particles.
- Chemical digestion primarily takes place in small intestine. Number of enzymes are found in small intestine. The **intestinal juice** secreted from intestinal mucosa, contains aminopeptidase, carboxypeptidase, carbohydrate splitting enzymes

(like amylase, maltase and sucrase) and lipolytic enzyme (like lipase). Secretin, a hormone secreted from the small intestine, stimulates the secretion of pancreas. The small intestine receives bile secreted from liver, and pancreatic juice secreted from pancreas. **Bile** contains bile pigments, bile salts, amylase and some mucin-like substances. Bile salts play a major role in fat digestion by emulsification of fat. **Pancreatic juice** contains amylolytic or carbohydrate splitting enzymes (like amylase and sucrase), proteolytic enzymes (like trypsin and chymotrypsin) and lipolytic enzymes (like lipase, dipeptidase, aminopeptidase and carboxy-peptidase). The pancreatic secretion also contains buffering compounds which neutralises the acid chyme and set pH approximately at 6–8. All the 3 types of feeds (carbohydrates, proteins and fats) are digested here by enzymatic action and converted into absorbable forms (e.g. proteins to amino acids, carbohydrates to glucose and fats to fatty acids and glycerols) (Table 11.1).

- A considerable microbial digestion occurs in caeca of which cellulose is important. Caecum is also believed to synthesise some B vitamins. Some of the water is absorbed through caecal wall.

The end products of carbohydrate, protein and fat digestion are abosorbed primarily from the lower part of small intestine (mainly from upper ileum).

Table 11.1: Process of digestion in chicken

Part of digestive tract where digestion occurs	Enzyme (Secreted from)	Substrate	End product
Mouth cavity	Amylase (salivary glands)	Starch	Maltose
Crop	Amylase (salivary glands)	Starch	Maltose
Stomach	Pepsin (proventriculus) It is secreted as pepsinogen, converted to active pepsin by HCl.	Protein	Proteoses, peptones
Small intestine	Enzymes secreted from intestinal glands/pancreas/liver		
	Amylase	Starch	Maltose
	Maltase	Maltose	Glucose
	Sucrase	Sucrose	Fructose, glucose
	Trypsin (it is secreted as trypsinogen, converted to active trypsin by enterokinase of intestine.)	Protein, proteoses, peptones	Polypeptides, dipeptides.
	Chymotrypsin (it is secreted as chymotrypsinogen, converted to active trypsin.)	Protein, proteoses, peptones	Polypeptides, dipeptides.

Contd.

Table 11.1:   Process of digestion in chicken *(Contd.)*

Part of digestive tract where digestion occurs	Enzyme (Secreted from)	Substrate	End product
	Carboxypeptidase	Polypeptides with free carboxyl groups	Lower peptides, free amino acids
	Aminopeptidase	Polypeptides with free amino groups	Lower peptides, free amino acids
	Dipeptidase	Dipeptides	Amino acids
	Lipase (bile salts help in emulsification of fat.)	Fat	Fatty acids, glycerols
Caeca	Microbial digestion	Cellulose, polysaccharides, starches	Volatile fatty acids, microbial protein and vitamins

11.2   SOME SPECIALITIES OF POULTRY DIGESTION

- Poultry can be classified as a simple stomached animal. They have two types of stomach, viz. proventriculus or glandular stomach (for enzymatic digestion) and gizzard or muscular stomach (for mechanical digestion).
- Teeth and lips are absent in the mouth cavity. They take feed with the help of beak and swallowed. So feed ingredients should be of proper size (710 millimicron). There is a problem of taking powdered feed or whole grains.
- Their digestion is quite rapid and metabolic rate is very high. They take less time to digest feed. Feed passes through the digestive tract in 3½–4 hours when it is empty while with continuous feeding it takes 12 hours. High quality feed should be fed to the birds to avoid nutritional imbalance leading to deficiency diseases.
- Urinary bladder is absent in poultry, and cloaca is the common opening of digestive, urinary and reproductive systems. Urine and faeces mixed together and passed through the cloaca and vent.
- Poultry are unable to synthesise essential amino acids, vitamin B complex, vitamin K, *etc.* Laying birds require high level of calcium through feed. These points are to be considered for proper feeding of poultry.

11.3   POULTRY FEED INGREDIENTS

Common poultry feed ingredients, their chemical compositions and maximum level of inclusion in various poultry rations are described in the following sections.

11.3.1   Common Poultry Feed Ingredients

Poultry feed ingredients are classified as energy-rich feedstuffs, protein-rich feedstuffs, vitamin and mineral sources, and non-nutritive feed additives. Many of such feed ingredients are mixed together to prepare commercial poultry feeds.

Energy-rich feedstuffs

About 45 to 65 per cent poultry feed is constituted by energy-rich feed ingredients. The common energy-rich feed ingredients are maize grain, jowar grain (sorghum), millets (bajra/pearl millet, ragi), oats, wheat, wheat bran, broken rice/rice kani, rice bran and rice polish, salseed cake, tapioca flour, molasses, *etc.*

Protein-rich feedstuffs

Protein-rich feed ingredients are mainly used to supply protein, but at the same time they also contribute some energy. They are divided into two groups, viz. vegetable protein and animal protein.

    The common **vegetable protein sources** are groundnut cake, linseed cake, sesame (*til*) cake, sunflower cake, mustard cake, cotton seed cake, soybean cake, coconut cake, maize gluten meal, guar meal, penicillium mycelium waste, *etc.*

    The common **animal protein sources** are fish meal, meat meal, blood meal, liver residue meal, silkworm pupae meal, poultry hatchery by-product meal, *etc.*

Mineral sources

The common mineral sources are common salt, oyster shell (37.4% Ca), limestone (37.5% Ca), bone meal (27% Ca and 12.11% P), dicalcium phosphate (23% Ca and 18.1% P), *etc.* Nowadays mineral mixtures are commercially available in the markets in many brand names (*See Chapter 13, Section 13.6: Poultry Drug Index*).

Vitamin sources

The feed ingredients used in the manufacturing of balanced poultry feed generally supply different types of vitamins. However, vitamin mixtures are commercially available in the markets, which may be used as per the requirements of birds (*See Chapter 13, Section 13.6: Poultry Drug Index*).

Feed additives

These are not essential nutrients, but their presence in feed in minute quantity increases the nutritive value of feed leading to increase feed efficiency, growth and production of the birds. The most common feed additives are antibiotic growth promoters, probiotics, antioxidants, enzymes, anticoccidials, antifungals and toxin binders, antistress medicines, anthelmintics, immunostimulants, electrolytes, *etc.* (*These are discussed in detail in the later part of this chapter.*)

11.3.2   Composition of Common Poultry Feed Ingredients

Composition of common poultry feed ingredients (moisture-free basis, in per cent) is presented in Table 11.2. This composition table is needed for formulation of poultry ration.

Table 11.2: Composition of common poultry feed ingredients (moisture-free basis, in per cent)

Sl no.	Feed ingredient	Dry matter (%)	ME (Kcal/kg)	Crude protein (%)	Crude fibre (%)	Ether extract (%)	NFE (%)	Calcium (%)	Phosphorus (%)	Manganese (mg/kg)	Zinc (mg/kg)	Lysine (%)	Methionine (%)
	Energy sources												
1.	Maize (grain)	89.5	3,309	9.2	2.4	3.9	82.8	0.25	0.4	4.8	12.1	0.18	0.15
2.	Jowar (grain)	87.3	2,645	10.3	3.6	4.6	78.1	0.18	0.32	16.3	15.4	0.35	0.18
3.	Bajra (grain)	89.6	2,642	12.7	2.2	4.9	78.2	0.13	0.72	–	–	0.43	0.2
4.	Oats (grain)	91.7	2,848	14.7	13.5	4.6	60.8	0.11	0.41	42.9	–	0.41	0.21
5.	Wheat (grain)	89.8	3,045	10.3	2.1	2.6	82.3	0.18	0.43	57	15.6	0.47	0.21
6.	Wheat bran	88.9	1,069	14.7	11.3	3.8	62.3	0.19	1.12	130	–	0.53	0.09
7.	Rice kani	90.7	2,345	7.9	1.4	1.7	87.1	0.11	0.48	–	–	–	–
8.	Rice polish	91.8	2,937	12.7	11.2	13.9	48.6	0.27	1.37	–	–	0.44	0.24
9.	Rice polish, deoiled	92.3	2,235	14.1	13.8	1.7	53.4	0.37	1.8	–	–	–	–
10.	Salseed cake, deoiled	90.4	3,096	10.4	3.4	2.9	79.6	0.24	0.16	–	–	0.6	0.38
11.	Tapioca flour	–	3,000	2.9	10.9	0.7	77	0.58	0.12	–	–	0.6	0.006
12.	Molasses	73.6	2,400	2.8	–	–	86.3	1.51	0.66	–	–	56.3	–
	Protein sources: Vegetable												
13.	Groundnut cake	91.5	2,596	40.9	8.9	7.9	36.4	0.23	0.59	27.7	–	1.24	0.57
14.	Linseed (Tisi) cake	90.7	1,671	29.6	11.1	10.4	42.6	0.48	0.98	43.3	–	–	0.59
15.	Sunflower cake	89.1	2,230	37.2	11.6	10.9	32.6	0.43	1.14	24.6	–	1.95	1.56
16.	Sesame (Til) cake	90.7	1,882	39.1	4.7	9.3	34.3	2.46	1.42	51.6	107.5	1.14	1.23
17.	Mustard cake	91.3	2,373	35.1	8.2	14.1	33.4	0.89	1.78	–	–	–	0.41
18.	Cottonseed cake	92.3	1,556	25.9	24.4	8.6	33.7	0.52	0.86	22.9	–	1.07	0.41
19.	Soybean cake	89.9	2,694	41.7	6.3	21.2	26.0	0.36	0.9	35.9	–	2.57	0.76
20.	Coconut cake	91	1,190	22.6	12.5	8.7	49.4	0.23	0.66	59.6	–	0.71	0.32
21.	Maize gluten meal	90.3	2,705	49.9	2.0	4.2	41.4	0.22	0.35	8.0	–	1.02	1.28

Contd.

Table 11.2: Composition of common poultry feed ingredients (moisture-free basis, in per cent) *(Contd.)*

Sl no.	Feed ingredient	Dry matter (%)	ME (Kcal/kg)	Crude protein (%)	Crude fibre (%)	Ether extract (%)	NFE (%)	Calcium (%)	Phosphorus (%)	Manganese (mg/kg)	Zinc (mg/kg)	Lysine (%)	Methionine (%)
22.	Guar meal	89.7	–	42.0	10.9	6.2	35.1	0.54	0.7	–	–	–	–
23.	Penicillium mycelium waste	91.8	–	31.9	8.4	6.7	34.5	3.97	1.12	–	–	1.24	0.46
Animal													
24.	Fish meal	93.8	1,834	43.1	3.6	4.3	11.5	7.16	1.67	38.9	–	4.17	1.42
25.	Meat meal	92.5	2,319	56.2	2.2	11.9	8.7	2.68	2.06	10.2	–	4.00	0.84
26.	Bone meal	95.5	1,044	14.6	2.5	3.1	5.6	27.0	12.11	32.0	447.0	–	–
27.	Blood meal	88.8	1,420	73.4	0.7	–	–	0.32	0.31	5.8	–	6.34	0.83
28.	Liver residue meal	90.9	3,000	65.4	1.3	15.8	11.9	0.54	1.35	9.5	–	4.72	1.28
29.	Silkworm pupae meal, deoiled	90.5	3,000	69.8	3.9	2.2	15.5	0.29	0.58	–	–	3.98	3.07
30.	Poultry hatchery by-product meal	93.0	–	56.4	0.9	17.8	10.2	3.95	1.73	–	–	–	–
Miscellaneous													
31.	Lucerne (Alfalfa) leaf meal, dehydrated	91	1,777	19.1	21.6	2.8	42.1	1.83	0.45	31.2	17.2	0.85	0.21
32.	Berseem leaf meal, dehydrated	89.7	180	15.3	23.5	3.7	42.8	2.6	2.2	–	–	0.66	0.30

Source: Singh and Panda (1988).

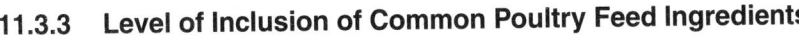
11.3.3 Level of Inclusion of Common Poultry Feed Ingredients

Maximum levels of inclusion of various poultry feed ingredients in chick ration and grower/layer rations are presented in Table 11.3.

Table 11.3: Maximum level of inclusion of common feed ingredients in poultry rations (in per cent)

Ingredients	Chicks	Growers/Layers
a. Energy sources		
Maize	60	65
Wheat	50	50
Barley	20	40
Oats	10	20
Jowar (white)	25	40
Molasses	5	10
Rice polish, fresh	40	40
Rice polish, deoiled	20	20
Tapioca meal	25	25
Wheat bran	10	15
Salseed cake	3	5
b. Vegetable protein sources		
Groundnut cake	40	40
Groundnut cake, deoiled	20	20
Soybean meal, heat-treated	40	40
Sesame (*Til*) cake	20	20
Linseed (*Tisi*) cake, water-treated	20	20
Cottonseed cake, degossypolised	5	5
Mustard cake	10	10
Maize gluten meal	15	15
Sunflower meal	20	20
Coconut meal	5	5
Guar meal	5	5
Niger cake	15	15
c. Animal protein sources		
Fish meal	10	10
Meat meal	5	10
Blood meal	3	3
Silkworm pupae meal	6	6
Poultry hatchery by-product meal	3	3
Liver residue meal	5	10
Penicillium mycelium waste	10	10

Contd.

Table 11.3: Maximum level of inclusion of common feed ingredients in poultry rations (in per cent) *(Contd.)*

Ingredients	Chicks	Growers/Layers
d. Miscellaneous		
Lucerne leaf meal	3	5
Berseem leaf meal	3	5
Bone meal	2	2
Limestone	2	6
Salt	0.5	0.5
Mycelium penicillin	2	2

11.4 NUTRIENT REQUIREMENTS OF POULTRY

The Bureau of Indian Standards (BIS) is a central government organisation that facilitates discussion between scientists and industry, and prepares guidelines and specifications. Table 11.4 shows the BIS specifications for nutrient requirements of poultry. The Compound Livestock Feed Manufacturers' Association (CLFMA) has prepared its own specifications which are shown in Table 11.5 for poultry. The specifications of both BIS and CLFMA are only guidelines and their use as standards is not compulsory. Nowadays the poultry feed business is very much competitive and feed manufacturers, therefore, try very hard to produce feed of the highest possible quality.

Table 11.4: BIS standards, nutrient requirements for poultry

Characteristic	Broiler (meat type chicken)		Layer (egg type chicken)			Breeder layer feed
	Broiler starter feed	Broiler finisher feed	Chick feed	Grower feed	Layer feed	
Metabolisable energy (minimum Kcal/kg)	2,800	2,900	2,600	2,500	2,600	2,600
Crude protein (N × 6.25) (maximum %)	23	20	20	16	18	18
Crude fibre (maximum %)	6	6	7	8	8	8
Acid-insoluble ash (maximum %)	3.0	3.0	4.0	4.0	4.0	4.0
Salt (as NaCl) (maximum %)	0.6	0.6	0.6	0.6	0.6	0.6
Moisture (maximum %)	11	11	11	11	11	11
Calcium (Ca) (maximum %)	1.2	1.2	1.0	1.0	3.0	3.0
Available phosphorus (minimum %)	0.5	0.5	0.5	0.5	0.5	0.5
Lysine (maximum %)	1.2	1.0	0.9	0.6	0.65	0.65
Methionine (maximum %)	0.50	0.35	0.30	0.25	0.30	0.30

Source: BIS Poultry feeds—specifications, fourth revision.

Table 11.5: CLFMA specifications for nutrient requirements of poultry

Characteristic	Chick feed	Grower feed	Layer feed I	Layer feed II	Broiler starter feed	Broiler finisher feed	Breeder chick feed	Breeder grower feed	Broiler breeder feed	Layer breeder feed	Broiler male breeder feed
Moisture (maximum %)	12	12	12	12	12	12	12	12	12	12	12
Metabolisable energy (minimum Kcal/kg)	2,600	2,300	2,500	2,300	2,600	2,700	2,600	2,400	2,500	2,500	2,400
Crude protein (minimum %)	18	14	16	14	20	18	18	14	16	16	14
Fat (maximum %)	2	2	2	2	3	3	3	3	3	3	3
Crude fibre (maximum %)	7	8	8	10	6	5	5	7	7	7	7
Acid-insoluble ash (maximum %)	4	4	4	4	4	4	4	4	4	4	4

Source: CLFMA Standards for compounded poultry feeds.

11.5 FEED FORMULATION FOR POULTRY

While formulating feed it should be kept in mind that a balanced feed should contain desired levels of energy, protein, crude fibre, moisture, vitamins, minerals, amino acids, fatty acids, non-nutrient feed additives and performance enhancers to help the birds to perform as per their genetic potentiality.

The following information are essentially required for formulation of poultry feed.

1. **Chemical composition of feed ingredients**

   Composition of feed stuffs may vary due to various factors like varietal variation of crop, soil type and environmental conditions in which the crops are grown, methods of estimation, *etc*. Chemical composition of common feed ingredients, as appeared in various literatures, is given in Table 11.2.

2. **Nutrient requirements of poultry**

   Fortunately, the nutrient requirements of chicken are known in much detail and accurately than other farm animals. Several standards are available like NRC (National Research Council, 1994), ARC (Agricultural Research Council, 1975), BIS (Bureau of Indian Standards, 1992), *etc*. Nutrient requirements may vary due to types of bird (broiler or layer or breeder), and their ages. For commercial layer chicken, three types of feed are commonly used, viz. **chick feed** (0–8 weeks), **grower feed** (9–20 weeks) and **layer feed** (21–72 weeks or during the laying period); and for commercial broiler chicken, two types of feed are commonly used, viz. **broiler starter** (0–4 weeks) and **broiler finisher** (5–6 weeks). Environmental conditions, system of housing (environmentally controlled house or open house), productivity level of birds, and stress factors are also to be considered in regard to nutrient requirements of birds. Nutrient requirements of various categories of chickens are given in Tables 11.4 and 11.5.

3. **Rate of inclusion of feed ingredients in compounded feed**

   Maximum level of inclusion of various poultry feed ingredients is given in Table 11.3.

4. **Cost, quality and availability of feed ingredients**

   About 70% of the total expenditure of poultry farming is mainly due to feed. So cost of feed ingredients should be considered while preparing feed for poultry. If feed ingredients are procured from the locality, the cost may be to some extent less. However, the quality of feed should not be compromised. The feed ingredients should be fresh and free from fungal contamination. Sometimes feed ingredients are adulterated, e.g. fish meal may be adulterated with urea, soybean meal is adulterated with rice bran, *etc.* So quality evaluation of feed ingredients is an important task in this regard. For this assistance of feed analytical laboratories may be sought.

5. **Method of feed formulation**

   The feed formulation can be done by hand calculation method or with the help of computer.

   a. **Feed formulation by hand calculation**

   It is also called **trial and error method**. It requires lot of time and labour, and only few ingredients can be considered for formulation of compounded feed. It is not always easy to maintain the desired levels of minor nutrients like vitamins, trace minerals, amino acids, fatty acids, *etc.* in this method. However, for formulating simple feed by considering major nutrients (like ME, CP, Ca and P) this method may be adopted.

   The steps are as follows

   1. Fix the desired levels of nutrients as per the requirements of a specific category of bird (like broiler starter or broiler finisher, *etc.*). The feed ingredients are to be added to provide the nutrients per kg or per 100 kg or per 1,000 kg compounded feed basis.

   2. Keep space for minor ingredients at the level of 5% of the compounded feed. Such minor ingredients are feed additives and supplements like vitamins, trace minerals, liver tonics, anticoccidial drugs, antibiotic growth promoters, *etc.* These can be added at the following quantities in broiler starter feed (per 100 kg)—trace mineral premix 100 g, vitamin premix 25 g, anticoccidial premix 50 g, antibiotic growth promoter premix 50 g, liver tonic 25–50 g, toxin binder 200 g, choline chloride 100 g and enzymes 50 g.

   3. Keep space for synthetic amino acids like lysine and methionine. However, cost of inclusion of such ingredients should be kept in mind. After calculating the level of amino acids contributed by protein sources especially animal proteins and soybean (rich in lysine) the required quantity of synthetic amino acids is to be added.

   4. Keep space for common salt (NaCl). The salt content is not usually calculated, and 0.5–0.6% salt is generally added in the feed.

5. Keep space for calcium and phosphorus. The phosphorus content of the feed should be calculated in terms of available phosphorus. Lime stone supplies calcium and bone meal supplies phosphorus.

6. Fix the level of animal proteins. These are generally added at fixed level because of cost, and these ingredients supply the limiting amino acids (lysine and methionine) at higher levels than other feed ingredients. It may be fixed up to 12%. However, fixing of animal proteins may be optional.

7. Fix the level of cereal by-products like rice bran, *etc*. It may be fixed up to the level of 10%.

8. Calculate the nutrients contributed from the above feed ingredients. Then subtract these values from the required values of nutrients for a specific category of chicken like broiler starter or broiler finisher, *etc*. The different nutrients (especially ME and CP) need to be supplied from the major feed ingredients like cereals and oil cakes. This can be done by trial and error method or Pearson's square method.

9. Finally calculate the ME, CP, lysine, methionine, calcium and phosphorus. At this stage, the ME and CP contents of the feed should be as per the recommended requirements.

10. If there is any gap between calculated and recommended values of calcium and phosphorus that can be met by adding dicalcium phosphate or rock phosphate in case of phosphorus, and by adding shell grit, marble chips or calcite powder, *etc*. in case of calcium. The differences in amino acids, if any, can be met by adding synthetic sources.

11. Now adjust the total quantity of feed by adding cereals or cereal by-products to make it 100%.

b. **Feed formulation with the help of computer**

Many software packages are available; they are Excel based or Visual basics. Least cost feed with several feed ingredients can be easily formulated with the help of computer. This method considers price variation and nutrient composition of feed ingredients as well as nutrient requirements of various categories of birds. In this method, feed formulation can be done at the quickest possible time with high degree of precision. One example of computer based software and how to prepare feed with the help of this is given below.

MakeFeed is a comprehensive feed formulation software, designed to combine the expertise, knowledge and standards of recent technologies in the field of poultry nutrition. It provides the integrated and efficient solutions for balanced formulation of rations for various categories of poultry, which would be of immense help for the poultry farmers, entrepreneurs, scientists, teachers and students alike. The software was developed by a team of scientists comprising Dr M Nath, Dr AV Elangovan, Dr AB Mandal and Dr TS Johri of Central Avian Research Institute (ICAR), Izatnagar, Bareilly, Uttar Pradesh.

Salient features of the *MakeFeed* software

MakeFeed is a Windows based unique software for efficient balanced formulation of feed. It is user-friendly and persons having little computer knowledge can utilise it effectively. It takes into account the nutrient requirements of a wide variety of poultry birds like layer and broiler chickens, ducks, turkeys, quails and Guinea fowls. It gives easy and quick access to feed ingredients and their inclusion or deletion from desired ration. It has unlimited and easy data storage facility for ingredients and nutrient specifications in ingredients database. It provides exhaustive information on nutritive values for a wide range of feed ingredients along with the maximum inclusion level for each ingredient. The user has options to edit the complete database of feed ingredients and modify it suitably. There is provision of simple and easy modification, addition or deletion of particular feed ingredient. The user can select a particular ration from the database and the nutrient requirement for that ration will be displayed automatically. The user also has the option to give own requirements in the custom ration and formulate accordingly. It has more than 75 readymade rations for easy reference and practical use. There are exhaustive help options to solve problems, if any, in ration formulation. Password security confirms the access to the programme only by the recognised user.

Steps for formulation of ration as per *MakeFeed* software:

It has three simple and easy steps in ration formulation. These are:

Step 1: Select the ingredients

Step 2: Select the ration specification

Step 3: Enter the choice of ration, viz. simple balanced ration or balanced least cost ration

All conditions for balanced ration formulation are made by default and no user intervention is needed. However, user has choice to modify default options on ingredient restrictions or nutrient restrictions. There are facilities of adding up to 50 ingredients in a ration; presentation of detailed as well as salient features on final formulated ration; and printing and saving the formulated ration.

The cost of the software package (compact disc plus a comprehensive user manual) is ₹ 2,600 including postal charges. For further information, the contact address is:

Dr AB Mandal, Principal Scientist and Head, N & FT Division, Central Avian Research Institute, Izatnagar, Bareilly, Pin 243 122 (UP), India.

Phone: 0581-2302004, 2303223. Fax: 0581-2301321.

E-mail: abmcari@rediffmail.com

Source: CLFMA of India; www.clfmaofindia.org.

11.6   ECONOMIZATION OF POULTRY FEEDING

Economization of feed is of utmost importance in commercial poultry farming, as feed cost alone accounts for about 70% of the total cost of poultry production. The first consideration in this regard is to formulate **least cost feed for poultry** with the help of computer by adding non-conventional feed ingredients without compromising the recommended nutrient requirements. Improved management practices can also reduce the feed cost as described below.

Feed restriction

The primary objective of feed restriction in poultry feeding is to maintain the uniformity of flock and its effect on economic returns. It is mostly practiced in growing pullets (9–20 weeks of age) to achieve the target body weight at specific age. In broiler breeder management the feed restriction is done in growing pullets to reduce the excessive fat deposition and to delay the sexual maturity by about 3 weeks. This in turn helps to extend the production life and check production of small sized eggs. The feed efficiency of the birds will also be increased.

The methods of feed restriction, as recommended by the NRC (1971), are (i) quantitative feed restriction, (ii) qualitative feed restriction, (iii) limited time feeding, (iv) nutrient dilution (like reducing dietary protein levels), (v) skip-a-day feeding, and (vi) elevation of environmental temperature (in case of environmentally controlled house). An experiment entitled 'studies on feed restriction in growing pullets on their subsequent performance' (Reddy and Eswaraiah, 1989) was conducted with seven different methods of feed restriction, viz. (a) *ad libitum* feeding (control), (b) low protein with normal lysine, (c) low protein with low lysine, (d) control diet diluted with sawdust to contain 17% crude fibre, (e) 70% *ad libitum* feeding, (f) limited time feeding (three hours in the morning and three hours in the evening), and (g) skip-a-day feeding once in a week. The results showed that birds which were fed *ad libitum* or fed low protein with normal lysine or low protein with low lysine diets from 7–20 weeks gained significantly ($P < 0.05$) better than those kept on 70% *ad libitum* diet or limited time feeding or skip-a-day feeding programme or control diet diluted with sawdust. The growers on 70% *ad libitum* feeding laid their first eggs 15 days later than full fed birds. There was no difference in age of sexual maturity as measured by first egg in all other feeding regimes. The egg weight was significantly ($P < 0.05$) better with 70% *ad libitum* fed birds than all other groups. No definite trend was observed in mortality in any of the groups. The results suggested that limited time feeding or skip-a-day feeding had no economic advantage over a full feeding programme in grower chickens; and growers fed diets diluted with sawdust or with 70% of *ad libitum* feeding or with low protein are more economical than feeding the birds *ad libitum*.

All the methods of feed restriction are not satisfactory. In practice, generally the total feed allowed per bird per day is restricted to about 70% of the feed that is consumed by a similar bird on an *ad libitum* feeding.

Minimising feed wastage

Proper feeding management including use of efficient feeders, filling not more than ⅓ to ½ levels of the capacity of feeders, use of pellet feeds instead of mash, *etc.* can reduce the wastage of feed. Rat control in poultry house and debeaking can reduce the feed wastage.

Nutrition adjustment during extreme weather conditions

Feed (especially the energy) requirement is increased in cold conditions below 13 °C, and total feed intake is reduced, if environmental temperature is high (above 30 °C) leading to less growth and production. Both the conditions are uneconomical. Suitable changes should be made in feed composition to overcome this environmental stress.

Maintenance of flock health

Any disease in a flock may reduce the feed efficiency of the birds. Subclinical level of disease (not showing symptoms) is more dangerous because the sick birds take more feed without efficient production. So prevention of disease indirectly reduces the feed wastage.

11.7 FEED FORMULAE FOR DIFFERENT AGE GROUPS OF CHICKEN

For commercial layer chicken, three types of feeds are commonly used for production of eggs, viz. **chick feed** (0–8 weeks), **grower feed** (9–20 weeks) and **layer feed** (21–72 weeks or during the laying period). For broiler chicken, two types of feeds are commonly used for commercial production of meat, viz. **broiler starter** (0–4 weeks) and **broiler finisher** (5–6 weeks).

Feed formulae for broiler and layer chickens are given in Tables 11.6 and 11.7 respectively. These rations, although typical, represent only few sets of examples. Depending on the price and availability of ingredients, many other combinations can be used to make up poultry rations for various categories of chickens.

Table 11.6: Feed formulae for commercial broiler chicken

Ingredients (kg/100 kg)	Broiler starter (0–4 weeks)		Broiler finisher (5–6 weeks)	
	1	2	1	2
Maize	43.75	57.10	65.10	44.10
Rice polish	10.00	–	–	20.00
Groundnut cake	14.00	–	–	11.00
Sunflower cake	14.00	15.00	12.00	11.00
Mustard cake	–	10.00	10.00	–
Fish meal (43% protein)	10.00	6.00	5.00	5.50
Meat meal (56% protein)	–	7.00	5.00	5.50
Silkworm pupae meal (40% protein)	–	3.00	1.20	–
Blood meal (73% protein)	3.50	–	.	–
Animal fat	3.00	1.00	.	1.25
Bone meal	1.15	–	0.60	0.60
Limestone	–	0.50	0.60	0.70
Common salt	0.50	0.30	0.40	0.25
Vitamin and mineral mixture	0.10	0.10	0.10	0.10
Total	100.00	100.00	100.00	100.00

1, 2— two different sets of feed composition of respective categories.

Table 11.7: Feed formulae for commercial layer chicken

Ingredients (kg/100 kg)	Chick mash (0 to 8 weeks)	Grower mash (9 to 18–20 weeks)	Layer mash (21 weeks and above)
Maize (yellow)	35	28	30
Jowar	15	20	17
Rice polish	10	5	8
Sunflower meal	5	5	5
Soybean meal	20	–	5
Groundnut cake	–	8	10
Rice polish (oil extracted)	5	25.5	9
Fish meal	6.7	5.7	6.7
Oyster shell	–	–	6
Mineral mixture	3	2.5	3
Vitamin mixture	0.3	0.3	0.3
Total	100.0	100.0	100.0

11.8 FEEDING OF POULTRY

Various aspects of feeding poultry are discussed in the following sections.

11.8.1 Feed Consumption of Poultry

The rate of feed consumption of broiler and layer chickens is given in Tables 11.8 and 11.9 respectively. These are only guidelines for feeding of chicken of high genetic merits. The actual performance may vary due to genetic make up of birds (strain variation), feed quality, environmental conditions, system of feeding and other management practices.

Table 11.8: Weekly feed consumption and FCR of broiler chicken

Age (in week)	Body weight (in g)	Feed consumption (in g per bird) Weekly	Feed consumption (in g per bird) Cumulative	Feed consumption (daily in g per bird)	Feed conversion
1	140	150	–	21.43	1.07
2	360	300	450	42.86	1.25
3	680	500	950	71.43	1.40
4	1,170	850	1,800	121.43	1.54
5	1,650	950	2,750	135.71	1.67
6	2,000	1,050	3,800	150	1.90

Total feed consumption up to 6 weeks of age is 3.8 kg per broiler (weighed 2 kg each) @ 1.9 kg/kg live weight (maximum) of which broiler starter feed (0–4 weeks)—1.8 kg and broiler finisher feed (5–6 weeks)—2.0 kg. FCR—feed conversion ratio.

Table11.9:   Feed intake of layer chicken

Age (week)	Body weight per bird (g)	Daily feed intake per 100 birds (kg)
1	70	1
2	120	2
3	170	3
4	230	3.5
5–8	310–580	4
9–12	660–900	6
13–16	970–1,110	6.5
17–20	1,160–1,360	7.5
During laying period	1,360	11

Total feed requirement up to 72 weeks of age is 47.5 kg per layer of which chick feed (0–8 weeks)—2 kg, grower feed (9–20 weeks)—5.5 kg, and layer feed (21–72 weeks) 40 kg @ 110 g/bird/day.

11.8.2   Feeding Systems of Poultry

The various systems of feeding poultry are:

1. Whole grain feeding
2. Grain and mash feeding
3. All mash feeding
4. Pellet feeding
5. Crumble feeding

Whole grain feeding system

This is also known as cafeteria or free choice feeding system. Feed ingredients (mainly grains) are kept in separate containers and offered to the birds. The birds take the feed ingredients according to their will.

This method is not suitable for commercial purpose. It takes more time and labour to fill different containers with different feed ingredients, and birds may not get all the essential nutrients due to selective feeding, leading to deficiency disease(s).

Grain and mash feeding system

In this system, both grains and mash are offered in the same container and allowed the birds to eat. Level of nutrients (like protein) may be increased or decreased easily on the basis of growth, egg production, environmental conditions, *etc.*, but it needs skill and experience. Here also birds may take feed ingredients selectively to some extent leading to deficiency of nutrient(s).

All mash feeding system

In this system, all the feed ingredients are usually ground to almost uniform particle size (710 millimicrons) and mixed together in the form of mash. This homogeneous mixture of feed ingredients, i.e. mash is offered to the birds, no other feed ingredients are offered to the birds separately, not even grit. There is no possibility of selective feeding by the birds.

All species and categories of poultry prefer their diet in the mash form. Generally, dry mash is offered to the fowl, but in summer months it is desirable to offer wet mash (mixing with water just before feeding) to increase feed consumption and to avoid wastage by dust. In case of duck, wet mash feeding is the only popular method of feeding.

All mash feeding system is the most popular, and used for commercial poultry production.

Pellet feeding system

Pellets are small cylindrical shaped feeds, made up of dry mash under high pressure. Pellets are of different sizes according to the age of birds. Generally, pellets are offered to the chicken/fowl.

Selective feeding is practically nil in this system, and hence all the nutrients including vitamins and minerals which are added in very small quantity are properly received by the birds. There is no choice, so rejection of unpalatable feed ingredients is also not possible. This system avoids the wastage of feed. The only disadvantage of this system is that pellet feeds are costlier than mash (about 10% more expensive). So this system is not generally followed for small scale poultry production.

Crumble feeding system

Crumbles are small and just like broken pellets. Consistency of crumbles is coarser than mash. Crumbles are generally offered to the starting chicken, because pellets are hard and over size during early part of birds' life.

11.8.3 Feeding Management of Poultry

Feeding management is of prime importance in poultry farming as feed cost alone constitutes on an average of 70% of the total cost of poultry rearing. Poultry growers in all over India tend to cite feed cost as the critical component of controlling and lowering production cost. Some management pointers regarding poultry feeding are listed below.

- Feed wastage must not be allowed by using proper feeders for different age groups of birds and by debeaking of birds at proper age especially in case of layer and breeder birds.
- Feed must be fresh (never use old, stale and mouldy feeds) and not left in the feeders and not stored in feed bags for long periods of time.
- Feed must be available to the birds all the time. Feeding during cooler part of the day should be encouraged especially during summer months.
- Feed should be offered to the commercial birds according to their physiological needs. When and how much to feed, and when to make changes in the daily feeding procedure depending on the seasons are important considerations.
- Birds should not move more than 8 ft for feed and water. To assure this, feeders and waterers should be distributed properly in the house (*See* Fig. 6.6).
- Feeders should not be filled more than ⅓ to ½ level of their capacities to avoid wastage. If hanging feeders are used, they must be shaken often.

[*Other aspects of feeding management are discussed in Chapter 7, Section 7.1*]

11.9   NON-NUTRIENT FEED ADDITIVES

Feed additives are not nutrients, but their presence in poultry feed in minute quantity increases the nutritive value of feed leading to increase in feed efficiency, growth and production of the birds. So they are called non-nutrient feed additives. Objective of using additives is to ensure tasty, safe and attractive feed that improves the performance of birds. Use and safety of feed additives is regulated by FDA under nation's food safety laws. Commonly used additives in poultry rations are categorised according to their functions. These are as follows:

a. **Additives that promote feed intake**, e.g. antioxidant, flavouring agents, pellet binders and antifungal additives or mould inhibitors.

b. **Additives that facilitate digestion and absorption**, e.g. grit, chelates, enzymes and probiotics.

c. **Additives that alter hormonal balance and metabolism**, e.g. hormones.

d. **Drugs added to poultry feed as additives**, e.g. (i) production promoting drugs like antibiotics and arsenicals and (ii) antiparasitic drugs like coccidiostats and anthelmintic drugs.

e. **Additives intended to improve the appearance of final products**, e.g. pigments.

f. **Miscellaneous additives**, e.g. tranquilisers, nitrovin and tissue preparations.

The most common poultry feed additives are described below.

Probiotics

Probiotics are not drugs, but mixed culture of living microorganisms (lactobacilli, yeasts, *etc.*) fed to the birds through feed, which helps them to improve the microbial environment of their digestive tract leading to better digestion and less disease incidence. Probiotics can act to some extent as antitoxic agent and immuno-stimulant. Cultures of *Lactobacillus acidophilus, L casei, Streptococcus faecium, Bacillus subtilis, Saccharomyces cerevisiae* (a yeast), *etc.* are commonly used in the feed as probiotics. Inclusion of probiotics in the feed improves live weight gain and FCR in broilers, and egg production and egg quality traits particularly egg size, albumen quality, reduced yolk cholesterol concentration, *etc.* in layers.

There are many ways by which probiotics can work.

i. Probiotics maintain useful microfloral concentration in the digestive tract. The Lactobacilli (lactic acid bacteria) inhibit the growth of many disease producing microorganisms (called pathogens) like *Salmonella sp, Staphylococcus sp, E coli, etc.* The Lactobacilli produce several bactericidal substances (like lactic acid, acetic acid, hydrogen peroxide, lysozyme, lactoferrin, lactoperoxidase, bacteriocin, lacticidin, acidolin and acidophilin) which kill the pathogens by competitive inhibition. Lactobacilli also compete with disease producing organisms for sites of attachment on the bird's intestinal surface. This attachment is needed for bacterial action. *Salmonella sp, E coli, Clostridium perfringens* and *Campylobacter jejuni* are inhibited by this competitive exclusion action of Lactobacilli. *Saccharomyces cerevisiae* releases metabolite mannan oligosaccharide which also acts against disease producing organisms.

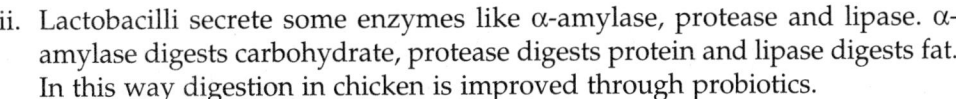

ii. Lactobacilli secrete some enzymes like α-amylase, protease and lipase. α-amylase digests carbohydrate, protease digests protein and lipase digests fat. In this way digestion in chicken is improved through probiotics.

iii. Probiotics containing *Lactobacillus acidophilus, Streptococcus faecium* and *Bacillus subtilis* suppress the ammonia production in the bird's intestine, thus improve the health and growth.

iv. *Lactobacillus bulgaricus* produces a metabolite which neutralises the enterotoxin produced by *E coli* in the bird's intestine.

v. Probiotics stimulate the bird's immune system, especially the immune system of intestine which responded to bacteria by secreting IgA (an immunoglobulin which protects the intestinal lining against bacterial infection).

Probiotics are to be used continuously and in adequate concentration in the feed to maintain the beneficial microflora in a healthy state, and this helps proper functioning of the intestine. On arrival of the day-old chicks, a probiotic may be given in the very first drinking water, even though the feed contains probiotics, and it should be continued for at least 5–7 days.

[For commercial probiotics, See Poultry Drug Index section, Chapter 13.]

Antioxidants

Antioxidants help to keep the feed fresh and prevent spoilage of fat and fat-soluble vitamins present in the feed. They also bind free radicals (which are produced in normal metabolism as well as coming directly from feed ingredients) and reduce the oxidative stress and potential damage caused by them. Some common antioxidants are vitamin E, selenium, ethoxyquin, santoquin, DPPD (Diphenyl-paraphenylene diamine), BHA (Butylated hydroxyl anisol), and BHT (Butylated hydroxyl toluene), propyl gallate, citric acid and ascorbic acid. Vitamin E is a powerful natural antioxidant. Most of the antioxidants are added at 0.01% level in poultry feed. They are normally incorporated in vitamin-trace mineral premix.

[For commercial antioxidants, See Poultry Drug Index section, Chapter 13.]

Enzymes

Enzymes are organic catalysts which cause normal hydrolysis of dietary proteins, fats and carbohydrates. Use of enzymes in the feed helps the birds to utilise the feed more efficiently. Its use is beneficial when the compounded feed contains poorly digestible ingredients. Enzyme supplementation results in better feed conversion and prevention of sticky wet droppings.

[For commercial enzymes, See Poultry Drug Index section, Chapter 13.]

Antibiotic Growth Promoters

Some antibiotics are used in feed continuously at a low level to improve growth and uniformity of the flock, health status and feed conversion of birds. The antibiotic growth promoters modify the intestinal microflora (by their antibacterial activities, particularly against gram-positive bacteria); they have no direct interaction with the physiology of birds. Beneficial effects of antibiotics may be through preventing bacterial destruction of feed proteins, by inhibiting toxin producing organisms, by preventing thickening of the gut wall and, thus permitting better absorption of amino acids, fatty acids and probably other nutrients. The most common antibiotics used in poultry feed as growth promoters are penicillin, streptomycin, erythromycin, bacitracin, lincomycin, virginiamycin, avilamycin, chlortetracycline, oxytetracycline, aureomycine, *etc.* Nutritional level of inclusion is 4 g per tonne of feed for narrow spectrum antibiotics like penicillin, streptomycin, *etc.* and 10 g per tonne of feed for broad spectrum antibiotics like tetracyclines, aureomycines, *etc.*

Nowadays use of antibiotic growth promoters in poultry feed is restricted due to their possible health hazards. In some countries their use is totally banned.

[For commercial antibiotic growth promoters, See Poultry Drug Index section, Chapter 13.]

Anticoccidial Drugs

Anticoccidial drugs are used to prevent coccidiosis, a protozoan disease which is common in deep litter housing. Anticoccidials are generally used in feed. Commonly used anticoccidials are amprolium, ionophore compounds (monensin, maduramicin, salinomycin), clopidol, robenidine, diclazuril, *etc.* Most of the coccidiostats (anticoccidial drugs) inhibit further proliferation of the parasites during their sexual cycles. As the coccidia tend to develop resistance to the anticoccidial drugs to which they are exposed over a long period of time, change to another drug will usually helpful to control the disease.

[For commercial anticoccidials, See Poultry Drug Index section, Chapter 13.]

Antifungals and Toxin Binders

Antifungals and toxin binders, when used as feed additives, inhibit the growth of fungi and their toxins. Certain organic acids are used as antifungals, and zeolytes (aluminosilicate) as toxin binders. Their use is desirable, if the feed ingredients contain more moisture (more than 10%) especially during rainy season.

[For commercial antifungals and toxin binders, See Poultry Drug Index section, Chapter 13.]

Arsenicals

Arsenicals may be added in broiler feed, but not in the layer feed. It promotes growth and yellow colour of shank and skin. Margin of safety is highest in chicken, which can tolerate 10 times the effective dose level. Dietary source of arsenicals, if any, should be withdrawn from the feed at least 5 days before the broilers are slaughtered. Arsenicals may be used at the rate of 22.5–50 g/tonne of feed (as 3-nitro-4-hydroxyphenylarsonic acid) or 45–90 g/tonne of feed (as sodium arsenite).

Immunostimulants

Immunostimulants stimulate the immune system of birds and facilitate digestibility and absorption of nutrients, and thereby enhance the performance of birds. Vitamin E with selenium, herbal liver tonics, *etc.* are very good immunostimulants.

Electrolytes

Electrolytes are recommended when there is loss of water from the body in certain diseases like coccidiosis, diarrhoea, *etc.*

[For commercial electrolytes, See Poultry Drug Index section, Chapter 13.]

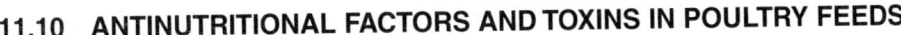

11.10 ANTINUTRITIONAL FACTORS AND TOXINS IN POULTRY FEEDS

The antinutritional factors are the substances, present in various feed ingredients, when introduced into the animal system beyond a certain level, produce some undesirable effects like reduced growth, poor feed conversion, hormonal changes and occasional organ changes. Many poultry feed ingredients incorporated in compounded feeds may contain antinutritional factors and toxins. These anti-nutritional factors and toxins may be endogenous or exogenous in nature and adversely affect the growth and production of birds. Removal of these toxicants is absolutely necessary to maintain the health and production of poultry. The common antinutritional factors and toxins present in various poultry feed ingredients, and their detoxification methods are inscribed below.

Table 11.10: Classification of common antinutritional factors and toxins present in feed ingredients

I. Endogenous antinutritional factors and toxins			
	Nature	Toxicants	Detoxification methods
a.	Proteins	i. Protease inhibitors/ trypsin inhibitor ii. Phytohaemagglutinins (lectins, ricins)	i. Atmospheric steaming (100 °C). ii. Autoclaving (1.055 kg/cm² at 122.2 °C for 30 minutes) or water-cooking (in boiling water, 1:5 w/v and heating for 30 minutes)
b.	Glucosides	i. Goitrogens (progoitrinin) ii. Cyanogens iii. Estrogens and iv. Saponins	i. Extraction with hot water, dilute alkali or acetone or decomposed with iron salts or soda ash. ii. Cooking of feed ingredients, followed by discard of cooking water or fermented or boiled then dried. iii. Dry or moist heat treatment or solvent extraction. iv. Saponins can be extracted with hot water followed extraction with ethanol or methanol.
c.	Phenols	i. Gossypol ii. Tannins	i. Solid substrate fermentation involving certain fungi is capable of reducing 90% of free gossypol. ii. Cold water processing, boil water processing, treatment with acids 0.1 N, HCl (1:10 w/v), 2.5% HCl, alkalies (0.01 N, NaOH, 0.1 N, NaHCO₃, 0.05–5% Ca(OH)₂), salt (3% NaCl), extraction with either acetone (30%) or ethanol (4%) or methanol and autoclaving.

Contd.

Table 11.10: Classification of common antinutritional factors and toxins present in feed ingredients *(Contd.)*

I. Endogenous antinutritional factors and toxins			
	Nature	**Toxicants**	**Detoxification methods**
d.	Others	i. Erucic acid and other fatty acids (responsible for fishy flavour to meat and eggs)	i. Solvent extraction
		ii. Non-starch polysaccharides (NSP)	ii. Water soaking, water treatment, enzyme supplementation, gamma irradiation, acid treatment and milling.
		iii. Oxalates and phytates	iii. Supplementation with adequate minerals, dietary supplementation of phytase enzyme (250–500 units/kg), autoclaving
		iv. Antivitamins	iv. Extraction with water and autoclaving, and supplementing with vitamins like pyridoxine hydrochloride with linseed meal for chicks.
II. Exogenous antinutritional factors and toxins			
		i. Mycotoxins (these are secondary metabolites of fungi that have the capacity to impair animal health and productivity, e.g. aflatoxins, ochratoxin A, T-2 toxin, rubratoxin B and citrin; aflatoxin B_1 is most pathogenic to poultry as compared to other aflatoxins, viz. B_2, G_1 and G_2.)	i. Given in the Tables 11.11 and 11.12.
		ii. Argemone (*Argemone mexicana*, a yellow flowered poppy, commonly used as an adulterant with mustard seed for oil extraction.)	ii. Heating of this oil to 240 °C for 15 minutes; proper processing of feed ingredients.
		iii. Pesticide and insecticide residues (like organochlorine, organophosphorus compounds, carbonate compounds and synthetic pyrethroids)	iii. Zeolite and activated charcoal (13.75:1) @ 2 kg/tonne of feed had a beneficial effect in protecting birds from lower levels of insecticide/pesticide toxicity.

Table 11.11: Dietary additives and their level of inclusion for protection of broilers against dietary aflatoxins

Dietary additives as detoxifying agents	Level of inclusion (g/q feed)
Activated charcoal	100–200
Hydrated sodium calcium aluminosilicate (HSCAS)	100–200
Esterified glucomannan (EGM)	50–100
Herbal mixture (*Acacia catechu* 25%, *Phyllanthus niruri* 400%, *Andrographis paniculata* 25%, base 10%)	50–75
Butylated hydroxyanisol	50–100
Butylated hydroxy toluene[*]	50–150
Dl-methionine[*]	100–200
L-lysine HCl	150
Selenium[**]	0.200–0.300
Water-soluble vitamins[*]	Double of the requirements
Dietary protein level to be increased	Up to 26–28%

[*] Growth sparing effect.

[**] Growth and mortality affect at higher level of aflatoxins.

Note: *Commercial antifungal and toxin binders commonly used in poultry feed are presented in Poultry Drug Index section of Chapter 13.*

Table 11.12: The physicochemical treatments for inactivation of preformed aflatoxins in contaminated maize and groundnut cake

a.	Raising the moisture content up to 20%. Autoclaving at 5 PSI for 1 hour followed by drying in an oven at 80 °C.
b.	Adding sodium hydroxide (15 g/kg) and mixing. Raising the moisture content up to 20%, autoclaving at 5 PSI for 1 hour and drying in an oven.
c.	Agitation of 1 kg of feedstuff with 20 g $Ca(OH)_2$ followed by addition and mixing of formaldehyde to raise the moisture content up to 15%. Autoclaving at 15 PSI for 1 hour and drying.
d.	Addition of liquor ammonia to yield 6% concentration. Raising of moisture content up to 20%. Storing airtight for 20 days. Heating at 35 °C and drying in an oven.

Table 11.13: Common poultry feed ingredients and respective antinutritional factors and toxins

Feed ingredients	Antinutritional factors and toxins
Raw soybean and its meal	Trypsin inhibitor, phytohaemagglutinin, antigenic protein, lipoxygenase, goitrogen, saponin, phytoestrogen, phytic acid and oligosaccharides (non-starch poly-saccharides, NSPs—30.3%)
Groundnut and its meal	Trypsin inhibitor, goitrogen, tannins, oligosaccharides and lectins

Contd.

Table 11.13: Common poultry feed ingredients and respective antinutritional factors and toxins *(Contd.)*

Feed ingredients	Antinutritional factors and toxins
Mustard or rape seed and its meal	Goitrogens (thioglucosides or glucosinolates), tannic acid, erucic acid, sinapine (cholinester), pectins and oligosaccharides (NSPs—46.1 %)
Safflower seed and its meal	Estrogenic factor, two phenolic glucosides (bitter flavour) and fibre
Sunflower seed and its meal	Chlorogenic acid, quinic acid and fibre (tannin-like compounds)
Sesame seed and its cake	Phytate (5 g/100 g) and oxalates (35 mg/100 g)
Linseed and its cake	Linamarin (cyanogenic glucoside), antipyridoxine (linatin) factor and mucilage
Kapok seed meal (seeds of silk cotton tree)	Tannins, tyrosine and fatty acids with cyclopropene rings
Copra meal (coconut meal)	Fibre (mannans) and estrogenic factor
Palm kernel meal	Fibre (half of the fibre–4NDF/ high levels of galactomannans, β-(1, 4)-D mannans) and sharp shells
Cotton seed and its meals	Gossypol (phenol-like compound), cyclopropenoid fatty acids, tannins
Guar meal	Guar gum (18–20%), antitrypsin factor and antivitamin E factor
Castor seed and its meal	Ricin (toxalbumin, a phytohaemagglutinin), ricinine (toxic alkaloid), ricinus allergen (protein polysaccharide)
Neem seed and its meal	Bitter principles: Protomeliacins, limonoids, azadirone, gedunin, vilasinin and secomeliacins. Non-isoprenoid polypenolics—flavanoids, tannins and coumarin, viz. nimbin, salannin and azadirachtin dried seeds—limonoids—0.001 to 0.1%, azadirone, 0.45% and epoxy azadirone 0.72%, azadiradione 0.7% and salanin 0.95%
Mahua cake	Mowrin (saponin) and tannins
Karanja cake	Fat bound toxic factors—karajnjin and pongamol (flavanoids) (NSPs—38%)
Lupin meal	Quinolizidine alkaloids, pectins, oligosaccharides, high manganese, saponin.
Peas	Protease inhibitors, tannins, lipoxygenase and lectins
Rubber seed meal	Hydrocyanic acid (20–40 mg/kg)
Maize	Selenoamino acids (seleniferous), estrogen (mouldy), trypsin inhibitor
Wheat	Tyramine, trypsin inhibitor, NSPs (11.4%)
Rice	Estrogen and haemagglutinins
Rye	Amylase and protease inhibitors and NSPs (13.2%)
Oats	Amylase inhibitor and estrogens

Contd.

Table 11.13: Common poultry feed ingredients and respective antinutritional factors and toxins *(Contd.)*

Feed ingredients	Antinutritional factors and toxins
Triticale	Trypsin and chymotrypsin inhibitors (NSPs)
Some varieties of barley	β-glucan (NSPs—16.7%)
Some varieties of sorghum	Tannins
Rice polish and rice bran	Trypsin inhibitor and antithiamine factor
Chunies	Antitryptic factor
Sal seed and its meal	Tannic acid (tannins)
Tapioca meal (Cassava)	Cyanogenic glucoside (HCN 1000–3000 mg/kg dry matter)
Fish meal and meat meal (prepared from spoiled or putrefied material)	Gizzerosine and histamine (biogenic amines)
Clover; lucerne	Phyto-oestrogens
Subabul seed and leaf	Mimosine (145 g/kg in seed and 25 g/kg in leaf)

Source: Poultry Nutrition Research in India and its Perspective by TS Johri (www.fao.org).

11.11 WATER MANAGEMENT FOR POULTRY

A safe and adequate supply of water is essential for efficient poultry production. Lack of water certainly reduces the performance of birds. Drinking water may act as a potential source of disease, if proper care is not taken. Water quality and quantity for poultry are discussed in this section.

11.11.1 Standards of Drinking Water for Poultry

Drinking water must be clear, colourless, odourless and without any sediment. In general, good quality water needs to be relatively low in total solid and low in sulphates, chlorides and sodium. It must be essentially free from pathogens, and have a pH of 6.8 to 7.5. Desirable quality of drinking water for poultry is detailed in Table 11.14.

Table 11.14: Drinking water quality for poultry

Characteristic or contaminants	Level considered average	Maximum permissible level	Remarks
Total solids			
Total dissolved solids	290 ppm		Over 500 ppm is considered as polluted.
Hardness	0–60 ppm	180 ppm	< 60 is unusually soft; > 180 is very hard; interferes with effectiveness of soap, disinfectants, medications.

Contd.

Table 11.14: Drinking water quality for poultry *(Contd.)*

Characteristic or contaminants	Level considered average	Maximum permissible level	Remarks
Bacteria			
Total bacteria	0/mL	50/mL	0/mL is desirable
Coliform bacteria	0/mL	0/mL	0/mL is desirable
Acidity			
pH	6.8–7.5	–	A pH of less than 6 is not desirable. Generally level below 6.3 may reduce performance. If medication is done through drinking water, preferably its pH should not be below 6.
Mineral levels			
Calcium	60 mg/L	75 mg/L	
Magnesium	14 mg/L	50 mg/L	Higher level has a laxative effect. Level greater than 50 mg/L may affect performance, if the sulphate level is high.
Copper	0.002 mg/L	1 mg/L	Higher level produces a bitter flavour.
Iron	0.2 mg/L	0.3 mg/L	Higher level produces a bad odour and taste.
Zinc	–	5 mg/L	Higher level produces toxicity.
Manganese	–	0.1 mg/L	–
Lead	–	0.02 mg/L	Higher level produces toxicity.
Sodium	32 mg/L	–	Level above 50 mg/L may affect performance, if the sulphate or chloride level is high.
Chloride	14 mg/L	200 mg/L	Level as low as 14 mg/L may be detrimental, if the sodium level is higher than 50 mg/L.
Sulphate	125 mg/L	200 mg/L	Higher level has a laxative effect. Level above 50 mg/L may affect performance, if magnesium and chloride levels are high.
Nitrate	10 mg/L	25 mg/L	Sometimes levels from 15 mg/L may affect performance; maximum ammonia level should be 0.5 mg/L.
Nitrite	0.4 mg/L	4 mg/L	Over 4 is toxic, and considered as polluted.
Fluoride	–	1 mg/L	–

Source: Waggoner R, Good R and Good R (1984). Water Quality and Poultry Performance, In: Proceedings of AVMA Annual Conference, July, 1984; Sharma *et al* (2008). Poultry Production in India, ICAR, New Delhi.

11.11.2 Water Requirement of Poultry

Drinking water should be kept clean and cool; if possible, its temperatures should be between 10 °C and 15 °C for the most comfortable consumption by mature birds. However, in some studies it is indicated that chicks prefer water, if its temperature is about 25 °C. Water temperatures over 30 °C will reduce consumption and birds will refuse to drink, if water temperature is more than 44 °C. In general a bird drinks 2–3 L of water for each kg of feed, it consumes. However, water intake increased by 2–3 times during summer months.

Water requirement of broiler birds is different from that of layer birds. It also depends on age of the birds, season, type of feed, *etc*. Water requirements for layer and broiler chickens are given in Tables 11.15, 11.16 and 11.17.

Table 11.15: Water requirement for layer chicken (agewise per 100 birds)

Age (week)	Water requirement (L/day)
0–3	3.5–5.0
4–6	6.5–9.5
7–10	15–16
11–20	18–20
21 and above	25–30

Table 11.16: Water requirement of 100 broiler chicken

Age (weeks)	Daily water intake (L)*
1	2
2	4
3	6
4	8
5	10
6	12

* Simply water requirement of broiler birds can be calculated in the following way: Daily water requirement of 100 broiler chickens = Age of birds in weeks × 2 (in L). For example, daily water requirement of 100 broiler chickens in 3rd week is 3 × 2 = 6 L.

Table 11.17: Water requirement for broiler chicken at various environmental temperatures

(Agewise per 100 birds at different room temperatures, L/day)

Age (weeks)	10 °C	15 °C	20 °C	25 °C	30 °C	35 °C
1	2.3	2.4	3.0	3.2	3.5	3.7
2	5.0	6.0	6.5	7.4	10.0	16.3
3	6.5	7.8	10.0	12.7	17.2	36.0
4	9.0	11.0	14.0	17.1	27.1	46.2
5	11.4	14.0	18.0	21.4	33.4	55.3
6	14.0	16.5	21.5	25.3	38.7	61.3

11.11.3 Diseases Spread Through Water Contamination and Prevention

Water may act as the potent source of many disease producing organisms and may spread the diseases, if cleanliness and hygiene of the drinking water is not maintained properly. The most common poultry diseases which may be spread through contaminated water are of bacterial origin like *E coli*, infectious coryza, ulcerative enteritis, pullorum disease, fowl typhoid, salmonellosis, fowl cholera and campylobacteriosis. Viral diseases like Ranikhet disease and infectious bursal disease may also be spread through contaminated water.

Always fresh and clean drinking water fit for human consumption must be given to the birds. Waterers should be cleaned and washed daily with an approved disinfectant. If earthen pots are used for drinking water, always two sets should be used so that one set can be put daily for airing and exposure to the sun. Strict water sanitation measures can prevent the waterborne diseases in poultry.

11.11.4 Water Sanitation

It is advisable to sanitise the drinking water on the basis of routine water analysis. Annual water analysis is must in every poultry farm, especially for *E coli* and other pathogens. Water sanitation is essential when the bacterial count is above the permissible limits (Table 11.9). However, water sanitisers should not be used 24 hours before and 24 hours after vaccination, if the vaccine is used through drinking water; as sanitisers reduce the efficacy of vaccine, sometimes making it completely ineffective.

Basic water treatment techniques are filtration (to remove organic matter and/or turbidity), chlorination (to remove bacteria, to prevent algae build-up in water lines, and to precipitate nitrite, iron, manganese and sulphur), and ozone treatment (to remove bacteria, taste and odour). To minimise hardness of water, softener like deionisation is done.

[For commercial water sanitisers, See Poultry Drug Index section, Chapter 13.]

EXERCISE

A. Objective Questions

i. **Indicate the correct answer by putting tick (√) mark (multiple choice).**

1. Glandular stomach of poultry is
   - (a) Crop
   - (b) Proventriculus
   - (c) Gizzard
   - (d) None of these

2. Muscular stomach of poultry is
   - (a) Crop
   - (b) Proventriculus
   - (c) Gizzard
   - (d) Duodenum

3. The largest single organ of the body of poultry is
   - (a) Liver
   - (b) Pancreas
   - (c) Gizzard
   - (d) Gall bladder

4. Crop is the enlargement of
   - (a) Proventriculus
   - (b) Gizzard
   - (c) Oesophagus
   - (d) Duodenum

5. Stomach of poultry is
   - (a) Proventriculus
   - (b) Gizzard
   - (c) Duodenum
   - (d) Both a and b

6. Which one of the following is known as crushing organ in poultry?
   - (a) Proventriculus
   - (b) Gizzard
   - (c) Oesophagus
   - (d) Duodenum

7. In poultry digestive system, feed goes from proventriculus to
   - (a) Small intestine
   - (b) Large intestine
   - (c) Gizzard
   - (d) Crop

8. In poultry, the part of digestive tract where feed is stored for brief period and softened is known as
   - (a) Proventriculus
   - (b) Caecum
   - (c) Gizzard
   - (d) Crop

9. The gastric juice secreted from proventriculus is highly acidic with a pH range of
   - (a) 0.5–2.5
   - (b) 3.0–4.5
   - (c) 5.0–6.5
   - (d) None of these

10. The main function of gizzard is
    - (a) To store feed temporarily and soften it
    - (b) To absorb digestible portion of feed
    - (c) To grind and crush the coarser feed materials
    - (d) None of these

11. Which of the following feed ingredients has the highest crude protein content?
    - (a) Mustard cake
    - (b) Groundnut cake
    - (c) Cotton seed cake
    - (d) Sesame cake

12. The approximate feed requirement of a layer (chicken) during its total economic life is
    - (a) 3.8 kg
    - (b) 7.0 kg
    - (c) 48.0 kg
    - (d) 70.0 kg

13. Approximate feed requirement of a broiler chicken up to the age of marketing is
    - (a) 4.0 kg
    - (b) 6.0 kg
    - (c) 8.0 kg
    - (d) 12.0 kg

14. Oyster shells in layer ration supply
    - (a) Fe
    - (b) Ca
    - (c) Vitamin A
    - (d) Vitamin C

15. Ca requirement in layer ration is
    (a) Less than 1%
    (b) 1.5%
    (c) 3%
    (d) None of these

16. Optimum Ca:P ratio in broiler starter ration should be
    (a) 1 : 1
    (b) 1 : 2
    (c) 2 : 1
    (d) 3 : 1

17. To protect fat and fat-soluble vitamins from rancidity in feed, the poultry feed contains
    (a) Toxin binders
    (b) Probiotics
    (c) Antioxidants
    (d) Antibiotics

18. Which one is used as antioxidant in poultry feed?
    (a) Ethoxyquin
    (b) Thyroxine
    (c) Levamisole
    (d) Terramycin

19. ME value (Kcal/kg) for laying poultry feed should be
    (a) 2,600
    (b) 2,800
    (c) 2,900
    (d) 3,000

20. ME value (Kcal/kg) of broiler finisher feed should be (as per BIS specifications)
    (a) 2,700
    (b) 2,800
    (c) 2,900
    (d) 3,000

21. ME value (Kcal/kg) of broiler starter feed should be (as per BIS specifications)
    (a) 2,700
    (b) 2,800
    (c) 2,900
    (d) 3,000

22. Minimum crude protein content of broiler starter and broiler finisher feeds should be (as per BIS specifications)
    (a) 23% and 20%
    (b) 22% and 16%
    (c) 19% and 22%
    (d) 16% and 18%

23. Maximum moisture content of poultry feed should be (as per BIS specifications)
    (a) 6%
    (b) 8%
    (c) 4%
    (d) 12%

24. Maximum salt (NaCl) content of poultry feed should be (as per BIS specifications)
    (a) 0.6%
    (b) 1%
    (c) 6%
    (d) 10%

25. Maximum crude fibre content of broiler feed should be (as per BIS specifications)
    (a) 4%
    (b) 6%
    (c) 8%
    (d) 10%

26. Maximum crude fibre content of layer feed should be (as per BIS specifications)
    (a) 6%
    (b) 8%
    (c) 10%
    (d) 12%

27. Minimum calcium content of layer ration (20–80 weeks) should be (as per BIS specifications)
    (a) 1.0%
    (b) 2.0%
    (c) 3.0%
    (d) 4.0%

28. The common mineral source(s) in poultry feed is/are
    (a) Limestone
    (b) Oyster shell
    (c) Dicalcium phosphate
    (d) All of these

29. Daily water requirement of layer chicken is (per 100 birds)
    (a) 5–10 L
    (b) 20–25 L
    (c) 25–30 L
    (d) 50–55 L

30. Daily water requirement of broiler chicken at the age of 6 weeks is (per 100 birds)
    (a) 2 L
    (b) 8 L
    (c) 12 L
    (d) 30 L

31. Which system of commercial poultry feeding is most popular in India?
    (a) Grain and mash feeding
    (b) All mash feeding
    (c) All grain feeding
    (d) Pellet feeding

32. To gain 1 kg weight a broiler chicken consumes
    (a) 1.2–1.5 kg feed
    (b) 1.7–1.9 kg feed
    (c) 2.5–3.0 kg feed
    (d) 3.5–4.0 kg feed

33. Cotton seed meal contains which of the following antinutritional factors?
    (a) Linamarin
    (b) Gossypol
    (c) Goitrogen
    (d) None of these

34. The nutrient requirements of chick ration are
    1. 20% CP
    2. 10% CF
    3. 2,600 Kcal/kg ME
    4. 0.9% lysine
    Select the correct answer from the code below:
    Code (a) 1, 2, 3 and 4 are correct
    (b) 1, 3 and 4 are correct
    (c) 2, 3 and 4 are correct
    (d) 1, 2 and 4 are correct

35. The nutrient requirements of layer ration are
    1. 18% CP
    2. 2,600 Kcal/kg ME
    3. 5% Ca
    4. 0.65% lysine
    Select the correct answer from the code below:
    Code (a) 1, 2, 3 and 4 are correct
    (b) 1, 2 and 4 are correct
    (c) 2, 3 and 4 are correct
    (d) 1, 3 and 4 are correct

ii. Fill in the blanks.

1. To improve shell quality of egg _____ is to be added in the layer feed.

2. The enlargement of oesophagus, which stores feeds temporarily, is known as _____.

3. The two blind tubes located at the junction of small and large intestines in poultry are known as _____.

4. _____ is the common opening of digestive, urinary and reproductive systems in poultry.

5. The stomach of poultry consists of _____ and _____.

6. In poultry _____ (gland) is located in between the two limbs of duodenum.

7. Bile is secreted by _____ and stored in _____.

8. _____ is known as glandular stomach of poultry.

9. _____ is known as muscular stomach of poultry.

10. Birds have no lips and _____ and, hence cannot chew their feeds.

11. Broiler chicken feed must not contain more than _____ per cent crude fibre.

12. Feeding alone costs about _____% of the total cost of poultry production.

13. _____ is located in between proventriculus and duodenum in the digestive system of poultry.

14. The very common method of poultry feeding in India is _____.

15. Fish meal is a _____ rich feed ingredient of poultry.

16. Silkworm pupae meal is a _____ rich feed ingredient of poultry.

17. Maize is _____ rich feed ingredient of poultry.

18. Cotton seed meal contains a toxic substance known as _____, which can be destroyed by steam cooking.

19. Shell grit supplies _____ in layer ration.

20. Moisture content of poultry feed should be _____% (maximum).

21. ME content of layer ration should be _____ Kcal/kg (minimum).

22. CP content of layer ration should be _____% (minimum).

23. According to BIS, ME content of broiler starter ration should be _____ Kcal/kg (minimum).

24. According BIS, ME content of broiler finisher ration should be _____ (minimum).

25. According to BIS, CP content of broiler starter ration should be _____ (minimum).

26. According to BIS, CP content of broiler finisher ration should be _____ (minimum).

27. Salt content of poultry feed should be _____ (maximum).
28. Vitamin E is used as _____ for stabilisation of fat and fat-soluble vitamins.
29. Broiler birds are marketed at the age of _____ weeks.
30. In broiler production, feed requirement per kg live weight should be _____ (maximum).
31. Total feed requirement per layer from day-old stage to the end of economic laying is _____ kg (approx)
32. A hybrid layer (chicken) needs _____ kg feed for egg production in a year.
33. A chick to become a laying pullet needs _____ kg feed.
34. _____ is the best animal protein source in poultry feeds.
35. The moisture content of broiler finisher feed should not be more than _____% (as per BIS specification).
36. Feeding of freshly harvested wheat grain to poultry may cause serious mortality due to presence of _____ in the endosperm protein.
37. _____ is the antinutritional factor present in subabul leaf.
38. Deoiled silkworm meal cannot replace 100% fish meal in broiler starter diet due to presence of high percentage of _____.
39. The low digestibility of feather meal is due to _____ .
40. Monensin is used as _____ drug.

iii. **Write True (T) or False (F) against each statement.**
1. The crop is the bulging portion of the oesophagus.
2. Shell grit is offered to poultry (layer) to provide calcium in laying stage.
3. Calcium requirement of growing birds is more than laying birds.
4. Broiler finisher feed contains more protein than broiler starter feed.
5. ME (Kcal/kg) requirement of layer feed is more than that of broiler feed.
6. Maximum salt (NaCl) content of poultry feed should be 0.6% (as per BIS specifications).
7. Maximum moisture content of poultry feed should be (as per BIS specifications) 8%.
8. Minimum calcium content of layer ration should be (as per BIS specifications) 2%.
9. Deoiled silkworm pupae meal is a rich source of limiting amino acids in poultry.
10. Feather meal is not very digestible unless cooked under pressure.
11. Pullorum disease may be spread through contaminated water.
12. Over 500 ppm of total solids in drinking water is considered as polluted.

13. Birds will refuse to drink, if water temperature is more than 44 °C.
14. Bile helps in fat digestion in poultry.
15. Caecum is the common passage for digestive, urinary and reproductive systems of poultry.

B. Subjective Questions

1. Describe the digestive system of chicken with the help of a labeled diagram. Discuss the function of each part.
2. How the knowledge of digestive system helps in diagnosis of disease?
3. Enumerate different feedstuffs and supplements used in preparation of poultry ration. What are the factors affecting selection of such feedstuffs?
4. Indicate the requirement of different nutrients for broiler and layer chickens.
5. Discuss various methods of feeding poultry. Which one is the best in your opinion? Give reasons.
6. What vitamins and amino acids are most critical in formulating chick ration?
7. Name two antibiotics used as growth promoters in poultry feed.
8. Discuss the role of antioxidants and probiotics in the nutrition of poultry.
9. Mention the important information needed for computation of ration for chicken. What points should be considered for low cost feed formulation for poultry?
10. What are feed additives? Classify them with examples. Discuss the feed additives that promote feed intake.
11. Write short notes on the following.
    (a) Non-nutrient feed additives
    (b) Antibiotic growth promoters
    (c) Feed restriction
    (d) All mash feeding of poultry
    (e) Standards of drinking water for poultry
    (f) Water requirements of poultry
    (g) Antinutritional factors and toxins in poultry feed

Answers of the Objective Questions

i. Multiple choice

1. (b) Proventriculus   2. (c) Gizzard   3. (c) Gizzard
4. (c) Oesophagus   5. (d) Both a and b   6. (b) Gizzard
7. (c) Gizzard   8. (d) Crop   9. (a) 0.5–2.5
10. (c) To grind and crush the coarser feed materials
11. (b) Groundnut cake   12. (c) 48.0 kg   13. (a) 4.0 kg
14. (b) Ca   15. (c) 3%   16. (c) 2:1
17. (c) Antioxidants   18. (a) Ethoxyquin   19. (a) 2,600

20. (c) 2,900 21. (b) 2,800 22. (a) 20% and 11%
23. (c) 10% 24. (a) 0.6% 25. (b) 6%
26. (b) 8% 27. (c) 3.0% 28. (d) All of these
29. (c) 25–30 L 30. (c) 12 L 31. (b) All mash feeding
32. (b) 1.7–1.9 kg feed 33. (b) Gossypol 34. (b) 1, 3 and 4 are correct
35. (b) 1, 2 and 4 are correct

ii. Fill in the blanks

1. calcium/Ca 2. crop 3. caeca
4. cloaca 5. proventriculus, gizzard
6. pancreas 7. liver, gall bladder 8. proventriculus
9. gizzard 10. teeth 11. 6
12. 70–75 13. Gizzard 14. all mash method
15. protein 16. protein 17. energy
18. gossypol 19. calcium/Ca 20. 11
21. 2,600 22. 18 23. 2,800
24. 2,900 Kcal/kg 25. 23% 26. 20%
27. 0.6% 28. antioxidant 29. 6
30. 1.7–1.9 kg 31. 48–50 32. 40
33. 7–8 34. Fish meal 35. 11
36. glutens 37. Mimosine 38. keratin
39. cystine disulphide bond 40. anticoccidial

iii. True or False

1. T 2. F 3. F 4. F 5. F
6. T 7. F 8. F 9. T 10. T
11. T 12. T 13. T 14. T 15. F

12

Care and Management of Poultry

This chapter deals with care and management of layers, broilers, pullets, cockerels, and breeder chickens.

12.1 IMPORTANT TIPS FOR CARE AND MANAGEMENT OF POULTRY

In this section, the discussion is confined to the special care to be taken before bringing chicks in the farm and care to be taken on arrival of the chicks in the farm.

12.1.1 Preparation Before Bringing Chicks in the Farm

- In case of existing poultry farm, the old litter should be discarded after the sale of birds.
- The farm and its surroundings should be properly cleaned. The floor, walls and roof of the shed should be cleaned with gushing water. Wire brush may be used for scrubbing and cleaning. Use of caustic soda helps in cleaning process.
- After cleaning the shed should be dried up in air.
- Walls, floor, roof, wirenets, electric and water lines may be repaired, if necessary.
- Lastly, one disinfectant should be used on the floor, walls, roof, cages, *etc.*
- Then the shed should be kept vacant for 10–15 days. This will decrease the possibility of germs in the farm by breaking their life cycle. The litter guard, waterer, feeder and other utensils used in the farm should be cleaned properly for the next lot of chicks.
- Litter materials (3–4 inches depth, minimum 2 inches) should be spread on the floor and brooder guard should be provided two days before bringing the chicks in the farm. Wooden or tin plank and cardboard may be used as brooder guard. Generally brooder guard is set in a circular manner away from the brooder. It is observed that, if the brooder guard is not used, the chicks assemble in a corner which results in the death of many chicks. New litter materials should be used for every lot of birds. Newspapers may be spread over the litter so that the chicks can not eat the litter materials.
- The desired temperature of the brooder should be maintained before keeping the chicks in the brooder. During the first week the brooding temperature should be 95 °F (35 °C). The old electric wire and bulb of the farm should be kept clean and in working condition.

12.1.2 Care of Chicks on Arrival in the Farm

- Electrolyte and glucose/sugar mixed water should be provided to the chicks in the brooder. Generally, 20 g of electrolyte powder and 50 g of sugar or glucose may be mixed with 1 L of drinking water. This reduces the tiredness of the chicks. Too much of stress of the chicks can be reduced by providing antistress medicine in the drinking water.
- While placing the chicks in the brooder they should be counted, and weaker ones should be segregated.
- Weight of the chicks should be judged. If the five chicks weigh 200 g (i.e. each chick weighs on an average of 40 g), then it may be assumed that their weights are all right.
- The chicks should be spread evenly in the brooder.
- After spreading the chicks they should be given water to drink for first 3–4 hours. Then they should be given starter mash to eat. This is done because the chicks should be introduced to water first.
- During the first 3–4 days the feed should be served on newspaper or brand new egg tray or plate, so that the chicks can eat the feed easily.
- If the newspaper, tray or plate gets soaked in water, immediately they should be replaced with new ones. The newspaper should be replaced with chick feeders after 4–5 days.
- At night during load shedding, if any necessary, lamps should be lighted. Otherwise the chicks will huddle close to each other in darkness and this will result in increasing death rate.
- The temperature of the brooder shed should be judged as per the activity of the chicks, and accordingly the temperature should be adjusted.

12.2   CARE AND MANAGEMENT OF LAYER (EGG TYPE) CHICKEN

Chickens purely reared for egg production are known as layers. These egg type chickens or layer birds are divided into three categories according to their physiological and production needs. These are **chicks** (0–8 weeks), **growers** (9–20 weeks) and **layers** (21 to 72–80 weeks). Tips for different stages of commercial layer management are described here.

12.2.1 Care and Management of Chicks

Brooding

The care and management of day-old chicks during early part of their lives is called **brooding**. This brooding management is provided to the chicks generally up to 4–6 weeks of age or until they are well-feathered. They require extra heat at this stage due to their ill-developed thermoregulatory mechanisms.

The brooder unit

It consists of the following arrangements.

1. A brooder with a heating source
2. Brooder guard
3. Feeders and drinkers

A **brooder** with a source of heat is the main item of brooder house. The brooding may be done on the floor (called floor brooding, in case of deep litter system) or in cages (called cage brooding, in cage system of rearing). Use of brooder depends on the system of rearing. In case of deep litter system **various types of brooders** may be bamboo basket, hover or canopy (round, conical or angular shaped structure usually made up of galvanised iron sheets fitted with bulbs), infrared lamps (electricity), infrared brooder (gas), and radiant brooder (gas). Cage brooders are used in case of cage system of rearing.

Brooder guard is provided in the brooder house to give them proper heat. A cardboard or a metal sheet or wire net may be used as a brooder guard. Its height should be about 18–24 inches. It is to be placed around the heat source (hover), generally 2–3 ft away from the edge of the hover. After the first few days, the area is to be enlarged gradually to provide more floor space, and after 7–10 days it can be removed completely.

A brooding unit with four 60-watt bulbs are suspended 6 inches above the floor and a brooder guard of 5 ft radius is sufficient for 250–300 chicks in deep litter system of rearing.

Proper type and quantity of **feeders and drinkers** are to be provided to the chicks in the brooder house. Four baby chick drinkers and three brand new egg trays (on which feed could be given) are sufficient for 250–300 chicks. Later, these would require to be increased gradually.

All the equipments should be in place in the brooder house, and brooder should be on at least 24 hours before arrival of the chicks.

Brooding requirements

These are proper temperature, ventilation, floor space, appropriate feeders and drinkers.

- Optimum brooding temperature during the first week is 95 °F, and then the temperature may be reduced at the rate of 5 °F on every successive weeks, until the room temperature of 60–70 °F (21 °C) is reached or the chicks are fully feathered (*See Table 6.2, Chapter 6*). However, chicks' behaviour is to be taken into consideration whether they are getting proper amount of heat or not. Since the temperature in our country varies a great deal, it is advisable to adjust the required comfortable temperature for the chicks as per their brooding behaviours.
- Fresh air should be available continuously in the brooding house. But ensure that there is no direct wind or draft that will chill the chicks.
- The minimum floor space in the brooder house should be 3–4 inches per chick. However, not more than 500 chicks should be placed under one brooder.
- During the first 3 days, feeds are offered on the newspaper or brand new egg tray. Regular chick feeders should be introduced after 3–4 days. Baby chick drinkers should be provided to the chicks.

Behaviour of chicks in the brooder, brooding of chicks with the help of electric bulb, arrangement of feeders and waterers in a brooder, chicks taking feed, and chicks taking water are shown in Figs. 6.4, 6.5, 6.6, 6.7 and 6.8 respectively (in Chapter 6 of this book).

Tips for brooding management

1. **Placing chicks in the brooder:** Chicks are to be placed in the brooder gently. Weak chicks should be separated from the others and placed in a separate brooder. They require more heat than other chicks.

2. **Offering drinking water to the chicks first:** Initially they should receive fresh water only (and no feed) for several hours. Sugar may be added to this water. The 8% sugar solution containing 1% sodium chloride is usually given for the first 15 hours after the chicks are placed in the brooder. Ensure that all the chicks are drinking water. Few chicks may be taught to drink water, by dipping their beaks.

3. **Offering antistress medicines, if needed:** If the chicks are under stress due to long journey or inclement weather conditions, antistress medicine (vitamins + electrolytes) may also be added to the drinking water for the first 3–4 days. Zeetress (Indian herbs @ 0.5 g/100 birds/day), Stressban powder (Zeus @ 0.5 g/100 birds/day), Stresroak (Dabur @ 5 mL/100 birds/day) are some brand names of antistress medicines available in the market.

4. **Feeding in early stages of chicks:** Generally three hours after placing the chicks in the brooder, maize grits (chick maize) are offered on the newspaper or on the brand new egg tray for them. Ensure that all the chicks are eating. Usually from 2nd day onwards, usual feed is given to the chicks. Chick mash is offered to the chicks up to the age of 8 weeks.

5. **Vaccination in early stages of chicks:** Vaccination is must against Marek's disease, Ranikhet disease, Gumboro disease and fowl pox at the early stages of egg type chicken. Marek's disease vaccine is given at the age of 0–3 days of age. Ranikhet disease vaccine is given first at the age of 5–7 days of age (F_1 or LaSota type), followed by booster dose at 5–6 weeks of age. Gumboro disease (IBD) vaccine is given at the age of 12–13 days of age followed by booster dose at the age of 6–7 weeks. Fowl pox vaccine is given at the age of 7–8 weeks of age. The vaccine is to be given at proper age with recommended dose (See Table 13.3, Chapter 13).

6. **Monitoring:** Constant round the clock monitoring is very essential during the first few days.

12.2.2 Care and Management of Growers

Egg type birds aged 9–20 weeks or up to the point of lay are called grower. During this growing period, care and management of birds is more or less or same as chick management; however, floor space requirement along with feeder space and waterer space are to be increased (See Table 10.1, Chapter 10).

No extra heat is needed during growing period. Twelve hours natural daylight is sufficient for them. Extra light, if provided to them at this stage, may lead to early maturity of pullets which ultimately result production of more numbers of smaller sized eggs, incidence of prolapse and egg bound conditions.

Grower mash is offered to the birds during this period.

Vaccination and other medication are to be followed as per the schedule with proper care. Generally, Ranikhet disease (R_2B) and infectious bronchitis vaccines are given during growing period. It is better to use one dose of anticoccidial drug and one dose of anthelmintics before laying starts.

Debeaking is a standard practice in layer type birds. Generally 1/3rd part of the upper beak (mandible) is removed and lower beak is trimmed in such a way that lower beak is slightly longer than the upper one. Debeaking reduces feed wastage and cannibalism. It may be done at 15–16 weeks of age. However, it can be done at 6–10 days (usually 10 days) of age during chick stage, followed by final debeaking at 15–16 weeks (usually 16 weeks) of age of pullets. It is easy to use electric debeaker for this purpose instead of manual one. While the debeaking operation is done, the cut beak should be in contact with the red hot blade of the debeaker for 2 seconds only. Holding of blade for longer duration may burn the beak and cause permanent damage; and if held shorter, the beak may grow again. A gentle pressure on the bird's throat during debeaking will pull back the tongue and prevent it from burning. In case of chicks, both the beaks are cut and cauterised in one step. In pullet stage, both the beaks are to be cut separately. New blade should be used for this purpose, and it should be changed for every 1,000 pullets or 2,000 chicks. Electrolytes, antistress vitamins including vitamin C (@ 20 mg/L), and vitamin K (@ 5 mg/L) should be given through drinking water for about 2 days before and 2–3 days after debeaking to facilitate blood clotting and to minimise stress. If bleeding is seen from the beak, that should be cauterised properly. Debeaking should be done gently, steadily and carefully by skilled personnel. Birds should not be subjected to any other stress during dekeaking. If possible, shifting from one house to other, vaccination, *etc.* should not be done for about 2 weeks after debeaking.

Weekly body weight of representative birds (5–10%) is to be taken to judge the growth of these birds. Culling is to be strictly followed during growing period; birds with lameness, retarded growth and ill-health are to be removed from the flock.

12.2.3 Care and Management of Layers

- **Transfer of birds from grower house to layer house:** Birds are to be transferred to the layer house at 18 weeks of age. If egg laying started in the grower house, birds feel more exhaustion during transfer process in laying period. Transfer of birds before 2 weeks of 1st laying gives the birds time to get accustomed to their new environment. It is better to transfer the birds during evening hours when it is cool. The birds should be carefully handled by skilled personnel during transfer process. Pullets should be transferred from grower house to layer house with the help of crates. A standard crate (measuring 100 cm × 60 cm × 25 cm) can accommodate 15–18 pullets, but in hot weather (when ambient temperature above 25 °C) it is better to move less number of pullets (say 12) in such a crate.

- **Floor space:** Overcrowding is strictly prohibited in the layer house. Floor space, waterer space and feeder space should be given as per requirement (*See Table 10.1, Chapter 10*). Besides these, laying nest is to be placed in the layer house @ 1 nest per 4–5 birds for clean egg production. At least 20 m gap should be there

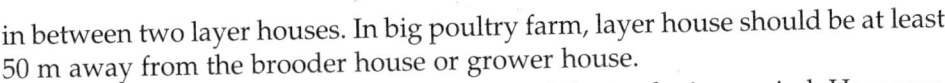

in between two layer houses. In big poultry farm, layer house should be at least 50 m away from the brooder house or grower house.

- **Light management:** No extra heat is required during laying period. However, presence of light in the layer house is very important. At least 16–17 hours light in a day (24 hours) should be present in the layer house. On the other hand, 7 hours complete darkness in layer house is also needed to allow the birds to take rest.

During growing period up to 20 weeks of age, 12 hours daylight is sufficient. From 20th week onwards, duration of light in the layer house is to be increased gradually by providing artificial light during evening or dawn hours till the total light duration in a day is 16–17 hours. Then 16–17 hours light duration is to be maintained. Light schedule in a layer house may vary from place to place or due to farmer's preference. One standard light schedule for a layer farm is depicted in Table 12.1 as a reference, which may be modified as per the need or local situation.

Table 12.1:   Light schedule in a layer house

Age of bird (week)	Light duration
20	6 am to 7 pm (13 hours)
21	5 am to 7 pm (14 hours)
22	4.30 am to 7 pm (14½ hours)
23	4.30 am to 7.30 pm (15 hours)
24	4 am to 7.30 pm (15½ hours)
25	4 am to 8 pm (16 hours)
26	4 am to 8.30 pm (16½ hours)
27 and above	4 am to 9 pm (17 hours)

Light intensity inside the poultry house is also important. Physiologically minimum light intensity is one foot candle (10 lux) at bird level. As a thumb rule, if one can read daily newspaper in the poultry house in standing position, the light intensity is considered as optimum. Generally one 40 watt bulb hung 7 ft above the ground is considered as sufficient for 100 sq ft floor area. The light source should have reflectors and bulbs should be kept clean. In case of incandescent light, 1 watt for every 4 sq ft area is sufficient.

- **Feed and water:** Layer mash is provided during laying period. On an average 40–41 kg layer mash is required for a bird during the first laying year. About 25–30 L of drinking water is needed daily for 100 layers. Fresh and clean drinking water is to be provided to the birds. [Details of feed and water management are given in Chapter 11.]
- **Vaccination and other medication:** During laying period various medicines are used routinely. These are anthelmintics, anticoccidials, antistress medicines, etc. In addition to these, after 35 weeks of age Ranikhet disease vaccine (F₁/LaSota strain) is given at an interval of 2–3 months in drinking water (in places where this disease is very prone). [Details of health management are given in Chapter 13.]

- **Stress management:** Stress management is an important consideration in poultry farming. Antistress medicines are to be used when the stress is unavoidable like severe cold or hot weather, vaccination, debeaking, *etc*; otherwise precautions are to be taken to reduce the stress on the birds especially during laying period for optimum egg production.

- **Culling:** It is must in economic poultry production. Culling operation based on physical and production performances should be done twice a month. The culled birds may be sold in the market for meat to earn something from this source.

- **Egg collection and handling:** Eggs can be collected manually or mechanically. In small or medium farms, egg collection is generally done manually. Eggs can be collected in baskets. However, in case of large farms, eggs can be collected directly in to trays which can be carried on a lorry hanging on a rail and mounted to the ceiling of the poultry shed. One such lorry measures about 130–160 cm × 35–65 cm × 85 cm, with space for empty trays and broken or discarded eggs. Manual egg collection may take about 2–3 hours per day per 10,000 layers.

  In very large layer farms, eggs can be collected mechanically. The mechanical system of egg collection may be semiautomated or fully automated. Eggs are collected directly from laying nests or laying cages to packing room with the help of conveyor belt.

  Eggs should be handled carefully to reduce the loss due to breakage.

- **Record keeping:** Various records of layer farm are to be maintained seriously. The most important records are flock strength, feeding, egg production, vaccination and other medication, death, culling, *etc*.

12.3 CARE AND MANAGEMENT OF BROILER (MEAT TYPE) CHICKEN

Chickens purely reared for meat production are known as broiler. These meat type chickens or broiler birds are divided into two categories according to their physiological and production needs. These are **broiler starter** (0–4 weeks) and **broiler finisher** (5–6 weeks or until they are marketed). Rearing practices of broiler chickens are different from that of layer chickens. Tips for broiler management are described in the following section.

- **Procurement of hybrid broiler chicks:** Broiler chicks are available in the market in various trade names. These are Hubbard, Vencob, Anak-2000, Kasila, CARI BRO-91, Pearlbro Samrat, Starbro, *etc*. Chicks are to be procured from reputed hatcheries and through known agents.

- **Preparation of house:** Generally deep litter system is followed for broiler rearing. Old litter materials should be replaced by new ones. Before bringing chicks the shed should be cleaned and disinfected properly to reduce the possibility of any infection. Proper floor space should be given to the birds (*vide Table 10.2 in Chapter 10*). Overcrowding is not desirable.

  Number of sheds in the poultry farm depends on the selling schedule of birds. If there is one shed, six batches of broilers can be sold.

- **Brooding:** Brooding is necessary generally up to 3–4 weeks. In the first week brooding temperature should be 95 °F, then it is to be reduced @ 5 °F per week (i.e. 90 °F at 2nd week, 85 °F at 3rd week and 80 °F at 4th week). Chicks' behaviour clearly indicates whether they are getting proper amount of heat or not (*See* Fig. 6.4).

- **Light management:** The basic principle of light management is to allow the birds to feed properly and to give them rest for feed utilisation. Continuous lighting is used in many farms from day-old stage to marketing age. It is more common when brooding is done with the help of electric bulbs. However, intermittent lighting is also being practiced in many places. It curbs the electricity cost, and feed efficiency is also good. The examples of intermittent lighting schedules may be 1 hour light followed by 3 hours darkness or 2 hours light followed by 2 hours darkness, *etc*. It is better to use a night bulb to avoid complete darkness.

- **Feed and water:** Broiler chickens are fed with high energy and high protein diets. Generally, two types of feed are offered to the broiler chickens. These are broiler starter feed from day-old stage to 3-4 weeks and then broiler finisher feed till marketing. Fresh and clean drinking water should be provided to the birds, and it should be available all the times. [*Details of feed and water management are given in Chapter 11.*]

- **Debeaking:** It is not generally required for broiler chickens due to their short life span. However, if it is done for better feed conversion efficiency, it should be carried out at the age of 9–10 days.

- **Culling:** Culling is an important operation in poultry farming. The birds of improper growth should be culled as and when identified on the basis of physical appearance and growth.

- **Vaccination and other medication:** Broiler birds are vaccinated against Marek's disease, Ranikhet disease and Gumboro disease. Various medicines are used routinely for maintenance of health as well as proper growth of the birds. These are antibiotics in old farms, antistress, anticoccidials, vitamins, liver tonics, *etc*. *Schedule of vaccination and other medication for broiler chickens from day-old stage to marketing is given in Tables 13.2 and 13.4 (Chapter 13).*

- **Record keeping:** Various records of broiler farm are to be maintained seriously. The most important records are flock strength, growth and feeding, vaccination and other medication, culling, death, *etc*.

- **Marketing of finished broiler:** Broiler chicken should be marketed at the age of 42 days. So prior arrangement should be made for efficient marketing of all the birds. The birds should be handled properly during shipment from farm, otherwise improper handling may cause excess bruises leading to lowering of quality. Feeding should be stopped about 2 hours before catching, and waterers should be removed during catching of birds. The birds should be caught and loaded properly. The birds may be grasped at their shanks, and not more than 4 or 5 birds should be carried by one attendant. This may be done preferably by experienced attendants and under a dim blue light at night. The birds should be protected from extremes of weather during transit; especially in hot weather they should be carried by using open crates and avoiding lengthy stops in route.

12.4   CARE AND MANAGEMENT OF PULLETS

Pullets are the young female chickens less than a year-old. The pullet rearing is same as that of grower management of egg type chickens. When pullets start to lay eggs, their management practices will be like layer management. They start to lay eggs at the age of 18–20 weeks, and weigh around 1.25–1.35 kg at this age. The pullets of broiler parents at this age weigh on an average of 2.1 kg.

12.5   CARE AND MANAGEMENT OF COCKERELS

Cockerels are the male chickens below one year of age. However, in commercial establishments cockerels are usually kept in the farm for 8 weeks only, i.e. 2 weeks more than broiler chickens. In some farms they are kept up to 12 weeks. Actually male chicks produced in the hatcheries dealing with layer chicks, are reared in India as cockerels. These are also called 'spring chicken'. In developed countries these egg type male chicks produced in the hatcheries are destroyed, as there is no market of such birds, and they are converted to meat meal by rendering process and used in animal feeds as a substitute of fish meal. In India, cockerels contribute a significant quantity of white meat and suitable for preparation of various poultry food products like *tandoori* and grilled chicken.

The care and management of cockerels are more or less similar to the egg type chicks. All-in all-out system or multiple-batch rearing system can be followed for commercial rearing of cockerels. The birds are fed chick mash *ad libitum* from day-old stage to marketing age. Vaccination must be done against Ranikhet disease and Gumboro disease (IBD). Initial LaSota strain RD vaccine may be given at 7 days of age, then IBD vaccine at 14 days and booster dose of RD LaSota at 28 days of age. Debeaking and deworming are not generally required. Some vitamins, minerals and liver tonics may be given to the birds for faster weight gain.

The capital investment and recurring expenditure in cockerel farming are lesser than those of broiler or layer farmings. So cockerel farming is more suitable for small farmers. The floor space requirement under deep litter system is less (½ sq ft/bird), total feed requirement during the 8 weeks period is around 2 kg and each bird weigh about 650 g at this age.

12.6   BREEDER FLOCK MANAGEMENT

Breeder flock is kept in the farm for production of hatching eggs. Breeder birds are generally kept in the farm for 60 weeks of age; and if the fertility level is high, they may be continued for another 3–5 weeks, maximum 70 weeks. A general principle of management for commercial layer flock and breeder flock is more or less same. However, special care is to be taken for maintaining breeder flock in regard to the housing requirement, nutritional requirement and feeding, breeding of male and females, vaccination and healthcare, and selection and culling. It is desirable to follow the breeder flock management guide provided by the concerned breeding companies.

12.6.1 Housing and Space Requirements for Breeder Flock

Breeder birds may be kept in deep litter house or in cages. However, deep litter system is practiced for both layer and broiler types of parent stock when natural mating is followed. If they are kept in breeding cages, artificial insemination is generally followed. The floor space requirement of breeder flock is more than commercial stock; and it is more in broiler type breeder flock than layer type breeder flock (Table 12.2).

Table 12.2: Floor space requirement for breeder flock

Types of breeder flock	Deep litter system (sq cm / bird)	Cage system (sq cm / bird)
Broiler male	3600	900–1125
Broiler female	2700	675–900
Layer male	2250	540–900
Layer female	1950	450–540

1 sq cm = 0.155 sq inch

In case of deep litter house, nest boxes should be provided for clean egg production. The nest materials should be clean and in adequate quantity. Generally, one nest box is required for five birds.

The performance of breeder flock is adversely affected when in-house temperature exceeds 30 °C. It generally produces heat stress leading to increased mortality, poor production and reduced hatchability. To avoid this problem in hot climatic zones, the breeder flock may be maintained in environmentally controlled house. If the birds are kept in open houses with more than 30 °C ambient temperature, weather control measures are strongly suggested to avoid this problem.

12.6.2 Light Management During Growing and Laying Periods

Light stimulation is very important for sexual maturity and egg production. Lighting programme to be followed in the grower/layer house depends on many factors, viz. age of the flock, body weight and uniformity of the flock, and natural day length.

Artificial light is not generally needed during growing period; and 12 hours daylight is sufficient. However, 16–17 hours light should be there during laying period and it should be gradually increased usually from 20 weeks of age (Table 12.1). However, in breeder flock light stimulation should not be given, if the uniformity of the flock is less than 85% and if more than 5% of the birds are weighing less than 1,850 g each.

12.6.3 Feeding of Breeder Flock

Breeder ration should be given to the breeder flock as per their nutritional requirements. In general, breeder ration should be rich in manganese, choline chloride, selenium, vitamin E, vitamin A, pantothenic acid, lysine and methionine. It is well-known that full feeding of breeder flock may cause problems with fertility and production; so restricted feeding is suggested. If male and females are fed separately, their performances will be increased.

12.6.3.1 Nutrient Requirements of Layer and Broiler Breeders of Different Age Groups

The nutrient requirement of layer type breeder birds is different from that of broiler type breeder birds. *The details of nutrient requirements of breeder birds are given in Tables 11.3 and 11.4 (Chapter 11).*

12.6.3.2 Separate Feeding for Male Breeders

For production of more semen of high quality, separate feeding for breeder male is suggested. The feed of breeder male should be comparatively low in protein (14%) and calcium, but rich in vitamin D_3.

Where male and female breeders are kept together for natural mating, separate feeders for males and females are provided in the shed. The feeders are covered with meshes, where smaller size meshes will allow only the heads of female birds to enter, as their heads are smaller than the males. The male feeders are hung at a height higher than female feeders, so that only male birds can take feed easily from these feeders, as males are taller than the females. If artificial insemination is followed, which is generally done in case of cage rearing, males are kept in separate cages and fed separately.

12.6.3.3 Feed Restriction

The main purpose of feed restriction in breeder birds is to keep the uniformity of the flock. A body weight between 10% above or below the average weight is called the flock uniformity. Full feeding may cause the birds becoming too heavy, leading to problems with fertility and production. It is specifically true in case of broiler parent stock. So feed restriction is must in broiler breeder flock and it is optional in case of layer breeder flock. Generally, 20% feed restriction is followed in breeding flock; however, care should be taken to provide all the nutrients to the birds as per their requirements.

For feed restriction in growing phase, body weight of the birds should be considered as a guide to determine the amount of feed to be supplied to the birds; and during laying phase, rate of egg production should be considered to provide the required feed to them. The desired weight at a specific age depends on breeds; so guidelines of breeding company in this respect should be given due consideration.

12.6.4 Breeding Management

Female birds may lay eggs without mating with their male counterparts. However, for getting hatching eggs (fertile eggs), breeding management is very important. Fertility of eggs depends on many factors like methods of mating, season of breeding, sex ratio, physical conditions of the parent stock, *etc.*

12.6.4.1 Methods of Mating

Various methods of poultry mating are flock mating, pen mating, stud mating, shift mating and artificial insemination.

Flock mating

In this method a group of two or more males are mated with a flock of several females. A ratio of one male to 12–15 females is a good proportion. Good hatchability percentage is obtained in this method. However, the males should not be used for longer periods and which should be changed, if there is a decline in fertility. This method is preferred where pedigree records are not maintained.

Pen mating

In this method only one male is used continuously for mating with 10–15 egg type females or 5–10 meat type females kept under trap nest system. This method of mating is used by the poultry breeders to know the sire and dam of each chick after hatching. Fertility is not as good as in case of flock mating. Sometimes the male may not like to mate a particular female and *vice versa*. In such cases, the females showing poor fertility are changed to another pen.

Stud mating

In this method a male is confined in a pen or coop and females are brought to the male's pen for mating purpose one by one. This method is followed to increase the use of outstanding males. However, labour requirement of implementing this method is more than flock mating or pen mating.

Shift mating

In this method male is shifted from one pen to another after a considerable period of time. In this way females are exposed to several males for mating and efficiency of the females can be thoroughly judged. In this method large number of males can be judged after a short span of time. Only problem is that after shifting of male to a new pen, eggs should be discarded for at least one week, because fertile eggs can be produced for at least one week after the last mating.

Artificial insemination

Artificial insemination (AI) includes various steps like semen collection, quality evaluation, extending and preservation (if needed) and deposition of semen in the female reproductive tract. It is not very common in poultry production; however, in commercial broiler breeding and turkey breeding it is becoming popular. It increases the fertility and hatchability, and increases the usefulness of superior sires. This method overcomes the problem of breeding in turkey and broiler breeders due to their over size and weight. The only limitation of AI in poultry breeding is that it requires skilled manpower.

Collection of semen from a cock is done by stimulating the copulatory organ to protrude by massaging abdomen and back over the testes. This is followed quickly by pushing the tail forward with one hand, and at the same time, using the thumb and forefinger of the same hand to 'milk' semen from the ducts of this organ. The semen may be collected with an aspirator or in a small tube or in any cup-like container. The frequency of semen collection should be once in 2 days. Average volume of cock semen per ejaculate is 0.1 mL. Usually undiluted semen is used. Cock semen can be kept for 4 to 5 hours in good condition. In poultry the AI is generally done in the afternoon (2–4 pm). For insemination, pressure is applied to the left side of the abdomen around the vent. This causes the cloaca to evert and the oviduct to protrude, so that a syringe or plastic straw can be inserted about 2.5 cm into the oviduct and the appropriate amount of semen deposited. As the semen is expelled by the inseminator, pressure around the vent is released, which assists the hen in retaining spermatozoa in the vagina or in the oviduct. Field experiments have demonstrated that over 150 hens per male can be successfully inseminated by the artificial method. In chicken, due to the lower spermatozoa concentration and shorter duration of fertility, 0.05 mL of undiluted pooled semen is required to be inseminated, at intervals of 7 days.

12.6.4.2 Season of Breeding

Birds can be bred throughout the year. However, fertility rate may be different in different seasons. In general, fertility is little bit less in summer than monsoon and winter in our country. Excessive heat in summer may reduce the breeding instinct leading to less fertility. In temperate areas, fertility percentage is found to be reduced in winter due to excessive cold.

12.6.4.3 Sex Ratio and Fertility

Male and female birds are to be kept together to obtain fertile eggs. The male-female ratio to be maintained depends on the body weight of birds. Light breeds male accommodates more females than the heavy breeds. In general, a ratio of one male to 10 females is a good proportion in case of broiler breeders. In case of layer breeders, one male for 15–16 females is taken as optimum for fertile egg production. About 3–5% extra males should be kept as reserve for future use.

The breeder males should be mixed with the breeder females at 18–20 weeks of age in egg type birds and 22–24 weeks of age in meat type birds in deep litter system of management. Hatching eggs are generally collected from 25 weeks of age onwards. In cage system of rearing, males should be prepared and trained for semen collection. Semen is generally collected from every male on alternate day. Care should be taken so that uniform body weight in male flock is maintained. Reduction in body weight adversely affects the mating ability of males, quality and quantity of semen, and fertility.

12.6.4.4 Egg Collection

Egg should be collected frequently to minimise breakage, cross-contamination among the eggs and to prevent preincubation of eggs which is happened very frequently in hot weather. Cell division in fertile eggs may continue, if surrounding temperature is more than 24 °C.

12.6.5 Healthcare

The breeder birds should be kept always in good health. Principles of health management of poultry irrespective of purpose of rearing them are same, which are discussed briefly in Chapter 13. Here the most important aspects in relation to health of breeder birds are indicated below.

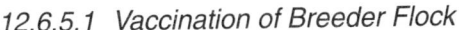

12.6.5.1 Vaccination of Breeder Flock

Vaccination schedule of commercial layer chickens and breeder birds are more or less or same. However, in case of commercial layers vaccination should be completed by 16–18 weeks of age; but in case of breeder birds vaccination schedule may be extended up to 22–23 weeks of age. The details of vaccination schedule for commercial layer chicken is given in Table 13.3. In addition to this schedule, one dose of Gumboro killed vaccine may be given at 18–22 weeks of age for long-term protection against this disease.

12.6.5.2 Common Diseases of Breeders

The pattern of diseases of breeder birds and commercial layers are more or less same. The details of the diseases and preventive measures are discussed in Chapter 13.

12.6.5.3 Fertility Disorder

Sometimes fertility disorder may be seen in breeding flock. The possible etiological factors for fertility disorder of breeder flock are preferential mating by male, improper sex ratio (more or less number of males in relation to females), stress especially the heat stress during summer months, lack of nutrients in the breeder ration, *etc.* Corrective measures are to be taken as per the predisposing factors concerned in each case.

12.6.6 Selection and Culling of Breeder Flocks

Growth and health condition, uniformity of the flock and egg production during laying phase are some of the factors which should be considered for culling of breeder birds. Selection and culling of female breeder birds can be done by score card method on the basis of physical characteristics. Male breeder bird selection should be carried out in 18 weeks of age. Uniformity of body weight and free from physical abnormalities are the two most important points based on which males should be selected. A good male breeder bird should have strong and straight legs, well-covered with feathers, proper height with muscle tone, and well-developed and bright red coloured comb and wattles. (*See Section 12.8 in this Chapter*)

12.6.7 Economic Parameters on Returns From Breeders

The target performance (i.e. saleable chicks/hen/production cycle) of a good layer type breeder bird may be as follows:

Total no. of eggs per hen (up to 70 weeks of age)	:	190
Total no. of fertile eggs (with egg weight 50 g or more)	:	180
Hatchability (%)	:	82–85
Total no. of saleable chicks	:	150

12.7 SPECIAL CARE OF BROILERS AND LAYERS DURING SUMMER, WINTER AND RAINY SEASONS

The most favourable temperature zone for chicken is 18–21 °C. High temperature and humidity produce stress to the birds leading to reduction in feed intake and loss of production, and in extreme weather conditions mortality may result. So special care of birds is to be taken during summer and winter months.

12.7.1 Special Care of Broilers and Layers During Summer

Summer stress on poultry leads to reduced feed intake, uneconomic feed conversion efficiency, loss of egg production including more numbers of thin shelled and small sized eggs, respiratory distress, loss of immunity and heat stoke.

To combat the ill-effects of summer stress the following measures are to be taken seriously.

i. **Housing management**
   - Height of the poultry shed should be 8 to 10 ft for proper ventilation in the poultry house.
   - Planting of shady trees in and around the poultry farm is necessary to reduce the ill-effect of hot summer.
   - Distance between the two poultry sheds in the farm complex should be at least 60 ft for proper air circulation.
   - East-west direction of poultry shed (lengthwise) is beneficial to reduce the direct sunlight entering inside the shed. Light reflectors may be used to reflect the light from the poultry shed. In some cases use of insulators at the roof and wall is recommended to reduce the heat effect inside the shed.
   - Depth of deep litter (in case of deep litter system of poultry keeping) is to be reduced.
   - Roof is to white washed (with lime), which will reduce the heat. Thatch type roof is beneficial in the summer months.
   - In extreme cases, pedestal or ceiling fans may be used to give comfort to the birds. Water sprinklers and foggers may be used to spread cold water to reduce the heat. Water sprinkling over the birds during extreme heat conditions may save the birds from heat stroke.
   - About 10% birds of the recommended strength is to be reduced in the poultry house.

ii. **Water management**
   - Chicken will not drink hot water leading to decreased feed consumption and less performance. They generally refuse to drink water at temperature above 38 °C (110 °F). So it is very important to provide cool drinking water during summer months. To cool the water ice cubes may be added in the water trough.
   - In general, feed and water intake ratio in chicken is 1:2, but during summer months it may be increased up to 1:4. So more water troughs are to be provided during summer months; and dose of medicines, if provided through drinking water, should be adjusted accordingly.

iii. **Feeding management**
   - Feeds should be given during the cooler part of the day, i.e. at early morning and at late evening. At noon hours wet mash may be given to the birds to increase the feed intake. However, the feed is to be mixed with water just

before offering the same to the birds; overnight soaking of feed is not desirable due to fear of fungal infestation (aflatoxicosis).

- More numbers of feeding troughs are to be provided than normal.
- Dietary modification may be done to minimise heat stress. If possible, the energy content of the compounded feed is to be reduced, and protein, vitamin and mineral contents of the feed are to be increased to some extent, with the help of Poultry Nutritionist. On an average energy of 100–150 Kcal/kg of feed is to be reduced and 2% protein is to be increased in the normal poultry feed.

iv. **Medication**

- During the noon hours glucose and electrolytes may be given in the drinking water (@ 8 g Glucose + 2 g Electral/Electrobion powder per 100 mL drinking water).
- Vitamin C may be added in the drinking water (@ 10 mg per bird for 2–3 days; Celin/Cell-C are available as 100 mg and 500 mg tablets).
- Multivitamin medicines may also be added in the drinking water, e.g. Vimeral or Vita-Dec @ 1 mL per 20 birds in drinking water for consecutive 7 days.

12.7.2 Special Care of Broilers and Layers During Winter

It is easy to combat winter stress in comparison to summer stress on poultry. Winter stress is severe on poultry when the ambient temperature goes below 10 °C. To counteract the ill-effects of winter stress the following measures are to be taken methodically.

- Extra heat is to be provided in the house with the help of electric heater or bulb (just like brooding management).
- Energy content of the feed is to be increased by about 100–150 Kcal/kg of feed.
- Depth of deep litter is to be increased (in case of deep litter system of management).
- About 10% of the recommended strength of birds is to be reduced in the poultry house.

12.7.3 Special Care of Broilers and Layers During Rainy Season

Birds feel fatigue and restless during hot-humid weather in rainy season; loss of appetite and drowsiness among the birds are also noticed. The floor and litter of the shed where the birds are kept becomes damp when humid air enters the sheds, this helps the ammonia gas to get accumulated in the shed. The pungent smell of the gas causes respiratory problem and panting to the birds. It also causes burning sensation in the eyes of the birds and they cannot see properly, and eat less, and become sick, and consequently, egg and meat production gets negatively affected. If rain water leaks inside the shed and dampens litter and floor of the shed then diseases like coccidiosis, and other bacterial diseases and worm infestation may occur and may cause death of the birds. Hence, the following special care must be taken to protect the birds from these diseases and to maintain growth and egg production.

- The shed of the birds must be kept clean and dry. Water can sip in through walls or roof of the room. Hence, leakage, if any, should be repaired well in advance. The overhang of the poultry shed should be 2.5–3 ft so that rain water does not sip in. The windows should be covered with polythene sheet so that water does not sip in. However, if all the windows are closed or covered then the shed may get suffocated and become stuffy. This condition is not good for health of the birds. So only those windows should be covered from where the rain water may sip in. They should be immediately opened after the rain stops, so that fresh air can let in. Under no circumstance should all the windows and doors be closed.

- The deep litter should be kept dry as far as possible (moisture should not be more than 25%). If the litter materials become wet, quick lime or super phosphate may be used to overcome this problem. Litter management should be done seriously especially during rainy season (*See section 10.3.1, Chapter 10*).

- Many a time the chicks may feel cold, if it rains throughout the night. In that case, artificial heat should be provided to keep them warm. Electric bulbs may help in this situation (just like brooding) or else coals may also be used for the purpose. The coal stoves free from smoke should only be let in the shed because the carbon monoxide gas emitting from the stove may be fatal to the chicks.

- The unwanted bushes surrounding the poultry farm should be cleared off.

- The feed of the birds must be stored in absolutely dry condition. Fungus may infest wet feed and can cause aflatoxicosis, a deadly epidemic to the birds which can kill hundreds of birds at a time. This fungus mainly infests feed ingredients like maize, groundnut cake, linseed cake, sesame cake, fish meal, *etc*. The moisture in feed must be below 14%. Some antifungal patent drugs available in the market may be used during this period.

- Water may get infected during rainy season. Therefore, water sanitiser should be used in the drinking water before offering it to the birds. Bacterial quality of the water must be judged frequently during this period.

- The layer chickens should be fed antiworm medicine at the onset and end of the rainy season specially in scavenging system and also in deep litter system of rearing. Various types of deworming medicines are available, viz. Piperazine, Levamisole, Fenbendazole, *etc*. Any one of these medicines may be used.

- They should be prevented from coccidiosis disease. For this, they can be given medicines beforehand in a regular basis. Codrinal, Esb$_3$, *etc*. may be given to the birds in the 3rd, 5th and 20th weeks of age of the layer chickens for 3–4 days. Dosage: 1 g/L of drinking water. The dose may be doubled, if coccidiosis breaks out in the farm.

- Antibiotics may be given to the birds to protect them from bacterial diseases. Tetracycline, Gentamicin, Ampicillin, *etc*. or sulpha drugs may be given to the birds as per need.

  Dosage of Tetracycline HCl water-soluble powder: 2.5 g per 4.5 L of drinking water, for consecutive 7 days.

- Multivitamins like Vimeral or Vita-Dec, *etc.* may be mixed with drinking water in this season to reduce the stress. Dosage: 1 mL per 20 birds for consecutive 5–7 days.
- In the hot and humid weather the birds become restless and tired and they get easily affected with deadly diseases like Ranikhet, Marek's, fowl pox, infectious bronchitis, Gumboro disease, *etc.* Therefore, they should be well-vaccinated as per the schedule in advance.

12.8   POULTRY JUDGING

The objectives of judging poultry are (a) to select good breeders as parent stock for future generations, (b) to cull unproductive birds in a flock and (c) to minimise cost of rearing by culling the non-performer in time.

Judging of poultry can be done on the basis of observing physical characters (by score card method) and on the basis of depigmentation.

I. Physical characteristics method

Judging is practiced on the basis of general appearance and body characteristics of birds for specific breeds and varieties of poultry. Usually, chicken attains sexual maturity at 20 weeks of age and judging is done at 26 to 28 weeks of age. Judging of layer chickens can be done on the basis of some characteristics as depicted in Table 12.3.

Table 12.3:   Characteristics of birds to be observed for judging good and poor layers

Characters	Good layers	Poor layers
• **Head**	Strongly feminine in females, well-proportioned, square and broad at the top	Tendecy to be masculine in female, crow headed or eagle headed, narrow and tapering at the top
Comb and Wattles	Ful, red, waxy and velvety	Dry, scaly, shriveled, cold, coarse
Beak	Stocky and well-curved	Long, thin and sharp-pointed
Eyes	Full, bright and alert	Dull and sleepy
Earlobes	Full, waxy and velvety	Shrunken, wrinkled and coarse
• **Neck**	Short and stocky	Long and thin
• **Body**	Capacious	Not so capacious
Back	Broad and straight	Narrow, pinched and crooked
Sides	Deep and straight	Shallow and barrel-shaped
Keel bone	Long and curved	Short and crooked
Pubic bone	Wide apart, thin and pliable	Thick, stiff and close together
Skin	Thin, soft and oily	Thick, dry and rough
Abdomen	Large, soft and free from lumps	Small, hard and full of fat
Vent	Full, large and moist	Small and dry
Feather	Compact	Loose

Contd.

Table 12.3: Characteristics of birds to be observed for judging good and poor layers *(Contd.)*

Characters	Good layers	Poor layers
• **Legs**		
Shank	Thin and soft in back	Thick and rounded in back
Toenails	Stocky and well-curved	Long, thin and sharp-pointed
• **Temperament**	Friendly and happy	Shy and nervous
• **Appetite**		
Crop	Full	Not full
• **Pigmentation**	Bleaching occurs as per laying age	Non-bleaching of body parts
• **Distance between two pubic bones**	At least 3 fingers	Less than 3 fingers
• **Distance between tip of breast bone and pubic bones**	At least 4 fingers, soft, pliable	Less than 4 fingers, not very soft

Score cards based on physical characteristics

Based on physical characteristics as well as sexes of bird, following score cards may be used to facilitate judging.

a. Score card for judging male birds

Particulars	Maximum score	Score obtained			
		Bird no. 1	Bird no. 2	Bird no. 3	Bird no. 4
Head	20				
Neck	5				
Body	40				
Legs	10				
Temperament	20				
Appetite	5				
Total	100				

b. Score card for judging female birds

Particulars	Maximum score	Score obtained			
		Bird no. 1	Bird no. 2	Bird no. 3	Bird no. 4
Head	10				
Neck	5				
Body	50				
Legs	10				
Temperament	10				
Appetite	5				
Pigmentation	10				
Total	100				

II. Depigmentation as a tool for judging layer birds

Depigmentation or bleaching acts as an index in assessing the persistency of egg production. The pigment, xanthophylls is derived from the feed (principally from yellow maize) and stored in different parts of body; the bird looses the pigment as the laying age progresses. At the last stage, i.e. in the last 20 weeks of egg production, when the production is less the pigments reappear in the same order.

Table 12.4: Order of depigmentation

Tissue bleached	Number of eggs
Vent	When first egg is laid
Eyelids	6–8
Earlobes	9–10
Beaks	11–35
Underside of feet	66
Front of shanks	95
Back of shanks	159
Top of toes	170
Hock joint	180

12.9 STRESS MANAGEMENT OF POULTRY

In poultry farm, birds are subjected to various kinds of stress. Some stress factors are avoidable and some are unavoidable.

Avoidable stress factors are overcrowding (giving less floor space per bird), housing excess chicks in brooder to save electricity, improper debeaking, sudden change in feed, poor quality of feed and irregular feeding schedule, inadequate ventilation, improper lighting schedule, *etc*. These types of stress can be reduced by improving the respective management practices.

The unavoidable stress factors in poultry farm are shifting of birds (from hatchery to farm, or from one house to another like from brooder house to grower house and from grower house to layer house), extremes in weather (heat stress in summer or cold stress in winter), vaccination, deworming and other preventive medication (use of anticoccidials, *etc*.), debeaking in layers or breeders and high egg production, *etc*. To minimise the action of these stressors, management practices are to be improved. Besides this, antistress medicines are to be used in proper dose rates. Vitamin C and other vitamins, liver tonic, glucose and electrolytes, *etc*. are used as antistress medicines.

[Commercial antistress medicines along with dose and administration are given in Poultry Drug Index section in Chapter 13.]

12.10 VICE IN POULTRY AND ITS REMEDIAL MEASURES

Vice means a bad habit or undesirable behaviour of animals. Some bad habits are occasionally seen in poultry. Once a bad habit is developed in a bird, it is copied by the others of the flock. Then it may become widespread and very difficult to control the problem. Some vices may be injurious to health; some may lead to death or make the birds almost useless. The most common vices of poultry are cannibalism, egg eating, egg hiding and pica.

Cannibalism

Literally cannibalism means eating of flesh of one animal by the other animal of its own type. In poultry, it is a condition in which some birds attack their flock mates and eat their flesh. This bad habit is generally developed when a hen attempting to lay too large egg leading to rupture of oviduct and protrusion of cloaca, and by seeing this red flesh other birds of the flock start to pick at it. Another possibility of developing cannibalism in poultry is—feather follicles and feet of young birds usually shine under bright light which attracts other birds of the flock. Being curious, some birds pick at feet or feather follicles, resulting in oozing of blood which attracts more birds to engage in this activity. Wounds caused by fighting among the birds may also serve as a stimulus for this bad habit. Cannibalism in chickens occurs in many forms. In chicks and growers, it is observed in the form of feather picking, toe picking and tail picking; and in layers as vent picking, feather picking, back picking, head picking or tail picking. A few cannibalistic birds may pass on this bad habit to others and soon the entire flock may be affected. Sometimes it may lead to death of birds and heavy mortality.

Causes: The most common causes of developing cannibalism are overcrowding, inadequate feeding and watering space, underfeeding, birds being without feed and water for too long period, excessive light in poultry shed, ill-ventilation and too much heat during brooding. Lack of nutrients in feed, especially deficiency of amino acids like arginine and methionine, and deficiency of minerals and salt (sodium chloride) may predispose the condition. Excess of maize in the feed may be an important contributing factor. Wounds caused due to fighting among the birds may lead to this bad habit. Irritation and oozing of blood from the skin caused by ectoparasitic (lice, mite, *etc.*) infestation may also predispose the cannibalistic activity.

Remedial measures: Good management practices including feeding of balanced ration can prevent the cannibalism. The following management pointers are considered as remedial measures against this bad habit of poultry.

1. Proper brooding temperature is to be maintained in brooder house. Offering feed on egg trays or chick box covers placed under the hover during the first few days is a good practice to prevent toe picking in chicks.

2. Proper space (for floor, feeders and waterers) should be provided according to the age of the birds. Overcrowding is not desirable at any point of time. This is especially important in broiler sheds when birds are approaching slaughter age; otherwise feather picking or feather pulling may develop among them.

3. Laying nests are to be provided in the layer house with proper bedding materials. If cannibalistic activity, especially vent picking is seen among the layer birds, red bulbs near laying nests may help to overcome the problem.

4. Light intensity is to be reduced. Darkening of windows and laying nests are recommended. Good ventilation in poultry house is also important.

5. Feed and water should be available all the times. Feeding finely ground oats to chicks and coarse-ground or whole oats to growers and layers may help to reduce the problem. Fresh green feeds or dry leafy lucerne may be given to the birds. In case of outbreak of cannibalism, vitamins and mineral mixture may be marginally increased in the ration. Likewise, increasing the methionine content of feed may be helpful to prevent the problem in layers. Salt deficiency should be corrected by supplying fish meal (2%) in the feed or by marginally increasing common salt content of the feed for 5–7 days. Alternatively finely ground salt may be sprinkled on the mash for 3–5 days.

6. Injured and crippled chicks should be removed from the flock as soon as they are discovered. Growers or layers or breeders with injuries in comb, wattles or earlobes should be isolated from the flock and wound should be treated properly. Birds showing this bad habit should be isolated from the shed, and may be kept separately in individual cages.

7. Measures are to be taken to keep the flock free from ectoparasitic infestation.

8. Debeaking or beak-trimming (removal of 1/3rd of the upper beak and trimming of lower beak, leaving the lower beak slightly longer than upper one) is the most important technological intervention to prevent cannibalism. It should be done first at 6–10 days of age and again at 15–16 weeks of age in layer flocks as a preventive measure. Therapeutic debeaking is also recommended, if an outbreak of cannibalism occurs.

Egg eating

Sometimes egg eating behaviour is seen in some layer or breeder flocks. This tendency is developed when there are cracked eggs or accidental breaking of eggs in the poultry shed. Once the birds develop taste for eggs, they start to break their own eggs; and then it is very difficult to control this bad habit.

Causes: Factors responsible for cracking or breaking of eggs are considered as the predisposing factors for egg eating behaviour. Soft- or thin-shelled eggs, broken or cracked eggs, insufficient space in laying nests, insufficient bedding materials, and delay in collection of eggs from the shed are important reasons for this bad habit.

Remedial measures: The following management pointers are helpful to control the egg eating behaviour of poultry.

1. The birds showing this bad habit should be immediately isolated. They may be kept in individual cages where eggs roll away just after laying, so they will be out of reach of the birds.

2. Sufficient number and space should be provided in laying nests. Darkness in the laying area may be helpful.

3. Calcium supplementation in layer ration is to be increased to reduce the egg abnormalities like soft- or thin-shelled eggs.

4. Eggs should be collected from the shed at frequent intervals.

5. Debeaking is also helpful to reduce the tendency of this bad habit.

Egg hiding

It is a bad habit of poultry, sometimes seen in scavenging system of management. In case of commercial egg production under deep litter or cage management, it is of no importance. Actually egg hiding is a maternal instinct of jungle fowl, and sometimes seen in domestic fowl. They generally lay and hide their eggs in bushes.

Remedial measures: Providing laying nests inside the poultry house is recommended. The laying nest should be provided with bedding materials like sawdust, soft straw, *etc.* It should be comfortable and placed in isolated place. Restriction in movement of birds may be helpful.

Pica

Eating of unusual materials like feathers, litter materials, *etc.* is called pica. Sometimes it is seen in poultry, though it is not a common problem in modern poultry farms. Phosphorus deficiency, parasitic infestation and new litter materials in the shed may predispose this bad habit.

Remedial measures: Good management practices including balanced diet can prevent the occurrence of pica in poultry.

EXERCISE

A. Objective Questions

  i. **Indicate the correct answer by putting tick ($\checkmark$) mark (multiple choice).**

  1. Removal of uneconomical birds from the flock is known as
     - (a) Brooding
     - (b) Caponisation
     - (c) Culling
     - (d) Cannibalism

  2. Broiler birds should be kept in the farm for a period of
     - (a) 6 weeks
     - (b) 8 weeks
     - (c) 10 weeks
     - (d) 12 weeks

  3. Recently the feed conversion efficiency of broiler chicken (kg feed required/kg live weight) is
     - (a) 3.8
     - (b) 3.2
     - (c) 2.7
     - (d) 1.8

  4. Egg type chickens are kept in the farm for the total period of
     - (a) 20–22 weeks
     - (b) 40–52 weeks
     - (c) 72–80 weeks
     - (d) 90–100 weeks

  5. A hen starts to lay egg at the age of
     - (a) 6 weeks
     - (b) 20 weeks
     - (c) 72 weeks
     - (d) 80 weeks

  6. A broiler chicken should have the following characteristic(s)
     - (a) May be of either sex
     - (b) Soft and pliable breast bone/cartilage
     - (c) FCR 1:1.9
     - (d) All of these

7. Desirable character(s) of egg type chicken
    (a) Feed consumption per pullet up to 20 weeks—7 to 8 kg.
    (b) Feed consumption per hen in a laying year—40 kg (maximum).
    (c) Annual egg production per hen housed—250 (minimum).
    (d) All of these.
8. In a layer house light should be present for (per day)
    (a) 24 hours   (b) 16 hours
    (c) 7 hours   (d) 12 hours
9. In a grower poultry house light should be present for (per day)
    (a) 24 hours   (b) 16 hours
    (c) 7 hours   (d) 12 hours
10. To avoid cannibalism of poultry the most appropriate measure is
    (a) Filling up the feeder up to 2/3 rd level
    (b) Debeaking
    (c) Increasing the stocking density
    (d) Culling
11. Breeders' ration should be fortified with which of the following vitamins?
    (a) Vitamin A   (b) Vitamin E
    (c) Pantothenic acid   (d) All of these

ii. **Fill in the blanks.**
1. The term 'broiler' is related to _____, and _____ is related to egg.
2. Layer type chickens are kept in the farm for _____ weeks (maximum).
3. Abdominal capacity is the distance between _____ and end of breast bone (keel bone).
4. In good layer (chicken), distance between pelvic bones and keel bone should not be less than _____.
5. In good layer (chicken), distance between the two pin bones should be _____ and above.
6. The male-female ratio of parent stock (chicken) should be _____ for production of fertile eggs.
7. Elimination of non-productive and uneconomical birds from the flock is called _____.
8. A hybrid layer (hen) starts to lay egg at the age of _____ weeks.
9. In layer house _____ hours light should be present daily (per day).

iii. **Write True (T) or False (F) against each statement.**
1. Depigmentation of beak, shanks and vent gives information regarding past production of birds.
2. Early feathering is a desirable feature in broilers to avoid problem of pin feathers at the time of processing.

3. Distance between pubic bones in good layer should be more than 2 fingers (3.3 cm).

4. Distance between keel bone and pubic bone in good layer should be 4 fingers (6.6 cm) or more.

5. Oval, large and moist vent is ideal for good layer.

6. In a layer house 24 hours light should be present for efficient egg production.

B. Subjective Questions

1. What is broiler? Discuss in brief the care and management of broiler chickens from day-old stage till marketing.

2. What is layer? Discuss in brief the care and management of a commercial layer flock from day-old stage to the end of laying.

3. What do you mean by breeders? Discuss in short the important points for breeder flock management.

4. How would you differentiate a layer hen from a non-layer hen?

5. What is culling? What are the advantages of culling in poultry?

6. When does a fowl start laying? Up to what age one should rear layers? How many eggs one can expect from a White Leghorn hen during the first laying year? When does a hen lay egg during the day?

7. What is debeaking? What is the proper age for debeaking of chicken? Describe in short the method of debeaking of chicken.

8. What are the vices of poultry? Mention the remedial measures to reduce this problem in a poultry farm.

9. What special care should be taken during rainy season for maintaining health and production of poultry?

10. Write short notes on the following.
    (a) Cannibalism
    (b) Debeaking
    (c) Poultry judging
    (d) Preparations before bringing chicks in the farm
    (e) Care of chicks on arrival in the farm
    (f) Brooding
    (g) Economic parameters on returns from breeders
    (h) Light management in layer house

Answers of the Objective Questions

i. Multiple choice

1. (c) Culling	2. (a) 6 weeks	3. (d) 1.8
4. (c) 72–80 weeks	5. (b) 20 weeks	6. (d) All of these
7. (d) All of these	8. (b) 16 hours	9. (d) 12 hours
10. (b) Debeaking	11. (d) All of these	

ii. **Fill in the blanks**

1. meat, layer
2. 72–90
3. pelvic/pubic/pin bones
4. 4 fingers/6.6 cm
5. 2 fingers/3.3 cm
6. 1:10
7. culling
8. 18–20
9. 16–17

iii. **True or False**

1. T   2. T   3. T   4. T   5. T   6. F

13

Healthcare of Poultry

13.1 COMMON POULTRY DISEASES

Disease is the greatest threat to the success of poultry enterprise either through loss of birds or through drop in production. There are many devastating poultry diseases by means of which a large number of birds may be affected at a time. Moreover, early diagnosis of disease and line of treatment are very difficult in case of poultry, as it gives practically no time to diagnose a disease and in maximum cases symptoms are overlapping. So the phrase **'prevention is better than cure'** is more relevant in maintenance of poultry health. Besides this, prevention is cheaper than treatment as nowadays the treatment is very costlier and involves many risk factors. Common poultry diseases are discussed below.

13.1.1 Classification of Common Poultry Diseases

A. **The poultry diseases on the basis of etiology (cause)**

   i. **Viral diseases**

   1. Ranikhet disease (RD) or Newcastle disease (ND)
   2. Marek's disease (MD)
   3. Gumboro disease or infectious bursal disease (IBD)
   4. Fowl pox
   5. Infectious bronchitis (IB)
   6. Avian leucosis complex (ALC) or lymphoid leucosis
   7. Infectious viral arthritis
   8. Inclusion body hepatitis (infectious anaemia)
   9. Egg drop syndrome (EDS/avian adenovirus)
   10. Avian encephalomyelitis (epidemic tremor)
   11. Avian influenza (bird flu)

   ii. **Bacterial diseases**

   1. Fowl cholera or pasteurellosis
      (the causal organism is *Pasteurella multocida*, a gram-negative bacteria.)
   2. Infectious coryza
      (the causal organism is *Haemophilus gallinarum*, a gram-negative bacteria.)
   3. Pullorum disease or bacillary white diarrhoea
      (the causal organism is *Salmonella pullorum*, a gram-negative bacteria.)

4. Fowl typhoid

(the causal organism is *Salmonella gallinarum*, a gram-negative bacteria.)

5. Fowl paratyphoid or avian salmonellosis

(the causal organisms are *Salmonella typhimurium* and other serotypes of Salmonella except *S pullorum* and *S gallinarum* which cause two distinct diseases of poultry.)

iii. Mycoplasmal diseases

1. Chronic respiratory disease (CRD)

(the causal organism is *Mycoplasma gallisepticum*.)

2. Infectious synovitis

(the causal organism is *Mycoplasma synoviae*. *M gallisepticum* and Reovirus are usually associated with this disease.)

iv. Protozoan diseases

1. **Coccidiosis (eimeriasis)**

The disease is caused by Eimeria protozoa. Nine species of Eimeria are recorded to cause this disease in chicken, viz. *E tenella, E necatrix, E acervulina, E brunetti, E praecox, E mitis, E hagani, E maxima* and *E mivati*. Out of these, *E tenella* causes caecal coccidiosis and *E necatrix* causes intestinal coccidiosis, and they are considered most pathogenic and sometimes cause disaster in poultry farms.

2. **Other protozoan diseases of poultry**

Avian trichomoniasis (*Trichomonas gallinae*), avian malaria (*Plasmodium gallinaceum*), Histomoniasis (*Histomonas meleagridis*), *etc.* These are less important in causing problems in poultry.

v. Fungal diseases

1. Aspergillosis (brooder pneumonia)

(the most important causal organism is *Aspergillus fumigatus*.)

2. Mycotoxicosis (aflatoxicosis)

(the causal organism is *Aspergillus flavus* which produces toxins.)

3. Other fungal diseases of poultry

White comb/favus (*Trichophyton megnini*)

Candidiasis/thrush (*Candida albicans*)

Mycotic dermatitis (*Rhodotorula mucilaginosa*), *etc.*

vi. Parasitic diseases

1. **Endoparasitic diseases/worm infestation**

a. **Roundworms (nematodes) of poultry**

1. *Ascaridia galli* (common roundworm of poultry, lives freely in intestinal lumen, migration of larvae in vital organs, as seen in other livestock, are not generally noted in poultry.)

2. *Heterakis gallinarum* (caecal worm of poultry, carrier of a protozoa *Histomonas meleagridis* which causes 'Blackhead disease' of turkey.)

3. *Capillaria annulata, Capillaria contorta* and *Capillaria hamulosa* (threadworm or crop worm)

4. *Gongylonema ingluvicola* (gullet worm)
5. *Tetrameres americana* (proventriculus worm)
6. *Cheilospirura hamulosa* (gizzard worm)
7. *Syngamus trachea* (gapeworm of poultry, mostly lives in trachea)

b. Tapeworms (cestodes) of poultry

1. *Choanotaenia infundibulum*
   (intermediate hosts: Flies, beetles, grasshoppers)
2. *Hymenolepis cantaniana*
   (intermediate hosts: Beetles)
3. *Davainea proglottina*
   (intermediate hosts: Slugs and snails)
4. *Amoebotaenia sphenoides*
   (intermediate hosts: Earthworms)
5. *Raillietina tetragona*
   (intermediate hosts: Ants)
6. *Raillietina echinobothrida*
   (intermediate hosts: Ants)

c. Flatworms (trematodes) of poultry

They are of little practical importance in India. Some pathogenic trematodes identified in birds in India are (1) *Echinostoma revolutum*, (2) *Echinoparyphium recurvatum*, (3) *Prosthogonymus macrorchis*, (4) *Prosthogonymus indicus* and (5) *Catatropis indica*. The intermediate hosts are mainly snails.

2. Ectoparasitic infestation

The ectoparasites of poultry are ticks, mites, lice and fleas.

a. Ticks of poultry

(1) Argas persicus (soft tick of poultry). They do not only suck blood, but are said to transmit *Borrelia anserina* (causing spirochaetosis) and *Pasteurella multocida* (causing fowl cholera). They also inject a toxin through their saliva causing paralysis in poultry.

b. Mites of poultry

1. *Dermanyssus gallinae* (red mite)
2. *Cnemidocoptes gallinae* (feather mite)
3. *Cnemidocoptes mutans* (scaly leg mite)
4. *Cytodites nudus* (air sac mite)

c. Lice of poultry

1. *Cuclotogaster heterographa* (head louse)
2. *Menacanthus stramineus* (body louse)
3. *Menopon gallinae* (shaft louse or small body louse)
4. *Lipeurus caponis* (wing louse)
5. *Goniocotes gallinae* (fluff louse)
6. *Goniodes gigas* (large chicken louse)

d. Fleas of poultry

1. *Ceratophyllus gallinae*
2. *Echidnophage gallinacea*

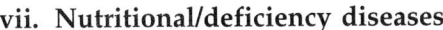

vii. **Nutritional/deficiency diseases**
1. Ricket (deficiency of vitamin D and calcium)
2. Polyneuritis or star gazing appearance (deficiency of vitamin B_1 or thiamine)
3. Curled toe paralysis (deficiency of vitamin B_2 or riboflavin)
4. Crazy chick disease or nutritional encephalomalacia (deficiency of vitamin E)
5. Nutritional roup (deficiency of vitamin A)
6. Perosis or slipped tendon (deficiency of choline, biotin and manganese)

viii. **Metabolic diseases**
1. Gout in poultry
2. Ascites (pulmonary hypertension syndrome, water belly)
3. Fatty liver and kidney syndrome
4. Sudden death syndrome (SDS)
5. Toxic fat syndrome (chick edema disease)

ix. **Miscellaneous diseases**
1. Cannibalism in poultry (a vice of poultry)
2. Cage layer fatigue (deficiency or poor utilisation of calcium, phosphorus and vitamin D_3; observed in modern layers kept in cages)
3. Egg bound condition (unusually large egg is found lodged in the cloaca in young pullet)
4. Heat stroke (heat stress, heat prostration)
5. Bumble foot (massive swelling of foot and lameness, caused by *Staphylococcus* bacteria)

B. **The poultry diseases according to the body systems affected**

i. **Respiratory diseases**
For example, Aspergillosis, Infectious bronchitis, Quail bronchitis, *E coli* infection, Fowl pox, Gapeworms, Infectious coryza, Mycoplasma, Newcastle disease, Pullorum disease, *etc.*

ii. **Digestive diseases**
For example, Ascarid worms, Blackhead, Capillaria, Caecal worms, Coccidiosis, Necrotic enteritis, Ulcerative enteritis, *E coli* infection, Fowl cholera, Fowl typhoid, Heximitiasis, Infectious bursal disease, Pullorum infestation, *etc.*

iii. **Skin and feather diseases**
For example, Cannibalism, Chiggers, Erysipelas, Fowl cholera, Fowl pox, Marek's disease, Omphalitis, Lice, Mite and Tick infestations, *etc.*

iv. **Nervous diseases**
For example, Aspergillosis, Botulism, Cage layer fatigue, Fowl cholera, Infectious bursal disease, Marek's disease, Newcastle disease, *etc.*

v. Diseases with non-categorised symptoms

For example, Blackhead, Botulism, Cage layer fatigue, Erysipelas, Fatty liver haemorrhagic syndrome, Fowl cholera, Fowl typhoid, Infectious bursal disease, Lymphoid leucosis, Marek's disease, Mycotoxicosis, Omphalitis, Pullorum disease, *etc.*

13.1.2 Description of Common Poultry Diseases

13.1.2.1 *Ranikhet Disease*

Synonyms: RD, Newcastle disease, Pneumoencephalitis, Avian distemper, Avian pest, Doyle's disease.

This disease was first reported from Newcastle town in England, UK, by Doyle in the year 1926, so the name is Newcastle disease or ND or Doyle's disease. In India, the disease was first reported from Ranikhet area in Kumaon hills, district Nainital of erstwhile Uttar Pradesh (presently Uttaranchal) by Edward in 1927, hence the name is Ranikhet disease or RD. It is an acute highly contagious viral disease of poultry. It affects birds of all age groups. The disease is mainly manifested with respiratory and nervous symptoms. All birds in a flock usually become infected within three to four days, with varying mortality. Human beings are also susceptible to this disease causing a mild form of conjunctivitis. It is worldwide in distribution. In India, it is the most dreadful disease of poultry, causing huge deaths every year leading to great economic loss in poultry industry.

Symptoms: There are three main forms of Ranikhet disease, viz. mild pathogenic form (lentogenic), moderately pathogenic form (mesogenic) and highly pathogenic form (velogenic). It is characterised by a sudden onset with hoarse chirps (in chicks), watery nasal discharge, sneezing, difficult breathing (gasping), facial swelling, cloudiness in the cornea of the eye, and paralysis of one or both wings and legs or a twisting of the head and neck (due to involvement of central nervous system). The head often is drawn over the back or down between the legs. In adult laying birds, symptoms may also include decreased feed and water consumption and a dramatic drop in egg production. Characteristic **postmortem symptoms** are pinpoint haemorrhages on the tips of proventricular glands and haemorrhagic patches in the mucosa of proventriculus. **Mortality** ranges from 10 to 80% depending on the pathogenicity of the disease. However, mortality may reach up to 100% in susceptible flock of chicks. **Incubation period** of the disease is short (2–5 days).

Transmission: The RD virus can be transmitted short distances by the airborne route or it can be introduced mechanically through contaminated shoes, caretakers, feed suppliers, visitors, vehicles, dirty equipment, feed sacks, crates and wild birds. The virus can be passed in the eggs, but RD infected embryos die before hatching. In live birds, the virus is shed in body fluids, secretions, droppings and expired air. Recovered birds are not considered as carriers and the virus usually does not live longer than thirty days on the premises.

Treatment and control: There is no specific treatment for this disease. Antibiotics may be given for 3–5 days to prevent secondary bacterial infections (particularly *E coli*). High levels of tetracyclines are contraindicated because they tie up calcium, thereby producing rickets. Increasing 5 °F brooding temperature may help to reduce losses in chicks.

Vccination is the recommended method of prevention, and it is practiced widely (*See* Tables 13.2 and 13.3). Good sanitation and comprehensive biosecurity practices will help to reduce the incidence of this disease.

13.1.2.2 Gumboro Disease

Synonyms: Infectious bursal disease (IBD), Infectious bursitis, Infectious avian nephrosis.

This disease was first reported from Gumboro district in Delaware state of the USA, in 1962, hence the name is Gumboro disease. In India, this disease was first recorded in Uttar Pradesh in 1971. Disease producing virus settles in Bursa of Fabricius, an organ of avian immune system and causes severe damage to it; so the name is IBD. The name 'avian nephrosis' is given because of the severe kidney damage it caused. It is an acute, highly contagious viral disease of young chickens. It is generally found in highly concentrated poultry producing zones. The disease is worldwide in distribution. In India, it causes a heavy loss in poultry industry every year.

Symptoms: In affected chickens aged more than 3 weeks, the important clinical signs are sudden drop in feed and water consumption, strained defaecation and watery droppings leading to soiling of feathers around the vent, vent pecking, ruffled feathers, listlessness, dehydration, tendency to sit and when forced to move, have an unsteady gait, initially high body temperature followed by subnormal temperature, prostration and death. Infected chickens aged less than 3 weeks, do not develop clinical disease, but their immune system becomes severely and permanently suppressed leading to vaccination failure, *E coli* infection, gangrenous dermatitis and inclusion body hepatitis-anaemia syndrome, which may be instrumental in causing death, and the rate of such death may be greater than Gumboro disease itself. **Postmortem findings** include dehydration and changes in the bursa, skeletal muscle, liver and kidneys. Bursal change is characterised by swelling, change in shape (oblong) and colour (pink, yellow, red or black), and formation of a gelatinous film around the bursa. Breast muscles are dark in colour. The **mortality** in affected flocks is 5–15%, although morbidity is very high. **Incubation period** of the disease is very short (2–3 days).

Transmission: The spread of the disease can occur by direct contact (bird to bird), contaminated litter and faeces, caretaker, contaminated air, equipment, feed, farm workers and possible insects and wild birds. The virus is shed in the birds' droppings and can be spread by air on dust particles. Dead birds are the good source of the virus.

Treatment and control: There is no specific treatment for this disease. Antibiotics may be given for 3–5 days to prevent secondary bacterial infections. Supportive measures such as increasing heat, ventilation, water consumption and vitamin-electrolyte therapy are helpful. Surviving chicks remain unthrifty and more susceptible to secondary infections because of immunosuppression.

Vaccines are commercially available which must be carefully used to prevent this disease (*See* Tables 13.2 and 13.3).

13.1.2.3 Marek's Disease

Synonyms: MD, Neural leukosis, Fowl paralysis, Range paralysis, Gray eye.

This disease was first described by the Hungarian veterinarian Dr J Marek in 1907, hence the name is Marek's disease. It is caused by a virus belonging to the Herpes virus group. It is a type of avian cancer. It is characteristically a disease of young chickens (8 to 32 weeks of age), but older birds may also be affected. Occasionally quail, turkey and game fowl are affected due to this disease. Marek's disease is distributed throughout the world including India.

Symptoms: Marek's disease may produce a variety of clinical signs, all lymphoids in character. These are acute neural, ocular, visceral, skin or combinations of these. Tumors in nerves cause progressive paralysis of the wings, legs and neck. When the eyes are affected it is characterised by the spotty depigmentation of the iris, irregular shaped pupils and blindness. The pupil fails to react to light. Tumors of the visceras like liver, kidney, spleen, gonad, pancreas, proventriculus, lungs, muscles, and skin can cause incoordination, unthriftiness, paleness, weak-laboured breathing, and enlarged feather follicles. Visceral form of the disease is often acute, with apparently healthy birds dying very rapidly with massive internal tumors. Skin lesion is characterised by enlargement of the feather follicles due to accumulation of lymphocytes in the typical lesion. The **mortality** rate may go as high as 60% in acute form of the disease. In chronic conditions one or two birds may die every day over a considerable period of time. **Incubation period** of the disease is approximately 2 weeks in experimental cases. In field conditions it is difficult to determine.

Transmission: The Marek's disease viruses are shed through the feather dander (minute scales from feathers or skin), poultry house dust and litter, faeces and saliva, and transmitted by air within the poultry house. Virus may stay in these materials in infective state for at least one year at room temperature. Infected birds carry the virus in their blood for life and act as a source of infection for other apparently healthy birds.

Treatment and control: There is no treatment for this disease.

Chicks can be vaccinated within 0–3 days, preferably at the hatchery. A vaccine is available in the market, which are extremely effective (90% +) in the prevention of Marek's disease. Vaccination must be carried out in commercial layer and breeder farms (*See* Table 13.3).

13.1.2.4 Fowl Pox

Synonyms: Avian pox, chicken pox (human chicken pox and poultry chicken pox are totally different), sore head, avian diphtheria.

Fowl pox is caused by a virus having three different strains, viz. fowl pox virus, pigeon pox virus and canary pox virus. All poultry species like chicken, duck, turkey, quail and ratite of all ages are susceptible to this disease.

Symptoms: Fowl pox may be appeared in two forms. These are cutaneous or skin form (dry pox) and diphtheritic form (wet pox). Birds may be affected with either or both the forms of fowl pox at one time.

The **cutaneous form** is characterised by wart-like lesions on unfeathered areas (head, neck, legs, vent, *etc.*). It is the most common form in disease outbreaks. It speads slowly and in some cases it may last several weeks. Healing of wounds take about 2 weeks; if the scab is removed before healing is complete, the surface beneath is raw and bleeding. Unthriftiness and retarded growth are common symptoms of fowl pox. In laying hens, there is severe decline in egg production.

The **diphtheritic form** is characterised by the canker-like lesions (small white nodules) in the upper digestive and respiratory systems, especially in the mouth, pharynx, larynx and trachea. It may cause respiratory distress by obstructing the upper air passage. Mortality is not usually significant unless the respiratory involvement is marked.

The **Mortality** rate is very high. The mortality in dry pox is usually low, whereas in wet pox (diphtheritic form) mortality is high, but it rarely exceeds 25%. The mortality is mainly due to secondary complication or blindness and starvation.

Transmission: Fowl pox is transmitted by direct contact (bird to bird), or by mosquitos. Virus-containing scabs, sloughed from the infected birds, served as a source of infection. The virus can enter the blood stream of apparently healthy birds through the eye, wounds or respiratory tract. Mosquitos are the primary reservoirs of fowl pox virus and spread the diseasse.

Treatment and control: There is no specific treatment for this disease. Fowl pox usually spreads slowly; it may be manifested in a flock for several months. The individual bird may take 3 to 5 weeks to recover. During this period supportive treatment may be provided.

In endemic areas, vaccination against fowl pox is recommended. The chicks may be vaccinated as young as day one by using the wing-web method using needle applicator. The commercial and breeder pullets should be vaccinated against fowl pox when they are 6 to 10 weeks of age. One application of fowl pox vaccine generally results in lifelong immunity.

13.1.2.5   Infectious Bronchitis

Synonyms: IB, Avian infectious bronchitis.

Infectious bronchitis is an extremely contagious viral disease of chickens. This disease affects chickens only; other birds or animals cannot be infected with this virus. This disease is worldwide in distribution. In India too, it is a serious problem in poultry industry, causing heavy economic loss mainly due to reduced egg production, watery albumen and poor eggshell quality.

Symptoms: This disease may affect the respiratory as well as reproductive systems of the birds. The involvement of respiratory system is characterised by coughing, sneezing and rales (rattling). The severity of infection is influenced by the age and immune status of the flock, environmental conditions, and presence of other diseases. There is loss of appetite and less water consumption. Other signs are chirping, watery discharge from the eyes and nostrils, and laboured breathing. Breathing noises are noticeable at night while the birds are taking rest. The involvement of reporoductive system is characterised by dramatical drop in egg production in layer flock with rough eggshell and watery egg white. The morbidity rate may be as high as 100%. The **mortality** may range from 25 to 60% in young chicks aged up to 6 weeks; however, mortality in adult birds is negligible. **Incubation period** of the disease is 18 to 36 hours.

Transmission: The disease is spread by air, or by mechanical means such as on clothing, poultry crates, equipment, feed bags, infected birds, infected houses, and rodents. The virus may not survive for probably more than one week in the house when birds are not there.

Treatment and control: There is no specific treatment for this disease. Antibiotics may be used for 3–5 days to check secondary bacterial infections. Brooding temperature 5 °F may be increased until symptoms subside.

Strict biosecurity programme should be in force. The virus is easily destroyed by heat and ordinary disinfectants. Vaccine is available to prevent this disease; however, the area specific vaccine should be used due to strain variation of the virus.

13.1.2.6   Egg Drop Syndrome

Synonyms: EDS, EDS-76.

Egg drop syndrome is an infectious viral disease of poultry affecting chickens of all ages and breeds. It is most severe in broiler breeders and brown egg layer strains. The first major problem was identified in broiler parents in the year 1976, so the name EDS-76.

Symptoms: The disease is characterised by sudden drop in egg production and shell-less or thin shell eggs in healthy flock. Other signs are not consistent; however, dullness, inappetance and diarrhoea are seen.

Transmission: The disease may be transmitted horizontally through direct or indirect contact with other birds like ducks, geese, *etc.* It is also spread vertically from infected breeders to chicks. Introduction of virus into chickens from contaminated vaccine is also reported.

Treatment and control: There is no specific treatment.

Prevention involves a good biosecurity programme in the farm. Recently a vaccine (oil adjuvant inactivated vaccine) is available which may be used at the age of 14–18 weeks of age in high challenge areas (i.e. in areas where this disease continues to pose a problem) to obtain satisfactory immunity against the disease.

13.1.2.7   Avian Influenza

Synonyms: Bird flu, Fowl plague.

Avian influenza or bird flu is a very contagious disease of poultry caused by Influenza virus type A (a single-stranded RNA virus). The H_5N_1 subtype is most harmful and may cause 100% mortality. The disease can occur in almost all species of birds including chicken and duck. Ducks may have yielded more virus than any other birds. It has a zoonotic importance too. This disease was first recorded in Italy in 1878. Then it was spread in various countries of America, Australia, Russia and Aisa. In India, it was recorded first time in the year 2006 at Navapur village under Nandurbar district of Maharashtra. Then it was reported from Manipur in 2007 and West Bengal in 2008.

Symptoms: Respiratory, digestive and nervous systems are affected due to Avian influenza. The disease may be of two types, viz. mildly harmful and extremely harmful. The mild form produces listlessness, loss of appetite, respiratory distress, diarrhoea, transient drops in egg production, and low mortality. In case of extremely harmful form of the disease, there is sudden onset of high mortality which may be 100% within a few days, and the symptoms in birds which may take some time to die, include stoppage of egg laying, facial swelling, bluish discolouration of comb and wattles, excessive lachrymation, and dehydration with respiratory distress. It may be noted that these symptoms may be seen in some other diseases also, so confirmation needs virus isolation and identification (in samples from faeces, intestinal contents and trachea). The disease must be differentiated from Ranikhet disease. **Incubation period** of the disease is few hours to 14 days.

Transmission: The Avian influenza virus can remain viable for long periods at moderate to low temperatures. The disease is spread directly from bird to bird through droplets or through contaminated feed and water. It may also be spread mechanically through contaminated equipment, clothes, delivery vehicles, insects, rodents, birds and mammals. Vertical transmission through eggs is not reported. Waterfowls including ducks are primarily responsible for introducing this disease in the domestic fowls.

Treatment and control: There is no satisfactory treatment of this disease.

Biosecurity measures are to be followed to prevent this disease. Till date vaccination against this disease is not recommended. Strict quarantine and rapid destruction of all infected flocks are the only effective methods of controlling an Avian influenza outbreak. If any flock is suspected to have this disease, it should be brought to the notice of Government Animal Health Centre for taking appropriate action. Quick and aggressive action is recommended even in case of mild form of the disease as this virus has the ability to readily mutate to a more pathogenic form and has zoonotic importance.

13.1.2.8 Fowl Cholera

Synonyms: Pasteurellosis, Avian Pasteurellosis, Avian Haemorrhagic Septicaemia.

Fowl cholera is a bacterial disease caused by *Pasteurella multocida*, a gram-negative bacteria. A wide range of bird species are affected by this disease. In India this disease occurs in sporadic forms, but in commercial poultry farms it is not a major problem.

Symptoms: Fowl cholera usually affects chickens aged more than 6 weeks of age. The common signs of this disease are fever, reduced feed consumption, mucoid discharge from the mouth, ruffled feathers, diarrhoea, and laboured breathing. In chronic form, loss of body weight, lameness due to joint infection, rattling noises from air passages due to presence of exudate, and swollen joints and foot pads are seen. However, in acute outbreaks, birds may die without showing any symptoms. The morbidity and **mortality** may be high. Sudden deaths may occur in healthy flocks. The disease may also appear in chronic form.

Transmission: The disease may be transmitted by various means. Addition of birds in the existing flock, free-flying birds, infected premises, predators, and rodents may be the sources of infection.

Treatment and control: Sulpha drug (sulphonamides, especially sulpha-dimethoxine, sulphaquinonxalene, sulphamethazine, and sulphaquinoxalene) or antibiotics may be used to treat the disease. Use of sulpha drug is not recommended in pullets older than 14 weeks of age due to possibilities of residues in the eggs. If the disease is treated with antibiotics, higher dose level and long-term medication are required to stop the outbreak.

In fowl cholera endemic areas, vaccination can be done. However, it is better not to vaccinate the birds, if it is not a serious problem in a farm. Strict biosecurity measures are to be followed to prevent this disease. Rodent control is essential in this regard.

13.1.2.9 Infectious Coryza

Synonyms: Cold, Infectious catarrh, Roup.

Infectious coryza is a bacterial disease caused by *Haemophilus gallinarum*, a gram-negative bacteria. A wide range of bird species including chicken may be affected by this disease.

Symptoms: Swelling around the face, foul smelling, thick and sticky discharge from the nostrils and eyes, laboured breathing and abnormal breathing sound are common signs of this disease. The eyelids may stick together. Diarrhoea may be seen in some birds. Growth (among grower birds) is stunted and egg production (in layers) is decreased due to this disease. Birds become prone to be affected with other diseases. The clinical symptoms may last from a few days to 2–3 months, depending on the virulence of the pathogen and the existence of other infections such as mycoplasmosis. **Mortality** is less (usually less than 20%). **Incubation period** of the disease is very short, i.e. 24–48 hours.

Transmission: Infected and carrier birds may transmit this disease directly to the apparently healthy birds. Birds recovered from this disease may remain as carriers throughout their lives and can spread the disease. Introduction of new birds in the existing flock, poultry shows, *etc.* are common sources of this disease. Most outbreaks occur as a result of mixing flocks. Within a flock, the disease may also be spread through inhalation of airborne respiratory droplets and contamination of feed and water. It is not transmitted vertically through egg.

Treatment and control: Water-soluble antibiotics or antibacterials can be used. Sulphadimethoxine is the preferred drug. If this is not effective, sulphamethazine, erythromycin or tetracycline may be tried.

Good management and biosecurity measures are the best ways to avoid infectious coryza. In high challenge areas, birds should be vaccinated against this disease to obtain good protection.

13.1.2.10 Pullorum Disease

Synonyms: Bacillary White Diarrhoea (BWD).

Pullorum is a bacterial disease caused by *Salmonella pullorum*, a gram-negative bacteria. Though a wide range of bird species may be affected by this disease, the chicken and turkey are mostly affected. It is primarily a disease of newly hatched chicks and poults.

Symptoms: Primary signs are huddling, droopiness, diarrhoea, weakness, pasted vent, gasping, and chalk-white faeces, sometimes stained with green bile. Affected birds do not eat and become unthrifty and stunted. Death of infected chicks begins at 5–7 days of age and reaches peak level of mortality in another 4–5 days. However, newly hatched chicks may die without showing any symptom. **Mortality** is very high in newborn chicks, which may be up to 50% or so. Survivor birds may become asymptomatic carriers.

Transmission: Pullorum disease is spread primarily by vertical transmission from hen to chick through the egg. Infected hens may lay up to 34% infected eggs. It can also spread by contaminated incubators, hatchers, chick boxes, equipment, feedstuffs and carrier birds. The disease may spread during chick sexing. Flies may help to spread the disease.

Treatment and control: Many sulphonamides and antibiotics are effective in reducing the mortality, but complete eradication of the disease from the flock is a problem.

Eradication requires destroying the entire flock. Strict biosecurity measures are to be adopted to prevent the occurrence of this disease.

13.1.2.11 Chronic Respiratory Disease

Synonyms: CRD, Avian mycoplasmosis, MG infection.

Chronic respiratory disease is a mycoplasmal disease caused by *Mycoplasma gallisepticum*. A wide range of bird species including chicken, duck and turkey may be affected by this disease. The disease is usually complicated with RD, IB and IBD viruses, disease producing strains of *E coli*, and *Haemophilus gallinarum* (cause of Infectious Coryza).

Symptoms: Usually no symptom is seen, if the disease is uncomplicated one. However, the disease is generally complicated with other organisms (like *E coli*) and infected birds may show sticky and serous exudate from nostrils, foamy exudate in eyes, swollen sinuses, respiratory rales and sneezing, *etc.* especially in broilers. The air sacs may become infected. Infected birds do not eat and become unthrifty and stunted. Broiler chickens aged 4 weeks and more are commonly affected due to this disease.

Transmission: CRD is usually transmitted vertically through the hatching eggs. The spread may also occur by carrier birds, contaminated dust, droplets, feathers, equipment and personnels working in the farm.

Treatment and control: Vaccine is not available in India. Outbreaks of CRD can be controlled with the use of antibiotics. Erythromycin, lincomycin, tylosin or spectinomycin may be used with good result. However, recovered birds may remain as carriers for life.

Eradication requires destroying the entire flock. Strict biosecurity measures are to be adopted to prevent the occurrence of this disease.

13.1.2.12 Coccidiosis

Synonyms: Eimeriasis

Coccidiosis is a protozoan disease of fowl caused by various species of *Eimeria* protozoa. Nine species of Eimeria are found to affect chickens. These are *Eimeria tenella, E necatrix, E acervulina, E maxima, E brunetti, E precox, E mitis, E hagani* and *E mitavi*. Out of these, *E tenella* (responsible for caecal coccidiosis especially in chicks) and *E necatrix* (responsible for intestinal coccidiosis especially in adults) are most dangerous and cause high morbidity and high mortality. This disease is worldwide in distribution. In India, it is very common and serious problem, and one of the biggest causes of economic loss in poultry production. It is mainly a problem in birds raised in deep litter as well as free range systems.

Symptoms: Caecal coccidiosis is commonly seen in birds aged 3–6 weeks and intestinal coccidiosis is seen in 8–18 weeks of age. The disease is characterised by diarrhoea, unthriftiness and variable levels of mortality. The common symptoms are loose droppings with blood, reduced weight gain and poor FCR, emaciation and mortality. In commercial flocks 25% mortality is seen due to naturally occurring infections. After an outbreak of a specific species of Eimeria, the flock will develop a resistance to the exposed species, but remain susceptible to other infective species. This means that a flock may experience several outbreaks of coccidiosis, each being caused by a different species of Eimeria.

Transmission: Coccidiosis is transmitted by direct contact or indirect contact with droppings of infected birds. The oocysts shed in the droppings and pass through a maturation process (sporulation) in the litter, which usually take 1–3 days or more. Ingestion of these sporulated oocysts (infective form) is the only natural method of spread of the disease. Mechanical transmission of oocysts is also possible through animals, insects, contaminated feed, equipment, dust, free-flying birds and rodents, *etc*. The spread of coccidiosis is more during cold, but humid weather, and less in hot dry weather. On **postmortem examination,** blood is found in caeca (in caecal coccidiosis). Lesions of intestinal coccidiosis vary from mild enteritis to a severe necrotic or haemorrhagic type.

Treatment and control: Many anticoccidial drugs are available commercially. It is very difficult to prevent coccidiosis by sanitation alone. It is best prevented by addition of a coccidiostat in the feed that controls the growth of protozoa in the digestive tract. However, the drug should not be used indiscriminately and proper recommendation must be followed. A vaccine is available against this disease. However, it is not used commonly.

13.1.2.13 Aspergillosis

Synonyms: Brooder pneumonia, Mycotic pneumonia, Bronchopneumonia, Fungal pneumonia.

Aspergillosis is a non-contagious fungal disease affecting all species of birds. This disease is called brooder pneumonia in chicks when the source of the disease is hatchery. In adult birds, it is called aspergillosis. *Aspergillus fumigatus* is the most common fungus causing this disease in poultry.

Symptoms: The common symptoms are inappetance, drowsiness, dyspnoea, gasping, increased respiration rate, increased thirst and diarrhoea. The disease occurs as an acute form in chicks and chronic form in adults. Deaths occur within 24–48 hours after appearance of symptoms. Chicks below 3 days of age are highly susceptible. Mortality in young birds ranges from 5 to 50%.

Transmission: The fungi produce spores on the litter, feed, hatching eggs, *etc.* Birds inhale these spores and fall sick. It is more prevalent in post monsoon season. Overcrowding, debility, dampness and wet litter condition, concurrent infections like RD, CRD, *etc.* are the predisposing factors of this disease.

Treatment and control: There is no successful treatment of this disease. However, one fungistat (mycostatin, sodium or calcium propionate, or gentian violet) may be added to the feed and/or copper sulphate or acidified copper in the drinking water for 3 days. Hamycin-AVS (Hindustan Antibiotics) may be tried to control the problem to some extent; it may be used at the rate of 10 mL suspension per litre of drinking water for 10–15 days.

The disease can be controlled by improving ventilation and eliminating the source of infection. The litter management is also very important in this regard. The infected litter and feed should be disposed off preferably by burning. Brooding area should be thoroughly cleaned and disinfected. Use of only fresh and clean litter materials, preferably soft wood shavings (not sawdust) is suggested.

13.1.2.14 Aflatoxicosis

Synonyms: Mycotoxicosis

Mycotoxicosis is one type of fungal toxicity. It may be aflatoxicosis, ochratoxicosis and T_2 toxicosis, out of which aflatoxicosis is the most common and dangerous. It may occur in all species of birds, but ducks suffer the most due to this disease. The more sensitivity of ducks is due to secretion of more liver microsomal enzymes which metabolized aflatoxins into more reactive products, aflatoxicol which produces toxicity. Aflatoxin is the most common mycotoxin or fungal toxin produced by *Aspergillus flavus* and *A parasiticus*. Both the fungi are widespread in the environment and produce aflatoxin in warm-humid conditions (30–35 °C temperature and 80–85% relative humidity). The name of the aflatoxin is given after the name of the fungus *Aspergillus flavus* (taking 'A' of Aspergillus and 'fla' of Flavus). Naturally occurring aflatoxins are B_1, B_2, G_1 and G_2, of which B_1 is the most common and most toxic.

Symptoms: Aflatoxins at high levels (> 10 ppm) are lethal to the birds. However, low levels in feed may lead to loss of appetite, dullness, lethargy, ruffled feathers, lameness, purple discolouration of legs, ascites, emaciation, dehydration and death within 1–5 days. In ducklings there may be convulsions and spasm of neck muscle with the legs stretched posterior. Multiple haemorrhages may be found in subcutaneous tissues and visceral organs. Chronic aflatoxicosis affects feed conversion efficiency, male and female reproductive performances and egg production.

Transmission: Growth of fungi is necessary for mycotoxin production in cereal grains or compounded feed. Fungi may grow in grains even before harvesting the crop, during storage or in compounded poultry feed, and produce toxins. Birds become infected through ingestion of these toxin infected feed.

Treatment and control: There is no specific treatment of aflatoxicosis. However, vitamin A, liver tonic and antibiotics may be used. Additional amount of choline may minimise the liver damage. Dietary level of protein may be increased. Supply of methionine and other sulphur-containing amino acids can protect the chicks/ducklings from growth depressing effects of aflatoxins. Supply of vitamin D$_3$ can minimise problems of lameness and poor eggshell quality caused by aflatoxins.

Retisol (Vets Farma, each mL containing 1,00,000 IU vitamin A) may be used @ 5 mL per 100 birds daily for 10 days. *Brotone* (Agrivet/Glaxo, as liver tonic) may be used @ 10 mL per 100 chicks/ducklings and 20 mL per 100 adults daily in drinking water for 10 days. *Neodox Forte* (Vetcare, containing neomycin and doxycycline) may be used as antibiotic @ 1 g per 5 L of drinking water daily for consecutive 4–5 days. Besides using these medicines, old feedstuffs should be discarded and uncontaminated feed should be offered to the birds.

To prevent this disease following guidelines should be followed:

- Clean feed ingredients should be used for preparation of compounded poultry feed. Proper storage of feed ingredients as well as compounded feed is must to avoid the mold growth. Moisture of grains should be kept less than 12%.
- Sun drying is very common and good method of preveting mold growth. However, it can not destroy the toxins which already liberated by the fungi.
- It is better not to store feed for more than a week.
- Pellet feed is better than mash feed in this regard, because pelleting may destroy fungal spores.
- Despite all precautions some mycotoxins may get entry into feed especially during rainy seasons. So to avoid any risk, mold inhibitors and toxin binders may be used in feed. Zeolytes and silica-containing compounds are used as feed additives which can reduce the effects of aflatoxins. Hydrated sodium calcium aluminosilicate can bind aflatoxin B$_1$ in the digestive tract and reduce toxicity.
- Fungistats may also be used in feed. e.g. Gention violet 2.05% or propionic acid 0.5%.

13.1.2.15 Parasitic Diseases

Parasitic diseases are of two types, viz. endoparasitic diseases (internal) and ectoparasitic diseases (external). These are described below.

13.1.2.15.1 Endoparasitic diseases

Endoparasitic diseases are caused by helminthes or worms. These worms are found inside the body of the birds. There are three different types of worms. They are roundworms (nematodes), tapeworms (cestodes) and flukes (trematodes).

Roundworms

These are the most important worms in poultry, so far the extent of damage they cause. The important roundworms of poultry are Ascarids (large intestinal roundworms), Heterakis (cecal worms), Capillaria (threadworms), and Syngamus (gapeworms).

Ascarids

The parasite *Ascaridia galli* is the most common of all roundworms in poultry and commonly known as Ascarid. The adult stages (male 50–76 mm and female 60–116 mm in length) are seen in the lumen of the small intestine and larval stages invade the intestine. Heavily infected birds show droopiness, emaciation, diarrhoea and reduced efficiency of feed utilisation. Death may occur in severe infestations. Chickens aged 3 months or more show a lot of resistance to the Ascaris infestation. Sometimes *A galli* is seen within the eggs; the parasite migrate up to the oviduct through the cloaca and is included in the egg contents as the egg in being formed.

Piperazine is the drug of choice for treating this parasite. It may be used in the feed (0.2–0.4%), water (0.1–0.2%) or as a single dose treatment (50–100 mg/bird). Drinking water application is the best in case of commercial flock; however, birds should drink medicated water in a period of few hours for maximum removal of worms from the intestine. Fenbendazole is also effective against *A galli* in chicken at the rate of 8–10 mg/kg body weight for 3–4 days. The parasite can be controlled by strict sanitation.

Heterakis (caecal worm)

The parasite *Heterakis gallinae* is found in the caeca of poultry and commonly known as caecal worm. It acts as a vector of a protozoa *Histomonas meleagridis* causing blackhead of turkey. Apparently, this protozoan parasite is carried in the caecal worm egg and is transmitted from bird to bird through this egg. However, the health of the birds is not seriously affected due to the caecal worm infestation. The life cycle of this parasite is similar to that of the common roundworms. The eggs are produced in the caeca and pass in the faeces. They reach to the infective form in about two weeks.

Fenbendazole is effective against the caecal worms. Chicken and turkey are to be kept separated to prevent spread of blackhead disease.

Capillaria (threadworms)

Various species of Capillaria may affect poultry. They are commonly known as threadworms. The most prevalent threadworms of poultry are *Capillaria annulata*, *Capillaria contorta* and *Capillaria hamulosa* found in the crop and oesophagus, and *Capillaria obsignata* found in the lower intestinal tract.

The life cycle of the parasite is direct. The adult worms may be embedded in the lining of the GI tract. They lay eggs which are passed in the droppings. The eggs become infective following embryonation that takes six to eight days, and infect any other birds that may eat them. The most severe damage occurs within 2 weeks of infection. These may cause thickening and inflammation of the mucosa, sometimes erosion of the intestinal lining leading to haemorrhage and death. Reduced growth, egg production and fertility are seen due to heavy infestations.

Capillaria infestation may be a severe problem in deep litter house. Scientific management of deep litter is very important to control this disease. Alternately raising of birds in cages may remove the threat of the infestation. Fenbendazole and leviamisole are effective dewormers against the Capillaria. Use of vitamin A may be of value.

Syngamus (gapeworms)

The parasite *Syngamus trachea* is found in the trachea (wind pipe) of poultry and commonly known as gapeworm. The parasite is also known as 'redworm' because of its colour, and 'forked worm' because of their presence in permanent copulation condition of male and female, just like the letter 'Y'. The infected birds show characteristic open-mouth breathing, hence the term is 'gape'. The worms can block the trachea, emit a grunting sound and may die from suffocation.

The life cycle of the gapeworm is more or less similar to that of the caecal worm. The female worms lay eggs in the trachea, the eggs are coughed up, swallowed, and pass out through the droppings. Within 8 to 14 days the eggs hatch and are infective when eaten by birds or earthworms. The earthworm, snails and slugs served as primary intermediate hosts for the gapeworm. Gapeworms in infected earthworms may remain viable for 4½ years while those in snails and slugs may remain infective for 1 year. After being consumed by the birds, gapeworm larvae hatch in the intestine and migrate from the intestine to the trachea and lungs. Young birds, reared under free range system, are at high risk.

Fenbendazole is an effective dewormer against the gapeworms. It may be used at an interval of 15 to 30 days to prevent this disease. Control of earthworms, snails and slugs by treating the soil is an effective method of control.

Tapeworms

Tapeworms are flattened, ribbon-shaped worms having numerous segments. They vary in size from very small to several inches in length. The anterior end of the worm is much smaller than the rest of the body. The common tapeworms of poultry are *Choanotaenia infundibulum, Hymenolepis cantaniana, Davainea proglottina, Amoebotaenia sphenoides, Raillietina tetragona* and *Raillietina echinobothrida*.

Postmortem examination by opening a portion of the intestine and placing in water may be helpful in finding the very small tapeworms. However, large worms can be seen easily with the naked eye. Young birds are more severely affected than adult birds. Heavy infestation may result in reduced efficiency and slower growth. Life cycle of tapeworms is intermediate host dependent. All poultry tapeworms apparently spend part of their lives in intermediate hosts, and birds become infected by eating the intermediate hosts. The common intermediate hosts are earthworms, snails, slugs, beetles, ants, grasshoppers and houseflies. The eggs, passed by the birds through their droppings, infect the intermediate hosts when they eat the eggs.

Fenbendazole or leviamisole may be used regularly to control the tapeworm infestation. Intermediate host control is the best method of preventing tapeworm infestation.

Flukes

They are also known as flatworms or trematodes. They are of little practical importance in India. Some pathogenic trematodes identified in birds in India are *Echinostoma revolutum, Echinoparyphium recurvatum, Prosthogonymus macrorchis, Prosthogonymus indicus* and *Catatropis indica*. The intermediate hosts are mainly snails.

13.1.2.15.2 *Ectoparasitic diseases*

The various ectoparasites of poultry are lice, ticks, mites and fleas. Out of these, lice infestation is the most common in poultry.

Poultry lice

Important poultry lice are *Cuclotogaster heterographa* (head louse), *Menacanthus stramineus* (body louse) and *Menopon gallinae* (shaft louse or small body louse). The head louse is very irritating and ranks first among lice of young chickens and turkeys. This head louse is oblong, grayish and about 1/10 inch long. The eggs are pearly-white in colour and attached singly at the base of the small feathers on the head. Body louse prefers to stay on the skin especially in the parts of the body that are not densely feathered like around vent. Body lice are straw-coloured which may be seen running rapidly on the skin in search of cover when the feathers are parted. Eggs are deposited in clusters near the base of small feathers, particularly below the vent. This body louse is the commonest louse in poultry. The shaft louse is similar in appearance to the body louse, but smaller. It has a habit of resting on the body feather shafts of chickens, where it may be seen running rapidly towards the body when feathers are parted suddenly.

The primary effect of lice on their hosts is the irritations they cause. The birds become restless and can not feed or sleep well. Birds may injure themselves or damage their feathers by pecking or scratching the areas irritated by lice. Body weight and egg production may be reduced.

Poultry ticks

Argas persicus is the most important soft tick of poultry. It is a blood-sucker, and when present in large numbers, it may result in reduced egg production, anaemia, emaciation and even death. They can transmit *Borrelia anserine* (cause of Avian spirochaetosis) and *Pasteurella multocida* (cause of Fowl cholera). The ticks may remain alive without food for more than three years. They feed on all birds. The poultry ticks spend most of their lives in cracks and hiding places, emerging at night to take blood of the birds. Larvae that hatch from the eggs in the hiding places crawl around until they find a host bird. They remain attached to the birds for three to ten days and then leave the birds for hiding places.

Poultry mites

The common poultry mites are *Dermanyssus gallinae* (red mite or chicken mite), *Cnemidocoptes gallinae* (feather mite), *Cnemidocoptes mutans* (scaly leg mite) and *Cytodites nudus* (air sac mite). All categories of poultry are susceptible to mites. The mites are extremely small and a microscope or magnifying glass may be needed to see them. Mites may be of different types. Some mites are blood suckers, some burrow into the skin or live on the feathers, and some may remain in the air passage and in the lungs, liver and other internal organs. Poultry mites may cause retarded growth, reduced egg production, lowered vitality, damaged plumage and even death. The red mite can transmit fowl cholera.

Treatment and control of Ectoparasites

Good hygiene and sanitation and use of insecticides form the basis of ectoparasitic control. Ectoparasites remain on the birds' as well as in the poultry houses and surrounding areas. So to treat the ectoparasitic infestations medicine should be applied on the birds body as well as in the poultry houses. In case of lice infestation it is more important to apply the insecticides directly to the birds' body rather than the premises. The most effective treatment for all mite species is a regular inspection and spraying programme of both the birds and their premises. Ticks are difficult to eradicate; and it is not necessary to treat the birds, but houses and surrounding areas must be treated thoroughly.

Many insecticides are available which may be used to control the external parasites of poultry. Cypermethrin, Deltamethrin and Cyromazine are found to be effective against all ectoparasites including mites that infest the birds. *Tikkil liquid* or *Clinar liquid* (Cypermethrin, 10% w/v) may be used by spraying with 1–2 mL medicine per litre of water. *Butox liquid* (Deltamethrin, 12.5% solution) may be used at the rate of 1 mL/L of water for birds and 2 mL/L of water for houses and surrounding areas. *Pestoban* (an ayurvedic preparation) may be used by spraying. Manufacturers' recommendations should be followed when using insecticides.

13.1.2.16 Ascites

Synonyms: Water belly, Altitude disease, Pulmonary hypertension disease.

Ascites is a cardiopulmonary metabolic disorder of young and rapidly growing broiler chickens. This disease is also seen in breeder birds. It is occurring worldwide, but seen especially at high altitude areas. The disease is predisposed by reduced ventilation, high altitude and respiratory diseases; and characterised by accumulation of fluid in the peritoneal cavity and death of the birds due to right-sided congestive heart failure. Morbidity is usually 1–5%; mortality 1–2%, but can be as high as 30% at high altitude. Peak mortality is seen in broiler chickens aged between 3 and 5 weeks. This disease is more common in males than in females. It is also more common in broiler chickens fed pellets compared to broilers fed mash which may be due to high energy content of pellet diets. It is mostly seen in flocks which are performing well. Inadequate ventilation is considered one of the major causes of ascites especially in winter months. Deficiency of selenium and vitamin E in diet may lead to ascites due to pulmonary hypertension. Sodium toxicity may cause ascites and right ventricular failure.

Symptoms: Two forms of ascites are common in chickens. These are acute form and chronic form. The most common symptoms are sudden death in rapidly growing birds, poor development, progressive weakness and abdominal distension (pot belly) and recumbency. They are reluctant to move and show dyspnoea and cyanosis of the skin of the head and abdomen. Panting and subcutaneous oedema are sometimes seen. **Postmortem lesions** reveal right-side cardiac enlargement, dilation of the ventricle, thickening of atrioventricular valve, general venous congestion, severe muscle congestion, congested lungs and intestines, liver enlargement, small spleen, and accumulation of ascetic fluid in the abdominal cavity which is straw coloured and more than 300 mL in volume with or without fibrin clots.

Treatment and control

The treatment is not satisfactory for the disease. However, the following therapeutic measures may be taken.

- Natural vinegar may be used once @ 25–50 mL/100 birds daily for 3 days. It reduces the problem of ascites because of its diuretic action.
- Furosemide along with L-arginine in diet reduces the incidence of pulmonary hypertension and ascites through pulmonary vasodilatation.
- Addition of 1% sodium bicarbonate in diet is helpful because it causes vasodilatation and, thus decreases the arterial pressure index.

The following preventive measures may be taken to prevent the ascites.

- Improvement of ventilation and lowering down the temperature of poultry sheds.
- Reduction of salt (NaCl) level in the diet.
- Improvement of protein quality of feed, and by lowering energy level of the feeds.
- Addition of urease inhibitor in the diet.
- Supplementation of vitamins and minerals in the diets including vitamin C, reduces the chance of the disease.
- Addition of antitoxic and antifungal agents in the diets.
- Rearing of birds which are resistant to hypoxia and ascites through genetic selection.

13.1.2.17 Sudden Death Syndrome

Sudden death syndrome (SDS) is a condition of broiler chickens of unknown cause, possibly metabolic. It may be induced by lactic acidosis. It is more common in males.

Symptoms: Convulsion and sudden death are the primary signs. Most of the birds are found lying on their back with lack of other pathology. **Postmortem lesions** reveal intestine filled with feed, haemorrhages in muscles and kidneys, the atria of the heart have blood, but the ventricles are empty, serum accumulation in lungs (may be little, if examined shortly after death), liver heavier than those of flock-mates (as a percentage of body weight).

Treatment and control: Treatment is not possible as death occurs suddenly.

The following preventive measures may be taken.

- Lowering of energy level of the diet
- Change of feed from pellets to mash
- Feed restriction
- Low intensity light
- Avoidance of disturbance

13.1.2.18 Gout in Poultry

Gout is generally characterised by swelling of joints and lameness due to retention of excess uric acid in the body. It is seen in man, apes and birds. In this condition chalk-like crystals of uric acid or urates of sodium and calcium are deposited in tissues. Gout may be occurred in two forms singly or in combination in birds. These are visceral gout and articular gout. In case of visceral gout, crystals of uric acid and urates are deposited in the visceral organs. In articular gout, crystals are deposited in the joints of wings, hock and feet and in the tendon sheath. Gout is seen in chicken of all ages. Mortality goes up to 5%.

The underline cause of gout has increased the rate of synthesis of purine precursors of uric acid and/or decreased elimination of uric acid by kidney. The factors that predispose this condition are renal diseases leading to failure of urinary excretion, vitamin A deficiency, high level of vitamin D_3 and calcium in the diet, excess salt in the diet, sodium bicarbonate toxicity, high protein diet leading to increased formation of purine precursors, excess sulpha drugs like sulphadimidine and sulphaguanidine leading to nephrotoxicity, mycotoxicosis and after infectious bronchitis and Gumboro disease outbreaks which lead to renal lesions, ammonia formation in the poultry shed, cold stress leading to less water intake, and hereditary cause.

Symptoms: Dull, ruffled feathers, loss of appetite, dehydration, swelling of joints, usually wing and leg joints, painful condition manifested as lameness, chalk-like crystals of uric acid and urates deposited in the kidneys, and surface of liver, heart, air sacs and muscles, white chalky synovial fluid, and death due to starvation as affected birds cannot move.

Treatment and control: Treatment is not satisfactory, and it is limited to supportive care and dietary management.

The following preventive measures may be taken:

- Change of quality of feed. Lowering of protein level of the diet may be helpful to reduce the condition. Gradual recovery is possible after reduction of protein level to 20%. Potassium and calcium levels should be reduced. Vitamin levels (except fat-soluble vitamins) should be increased. Vitamin A supplement through drinking water is useful.
- Diuretics may be used.
- Jaggery may be used in drinking water @ 5 g/L of water.
- After arrival of chicks in the farm, lukewarm water should be provided with electrolyte powder @ 1 g/2 L of water and antistress medicine like Zeetress @ 1 g/2 L of water. Hard water should not be used.

13.1.2.19 Nutritional/Deficiency Diseases

Some diseases occur due to deficiency of nutrients in poultry feed. The important nutrients are proteins, energy (fats and carbohydrates), fibre, moisture, vitamins and minerals. Out of these, vitamins and minerals are required in minute quantities, and if their incorporation in the feed is not proper, deficiency symptoms are commonly developed. Their deficiency is generally manifested by a specific symptom. On the basis of observing specific symptoms, the deficiency diseases can be diagnosed. In addition to that after incorporating the specific nutrient in the diet the symptoms will be disappeared, this confirmed the diagnosis. Besides this, the basic feature of nutritional disease is that many of the birds in a flock show similar type of symptoms as they are taking the same type of feed in a flock.

General symptoms of nutrient deficiency are weakness, stunted growth, loss of productivity, *etc.* Some specific deficiency diseases of poultry along with their symptoms are depicted in Table 13.1.

To combat the deficiencies, mineral and vitamin supplements are to be used judiciously either in feed or in drinking water. (*Commercial preparations of vitamins and minerals are given in the Poultry Drug Index section of this chapter.*)

Table 13.1: Important nutrients (vitamins and minerals) and their deficiency symptoms in poultry

Sl no.	Nutrients	Specific deficiency symptoms
Vitamins		
1.	Vitamin B$_1$ (Thiamine)	**Polyneuritis** (inflammation of many nerves), leg weakness, emaciation, tremors, paralysis and convulsion. They sit characteristically on legs with retraction of head to backside called '**star gazing appearance' or opisthotonus**. Birds respond within a few hours after oral administration of vitamin B$_1$.
2.	Vitamin B$_2$ (Riboflavin)	Weakness of legs and inability to extend digits called '**curled toe paralysis'**, normal appetite, but having diarrhoea. Toes are curled inward while both walking and resting. The sciatic and brachial nerves are swollen four times than normal size.
3.	Vitamin B$_6$ (Pyridoxine)	Reduced feed intake, slow growth, poor feather growth, **nervous sign and chondrodystrophy** (a bone disorder, earlier known as **perosis**). Jerky movements of legs while walking, flapping of wings, aimless running are some peculiar signs. Symptoms are less severe in grower and adult birds.
4.	Choline	**Chondrodystrophy (Perosis**, legs become bowed and **slipped tendon**)—it leads to inability to bear body weight, severe in chicks and especially in poults; adults are rarely affected as they can synthesise it.
5.	Vitamin H (Biotin)	Dermatitis in skin and legs, deformed hock joints, slipped tendon, reduced egg size and poor hatchability. Diets slightly deficient in this vitamin may cause a metabolic disorder known as '**fatty liver and kidney syndrome'**, it responds well in biotin treatment.
6.	Vitamin C (Ascorbic acid)	Normally chickens do not require external vitamin C, as they can synthesize it from glucose. Chickens synthesise this vitamin in the kidneys, not in the liver.
7.	Vitamin A (Retinol)	Loss of appetite, retarded growth, ruffled feathers, bleached beak, staggering gait, oculonasal discharge with swollen eyelid, drowsiness and weakness. Reduced egg productions in layer, very susceptible to infection, gout, night blindness are the consequences.

Contd.

Table 13.1: Important nutrients (vitamins and minerals) and their deficiency symptoms in poultry *(Contd.)*

Sl no.	Nutrients	Specific deficiency symptoms
Vitamins		
8.	Vitamin D (vitamin D$_3$ is essential in poultry)	**Rickets** in young and **osteomalacia** in adults; reduced production of egg with **thin or soft shell** and poor hatchability; **rachitic rosary** (beading of ribs at their junctions with the spinal column and formation of well-defined knobs on the ribs at the costochondral junction); bones, beaks, shanks and claws become soft and rubbery.
9.	Vitamin E	**Encephalomalacia** (**Crazy chick disease**, a nervous disorder); **exudative diathesis** (oedema of subcutaneous tissue); **nutritional muscular dystrophy** (generally seen when vitamin E deficiency is accompanied by deficiency of sulphur-containing amino acids like methionine and cysteine); sterility in males.
10.	Vitamin K	Large haemorrhages on the areas prone to be damaged from rubbing or scraping like breast, legs, wings and in abdominal cavity due to rubbing; petechial (pinpoint or minute) haemorrhages in liver and gizzard; high embryo mortality.
Minerals		
11.	Calcium and phosphorus	Rickets in young growing birds and osteomalacia in the layer birds; cage layer fatigue in caged hens (this problem is mainly due to osteoporosis).
12.	Manganese	**Chondrodystrophy (Perosis**, legs become bowed)— deformity of one or both the hocks with enlargement, twisting and slipping of gastocnemius tendon from condyles. High dietary calcium and phosphorus, low level of vitamins like choline, biotin, niacin, pantothenic acid and folic acid predispose this condition.
13.	Iron and copper	**Nutritional anaemia**, loss in body weight, ruffled feathers, reduced egg production and low hatchability.
14.	Iodine	**Goitre**, poor growth and low hatchability.
15.	Zinc and magnesium	**Goose stepping appearance**—abnormal bone formation; thin-shelled egg and low hatchability, dermatitis, poor feathering.

13.2 VACCINE AND VACCINATION SCHEDULE FOR POULTRY

13.2.1 Types of Vaccine

Vaccines are the biological agents containing modified form of microorganisms like bacteria or virus, which when introduced into the body induce antibody formation against that particular disease producing organism. Vaccines contain small, carefully measured quantities of the bacteria or virus that causes a particular disease, either in live or attenuated form.

The poultry vaccines are mainly of two types. These are (a) live vaccine and (b) killed or inactivated vaccine.

Live vaccine: The live vaccine usually contains only antigen, either a virus or a bacterium. The antigen may be naturally occurring mild strain or attenuated. Live vaccine is generally administered through ocular or nasal drop, through drinking water (oral route) or through aerosol route (by spray). The exception is Marek's disease vaccine, which is a live vaccine, but should be administered by injection only. Ranikhet disease R_2B live and fowl pox live vaccines are also given through injection. The immunity produced by live vaccine is generally short-term; so it needs repetition of vaccination. A live vaccine provokes a more rapid response than a killed vaccine. Use of live vaccine should be avoided in laying hens, as they may cause problems in egg production.

Killed vaccine: Killed vaccine is composed of concentrated antigen combined with an oil emulsion or aluminium hydroxide adjuvant (adjuvant increases the immune response of antigen). Killed vaccine may contain more than one antigen. Such vaccines are always administered by means of injection (through subcutaneous or intramuscular route). Killed vaccine always produces long-term immunity. One or two priming (1st vaccinating) with live virus vaccine followed by oil emulsion killed vaccine gives long-term high level immunity in the flock, especially in case of layer and breeder flocks. A killed vaccine performs better when given after a live vaccine prime. Duration of immunity endowed by a killed vaccine is usually longer than a live vaccine.

[A list of various poultry vaccines available in the market, along with their dose and route of administration, is given in Poultry Drug Index section of this Chapter.]

13.2.2   Vaccination Schedule for Broiler Chicken

Nowadays broiler chickens are marketed any time between 35 and 42 days of age; so vaccine requirements may vary to some extent. However, vaccination is must against Ranikhet disease and Gumboro disease. The immunity status of the day-old chicks should be known before a vaccination programme is implemented. Maternal antibody interfere in the vaccination response. In case of Gumboro disease, it is not desirable to vaccinate the chicks in the face of high maternal antibody. Ranikhet disease's 1st vaccine is generally given with a mild strain like F_1 followed by 2nd vaccine with stronger strain like LaSota. Marek's disease is given routinely in areas with a high challenge or where birds are kept up to 55 days of age or more. Marek's disease vaccine is generally given at day 1 by the reputed hatcheries; though it can be given up to the age of 3 days, with live HVT MD vaccine @ 0.2 mL through I/M or S/C route. A model vaccination schedule for commercial broiler chickens is presented in Table 13.2.

Table 13.2: Common vaccination schedule for broiler chicken

	Age	Disease	Vaccine	Dose and route of administration	Remarks
1.	4–7 days	Ranikhet disease	RDF$_1$ or LaSota strain (live)	1 drop, nasal or ocular route; or oral through drinking water.	Booster dose is to be given at 21–23 days of age.
2.	12–14 days	Gumboro disease (IBD)	IBD/Gumboro vaccine (live)	Oral through drinking water	May be repeated at 28–30 days of age.
3.	21–23 days	Ranikhet disease (booster dose)	LaSota vaccine (live)	1 drop, nasal or ocular route; or oral through drinking water.	–

NB: This is a typical vaccination programme in broiler chicken production areas. Individual programmes are highly variable and reflect local conditions, disease prevalence, severity of challenge, and individual preferences. Some vaccines may be combined in some areas. Vaccination for some diseases depends on local requirements. However, modification of this schedule, if needed, should be done with the help of experienced veterinarians or poultry specialists.

13.2.3 Vaccination Schedule for Layer Chicken

Vaccination of commercial layer chickens is must against Marek's disease, Ranikhet disease and Gumboro disease (IBD). Vaccination against infectious bronchitis (IB) and fowl pox is also common in endemic areas (i.e. in areas where these diseases are regularly found). Egg drop syndrome (EDS) and infectious coryza vaccines are required in areas of high challenge (i.e. in areas where these diseases continue to pose a problem). EDS vaccine, if required, is generally given by injection at 16 weeks of age as a single dose. Gumboro disease vaccine (intermediate strain) is generally given orally through drinking water. In case of high level of infection of this disease, a single dose of Gumboro killed vaccine may be tried at 4–7 days of age. Ranikhet disease (RD) killed vaccine is commonly given at 18 weeks of age to provide protection through out the laying period; however, to avoid any risk, at 35 weeks and then at every 8 weeks LaSota vaccine is repeated for maintaining antibody titre. IB vaccine is generally given at 15–16 weeks of age; however, in endemic areas this vaccine may be started at 4–5 weeks of age, with a booster dose at 13 weeks. RD, IB and IBD killed vaccines may be given in one combined injection at 18 weeks of age for long-lasting protection. A model vaccination schedule for commercial layer chickens is presented in Table 13.3.

Table 13.3: Common vaccination schedule for layer chicken

	Age	Disease	Vaccine	Dose and route of administration	Remarks
1.	1 day	Marek's disease	HVT MD vaccine	0.2 mL/bird, I/M injection	Generally it is given at hatchery level; it can be given up to the age of 3 days.
2.	4–7 days	Ranikhet disease	RDF$_1$ or LaSota vaccine	1 drop, nasal or ocular route; or through drinking water	Booster dose to be given at 5–6 weeks of age.
3.	12–14 days	Gumboro disease (IBD)	IBD/Gumboro vaccine	Oral through drinking water	Booster may be given at 6–7 weeks of age.
4.	5–6 weeks	Ranikhet disease (booster dose)	RDF$_1$ vaccine	1 drop, nasal or ocular route; or through drinking water	–
5.	6–7 weeks	Gumboro disease (booster dose)	IBD/Gumboro vaccine	Same as Sl No. 3	–
6.	7–8 weeks	Fowl pox	Fowl pox vaccine	0.01 mL/bird, injection at wing web or 1 drop by picking of feathers	One vaccine is sufficient for bird's life. However, it may be repeated at 14 weeks of age.
7.	8–10 weeks	Ranikhet disease	RDR$_2$B or Mukteswar strain vaccine	0.5 mL/bird, S/C at wing web	In endemic area, LaSota vaccine is given at this age followed by R$_2$B at 13 weeks of age.
8.	15–16 weeks	Infectious bronchitis	IB vaccine	0.5 mL/bird, S/C or I/M at wing web	Booster dose at 40 weeks of age.
9.	18 weeks	Ranikhet disease (booster dose)	RDR$_2$B vaccine (killed)	0.5 mL/bird, S/C at wing web	Then it is repeated at 35 weeks of age, and then LaSota vaccine at the interval of 8 weeks.

NB: This is a typical vaccination programme in layer chicken production areas. Individual programmes are highly variable and reflect local conditions, disease prevalence, severity of challenge, and individual preferences. Some vaccines may be combined in some areas. Vaccination for some diseases depends on local requirements. However, modification of this schedule, if needed, should be done with the help of experienced veterinarians or poultry specialists.

13.2.4 Factors that Govern Vaccination Schedule

It is not possible to formulate a universal vaccination schedule for all poultry farms in all areas. It depends on many factors as described below.

i. Vaccination schedule primarily depends on the categories of birds for which it is to be planned. Broiler chickens are kept in the farm only for 6 weeks, whereas layer chickens are kept in the farm for about 72 weeks. So long-term protection is required in layer birds than broiler birds. Broiler birds are essentially vaccinated against Ranikhet disease, Gumboro disease and Marek's disease; but in addition to these layer birds are should also be vaccinated against fowl pox and infectious bronchitis.

ii. Vaccine itself induces stress to the birds. So use of all available vaccines for a particular bird is not generally recommended, and it should depend on the incidence of a particular disease in the farm and its surrounding areas; in other words, local pattern of diseases must be kept in mind for formulating vaccination schedule.

iii. Maternal antibodies influence the response of vaccines used in early part of bird's life. Vaccines may be less effective when administered to chicks possessing maternal antibodies specific to the vaccine, through the process of neutralisation. It is known that high levels of maternal protection not only stop diseases, but also can stop live vaccines from working. For example, in case of Gumboro disease, it is not desirable to vaccinate the birds in the face of high maternal antibody. So monitoring of maternal antibody level is important to decide the age of birds for a particular vaccine in a flock. For measuring maternal antibody level, 20 day-old chicks may be sacrificed. However, sometimes vaccines are given irrespective of maternal antibody level. The possible reasons for such use are (a) when early exposure to the disease is anticipated, or (b) when maternal antibodies may not give reliable protection, as is seen in case of infectious bronchitis, or (c) maternal antibodies may help to reduce reaction after a live vaccination.

iv. The genetic type of the birds is also a considerable factor that govern vaccination schedule.

v. Experts' comment for developing vaccination schedule is very much important. It should not be compromised.

vi. The farms where all-in all-out system of rearing is followed, the vaccination schedule may be simple. But, if multistage rearing with different age groups of birds is followed in the farm, the vaccination schedule should be followed more strictly.

13.2.5 Pre- and Post-Vaccination Cares

i. Vaccines should be procured only from reliable sources. Quality and standard of vaccine should not be compromised at any cost.

ii. Cold chain of the vaccine should be maintained properly. The vaccines are to be stored under refrigeration until use at the temperature of 2 °C to 8 °C, if otherwise not instructed by the manufacturer.

iii. Proper vaccination schedule including accurate dose of vaccines and proper age of birds are to be followed preferably as recommended by the manufacturer.

iv. Expired vaccines and left-over vaccines should never be used. The left-over vaccines and the used vaccine vials should be disposed off properly.

v. It is desirable to vaccinate the birds during the cooler part of the day, i.e. either in the early morning or in the late evening especially in summer months.

vi. Vaccination must not be done to the sick birds. Only healthy birds are to be vaccinated at their recommended ages.

vii. It is desirable to provide a dose of anthelmintic drug (against worm infestation, if any) at least a week before the vaccination to overcome reaction, if any. Medication with antistress vitamin before and after vaccination is beneficial for better response or to reduce vaccine-induced stress.

viii. For vaccination through drinking water, birds are to be kept thirsty for a few hours before giving vaccine containing water. Clean and cold drinking water should be used for this purpose and it should be free from chlorine or any other water sanitiser.

ix. Minimum 5 days gap should be there between two vaccinations. It takes few days before adequate immunity is obtained. So good hygiene and sanitation should be maintained in the farm.

x. Sterilised syringes and needles and other equipment should be utilised for vaccination purpose to reduce the chance of secondary infections.

xi. Reconstitution of vaccine should be done by following the manufacturer's instructions. Clean sterilised containers should be used for this purpose. Reconstituted vaccine should be kept in ice bucket and should be used within 1–2 hours.

xii. Vaccinated birds should be observed for any adverse reaction or abnormal behaviour, and they should be monitored for vaccination response.

13.3 DISINFECTION

Disinfection simply means killing of microorganisms. This procedure must be done to reduce the disease risk in poultry farm. The chemical used for this purpose is known as disinfectant.

Disinfection reduces the pathogens in the poultry farm, which thereby reduces the risk of disease. Disinfection involves two steps: Cleaning and applying a disinfectant. Always proper cleaning should be done first, followed by disinfection. If the area is not cleaned thoroughly, the disinfectant will not work. Disinfection is a very important aspect to maintain the sanitation and hygiene of the poultry farm.

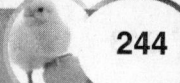
13.3.1   Routine Disinfection Work in a Poultry Farm

- Poultry house is to be cleaned daily to remove dirt, dust and filth, if any.
- The feeders and waterers are also to be cleaned daily before giving feeds and water in the morning. The feeders should be periodically scraped (once a week) to remove cakes of feeds, if any, in order to prevent fungal growth.
- Electric bulbs in the poultry shed should be cleaned once in a month.
- Cleaning is the prerequisite of disinfection, because presence of organic matter reduces the action of disinfectants. After proper cleaning of poultry houses and poultry equipments, *etc.* disinfectant is to be applied. Poultry house and its equipments should be thoroughly disinfected between the batches.

13.3.2   Steps of Disinfection

Step 1: Cleaning

- Remove all bedding, feed and manure.
- Sweep out loose dirt, cobwebs and other loose materials.
- Scrub all surfaces with a detergent or disinfectant cleaner. A high-power spray may be helpful for this purpose.
- Rinse away all detergent and organic matter (a high-power spray may be helpful).

Step 2: Applying a disinfectant

- Follow the directions on the disinfectant container, and use only the appropriate disinfectant.
- Disinfectants will not be as effective, if they are excessively diluted to cut costs, or if they are used improperly. Improper mixing decreases the effectiveness of the disinfectant and increases the probability of a disease outbreak.
- Allow the disinfectant to dry completely.
- Reapply the disinfectant second time and allow it to dry (optional).

After application of disinfectant (as per manufacturer's direction), rest is to be given for at least 2–3 weeks to break up the life cycle of disease producing organisms in the poultry house.

13.3.3   Types of Disinfectants, Indication, Mode of Action and Recommended Procedure

Disinfectants can be divided into many classes based on their chemical compositions. These are:

1. **Phenol:** It is a coal tar derivative having **carbolic acid** as base. This disinfectant has a characteristic pine tar odour and turns milky in water. It retains its more activities in the presence of organic matter than disinfectants containing iodine or chlorine. This disinfectant is effective against bacteria, fungi, and many viruses. It is generally used at a dilution of 1:1,000.
2. **Cresol and Lysol:** These disinfectants are commonly called as **phenyl**. These are most popular for general use. They are commonly used in footbaths and to sanitise hatcheries and equipments. They are used for washing of floor,

washing and dipping of shoes as 5% solution in water. These are not well-suited for using near eggs or chicks due to noxious gases. These are moderately expensive.

3. **Formaldehyde:** It is a very good disinfectant both in aqueous and gaseous forms. It is cheap and easily available in the market. It is available commercially as 40% solution of formaldehyde in water, which is known as formalin. It is very much effective against bacteria and fungi.

Formalin can be used in aqueous form by dissolving in water. It is widely used at 5% strength as a general disinfectant.

It is also used popularly for fumigation of brooder and hatchery along with potassium permanganate. Formaldehyde gas is liberated by action of formalin on $KMnO_4$. Gas should be allowed to remain for half an hour in the rooms, incubators, brooders, *etc*. The gas is very corrosive, and should not be inhaled by birds or human. Direct contact of formalin may cause burning of skin also.

For routine disinfection purpose 20 g $KMnO_4$ and 40 mL of formalin (40%) are required for 2.80 m^3 (100 ft^3) area. In case of disease outbreak and for disinfection of hatchery room, vehicles, *etc*. the concentration can be increased 2 to 3 times as needed. Nowadays the traditional use of formaldehyde fumigation is getting replaced by safer chemicals.

4. **Quaternary ammonium compounds:** These are effective against bacteria and partially effective against fungi and viruses. These are generally odourless, colourless, non-irritating, and deodorising. They also have some detergent action. However, their antibacterial activities are reduced in the presence of soap and soap residues and organic matter. They are non-irritating, non-corrosive and low toxicity. These are widely used in commercial hatcheries. Cost is low.

5. **Iodophors:** These compounds combine elemental iodone with a substance that increases its water solubility. These are effective against bacteria, fungi, and many viruses. They are commonly used to disinfect equipment, walls, and water. Their efficiencies are reduced in the presence of organic matter. It acts best at low pH (6 or below).

6. **Lime:** It is used for disinfection of litter, floor and poultry carcass @ 4–7 kg/100 sq ft. It generates heat, absorbs moisture, and liberates oxygen which destroys coccidia and eggs of parasites and even bacteria, and keeps fungi under control. A lime solution containing 38 parts lime and 15 parts sodium chloride may be used to disinfect wall and crevices in poultry sheds.

7. **Copper sulphate:** It is generally used to destroy fungi. A 0.5% solution is used to destroy fungi on poultry utensils and surrounding areas associated with outbreaks of fungal diseases.

8. **Bleaching powder:** It is also called chlorinated lime. A 20% solution of bleaching powder is used for disinfecting floor and poultry equipments (feeders, waterers, *etc*.). It has corrosive effect on skin and metals. Nowadays it is largely replaced by hypochlorites for disinfecting incubators, trays, brooders and waterers and feeders.

9. **Caustic soda (sodium hydroxide):** It is used as 2% solution for cleaning of waterers, feeders, metallic fittings, brooders, floor, *etc.* It is to be applied cautiously by gloved hands.

10. **Oxidising agents (hydrogen peroxide and potassium permanganate):** They have moderate to wide germicidal activity, having no sporocidal action. Efficacy is reduced due to presence of organic matter. These are moderately corrosive. Mainly used as a cleansing and deodorising agent. Cost is moderate.

11. **Natural agents:** These are effective against some microorganisms. Sunlight, heat, cold, and air can inhibit the growth of some microorganisms. The ultraviolet rays of sunlight are tremendously effective in killing micro-organisms. They are mainly helpful on the exterior of buildings. Fire in form of blow lamp is effective for disinfection of metallic fittings (poultry cages), floor, walls, *etc.*

12. **Commercial disinfectants:** Nowadays various commercial preparations are available in different trade names, which are mostly organic compounds. These are detailed in later part of this chapter under Poultry Drug Index section.

13.4 MEDICATION

Medication is a common practice in poultry rearing. Both preventive and therapeutic medications are in use for maintenance of poultry health.

13.4.1 Routes of Administration of Medicines and Vaccines

Different routes of administration of medicines and vaccines in poultry are:
1. Oculonasal route (drop into eye/nostril)
2. Oral route (in drinking water or in feed)
3. Aerosal route (spray)
4. Parenteral route (injection)

1. Oculonasal route (drop into eye/nostril)

Some medicines are applied through eye or nostril with the help of dropper. This intraocular/nasal route is generally used for application of vaccines at the early part of bird's life. General dose is 1 drop into eye/nostril.

This route is easy to apply and a satisfactory one. Several vaccines which can be applied through this route are available in the market, e.g. Ranikhet disease (F_1) vaccine, Gumboro vaccine, infectious bronchitis vaccine, *etc.*

2. Oral route (in drinking water or in feed)

Oral route is a very easy route of administration of medicines and vaccines, and commonly used. Various medicines that are commonly applied through feed are antioxidants and antibiotics, liver tonics, mineral mixtures, vitamin supplements, anticoccidial drugs, *etc.* For effective use of this route of administration of medicines, it must be kept in mind that the medicines should be well-mixed with feed. Some of these medicines can also be used through drinking water. In addition to this, various vaccines are commonly used through drinking water. However, the following points are to be kept in mind for application of vaccines through this route.

- Birds should be kept thirsty for 1–2 hours before application of vaccines in the drinking water. But, if water is withheld for too long period, birds may fight and splash the medicated water.
- The water should be free from chlorine or any other water sanitiser. Routine use of water sanitiser, if any, should be stopped at least for 24 hours before drinking water vaccination.
- Waterers must be thoroughly cleaned and washed with clean water to remove disinfectants, if any.
- It is better to add skim milk powder to water for vaccine administration (@ 5 g/L). The milk protects the vaccine against residues of disinfectants and adverse pH reaction. Pasteurised fat-free milk may also be used for this purpose (@ 30–50 mL milk/L of water). It is better not to use ordinary milk.
- Cold/chilled water is desirable for application of vaccine. Ice cubes may be added in the drinking water for this purpose. However, it should be ensured that ice cubes are prepared from borewell water having free of chemicals and sanitiser.
- In general the water requirement for drinking water vaccination is as follows:

Age (weeks)	Quantity of water (L/100 birds)
4–5	1.5
15–16	2.0–2.5
Adults	3.0–5.0

Vaccines which can be applied through oral route are available in the market, e.g. infectious bronchitis vaccine, Gumboro vaccine, Ranikhet disease vaccine, Avian encephalitis vaccine, *etc.*

3. Aerosol route (spray)

Vaccines may be used through aerosal route, i.e. by means of spraying within the poultry house when the air is still. Birds inhale the vaccine in the form of dust or spray. This is an easy and very effective method of vaccine administration. However, in small establishment use of this route is not common.

Vaccines which can be applied through this route are available in the market, e.g. Ranikhet disease (LaSota/F_1) vaccine.

4. Parenteral route (injection)

Some medicines and vaccines are applied through parenteral route, i.e. intramuscular injection (I/M) or subcutaneous injection (S/C), *etc.*

Marek's disease vaccine, fowl pox vaccine, egg drop syndrome vaccine, infectious coryza vaccine, Ranikhet disease (R_2B) vaccine are generally given by means of injection.

S/C injection is generally given at wing web or back of the neck, and I/M injection is generally given at thigh muscle.

13.4.2 Common Medication Schedule for Broiler Chicken

In addition to routine vaccination, preventive medication is also of value for proper growth and health maintenance in poultry (Table 13.4).

Table 13.4:   Preventive medication schedule for broiler chicken (0–42 days)

Age	Medicines/Vaccines
1st week	
Day 1	• Glucose—50 g, electrolyte powder—20 g and Zetress powder—0.5 g per 100 chicks • Marek's disease vaccine by intramuscular injection at thigh muscle at the recommended dose (this vaccine is generally given at the hatchery level.)
Day 2–4	• Vitamin in morning water and antibiotic in afternoon water [Vitamin: Bivinal liquid @ 10 mL and Recovit 5 mL per 100 chicks; Aitibiotic: Tetracycline water-soluble powder @ 2.5 g per 4.5 L of water]
Day 5–7	• Vitamin A and B complex in drinking water [Bivinal liquid @ 10 mL and Recovit 5 mL per 100 chicks] • At 5th or 6th or 7th day, RDF_1 vaccine through ocular or nasal drop [Ranikhet disease F_1 vaccine @ 1 drop in nose per bird]
2nd week	
Day 8–11	• No medicine/vaccine
Day 12–14	• Vitamins in drinking water [Bivinal liquid @ 10 mL and Recovit 5 mL per 100 chicks]
Day 12 or Day 13	• Gumboro/IBD vaccine through ocular drop or in drinking water at the recommended dose
3rd week	
Day 15–21	• Liver tonic in drinking water [Brotone @ 5 mL per 100 chicks in drinking water]
4th week	
Day 22–28	• Anticoccidial drugs. [Codrinal @ 1 g/L of drinking water for 100 chicks]
Day 21 or 22 or 23	RDF_1 vaccine (booster dose)—ocular drop or in drinking water
5th week	
Day 29–32	• Vitamins in drinking water and liver tonic in feed [Vitamin: Bivinal liquid @ 10 mL and Recovit 5 mL per 100 chicks. Liver tonic: Livol powder @ 5 g/kg of feed]
Day 33–35	• Liver tonic in drinking water or in feed [Brotone @ 10 mL per 100 chicks in drinking water, or Livol powder @ 7.5 g /kg of feed]
6th week	
Day 36–37	• Liver tonic in drinking water or in feed [Brotone @ 10 mL per 100 chicks in drinking water, or Livol powder @ 7.5 g /kg of feed]
Day 38–42	• No medicine/vaccine

Note: Broilers are marketed at the age of 42 days. The above medication schedule may be altered, if necessary, as per suggestion of a Poultry Specialist or a Veterinarian.

13.4.3 Deworming

A measure against endoparasitic (worm) infestation by using anthelmintic drugs is known as deworming. Roundworms are commonly seen for infesting poultry; however, tapeworms and flatworms may also be seen to infest the birds. The most common symptoms of worm infestation in poultry are unthriftiness in spite of increased feed intake, enlargement of abdomen, anaemia and appearance of worms in the droppings in case of excessive worm load.

Worm infestation is common under free range system as well as deep litter system of rearing, and rarely encountered in cage system of rearing. So in case of poultry keeping under free range system deworming is must and it should be repeated once in a month. In case of broiler farming deworming is not generally done as the birds are kept under sophisticated conditions only for 42 days or so. In case of layer farming and rearing of breeder birds, deworming is necessary irrespective of system of rearing as they are kept in the farm for longer duration of about 72 weeks or more. Grower birds are generally dewormed for one week before giving R2B vaccination at 8–10 weeks and again at 16–18 weeks of age. In case of adult birds the common practice is to deworm them once in a month under deep litter system and once in three months under cage rearing.

The common anthelmintic drugs used for deworming of poultry are piperazine, albendazole, fenbendazole, levamisole, etc. Antistress medicine may be used from the following day of deworming to combat deworming related stress.

[Commercial preparations of various anthelmintics are given in Poultry Drug Index section of this Chapter.]

13.5 BIOSECURITY

Biosecurity = Bio (Greek origin, means life) + Security (means protection). So the term 'Biosecurity' indicates protection of life. It is a set of management practices to reduce the risk of introducing and spreading diseases. It is the most efficient and cost effective method of disease prevention. The farm's performance is directly linked to good biosecurity measures. The fundamentals of biosecurity in poultry farm are outlined in this section.

13.5.1 Farm Fencing

Farm fencing is important for protection of farm as well as from biosecurity point of view. A buffer zone is to be established around the farm and perimeter fencing is to be used to keep people and other vectors out. It is better to use 'Biosecurity Area' and 'No Trespassing' signs at farm entrance. There should be provision of locks at gates, houses, and main entrance of the farm, if possible.

13.5.2 Disinfectant Pits

Disinfectant pit (i.e. footbath with disinfectant) is to be used at the entrance of poultry farm as well as at the entrance of each house to prevent the introduction of organisms by the movement of working personnel.

13.5.3　Personnel Management

All workers should be trained to maintain biosecurity measures. They should practice good sanitation. They should follow the following guidelines.

- They should always wear boots and coveralls on the farm.
- They should never wear hats and caps on the farm.
- They should clean footbaths daily, and fill them with fresh disinfectant. Footbaths are effective only if managed correctly.
- They should handle equipment carefully. All equipments should be cleaned and disinfected on a regular basis.
- They should not keep birds as pets including parrots, fighting cocks, or any type of backyard birds at their residence.
- Routine inspection of work areas and the entire farm should be carried out.

13.5.4　Restriction of Movement of Visitors and Vehicles

Unfortunately, visitors are one of the major causes of disease outbreaks. In an integrated poultry farm operation, many people move between poultry houses and farms. They are farm managers, supervisors, veterinarians, farm workers, electricians, feed truck drivers, and other similar visitors. It is better to keep their visits to a minimum. Visits should be planned for a reason, not as a pastime.

Casual visitors should not be allowed to enter the farm. They can transmit diseases from one farm to another via dust on hands, hair and clothing. Technical persons and some selected visitors/farmers should be asked to make use of footbath provided with disinfectant before entering in the farm and moving from one area of the farm to another.

All employees of the farm should be aware about how to handle outside visitors.

Traffic should be kept under strict control. In case of large establishment, a spray station may be installed for use on traffic entering and leaving the farm. In case of biosecurity control of feed trucks, it is must to disinfect all trucks entering the farm, not to allow the driver to leave the truck or wander around the farm, and to take a feed sample from each truckload for future reference in case of disease incidence or performance problems, if any.

13.5.5　Disposal of Poultry Wastes

Various poultry wastes are poultry droppings, dead birds, dressing waste and hatchery waste. Proper disposal of these poultry wastes is essential to prevent the spread of infections. The poultry farm wastes can be effectively used as a fertiliser, as an ingredient of ruminant feed, in fish pond and also for production of biogas.

- Poultry droppings are mixed with deep litter materials in the deep litter system of poultry rearing. This deep litter should be maintained properly and generally after rearing of each, a lot of birds in this deep litter should be removed from the poultry house before introduction of a lot of new birds. In case of cage system of rearing, poultry droppings should be removed daily or periodically as per the design of cages, and these may be collected in a manure pit and converted into high quality organic manure.

- The dead birds should be deeply buried in the soil or fully burnt in the incinerator. To ensure safety, dead bird disposal pits should be located away from the poultry house.
- The dry non-edible parts (dressing wastes) like feathers, feet, *etc.* should be burnt, and wet non-edible parts like digestive system, *etc.* should be dumped into deep manure pit.
- The common hatchery wastes are infertile eggs, dead embryos, eggshells and dead chicks, *etc.* These can be effectively converted into hatchery by-product meal. This hatchery by-product meal can be used as protein-rich feed item of poultry. During handling of hatchery wastes, care should be taken to avoid spread of infection. To overcome the strong objectionable odour from these wastes, chemical treatments may be required using gaseous sterilents like methyl bromide and ethylene oxide.

In India, the excreta of birds, in intensive system of management is used as fertiliser by the farmers for crop production and in aquaculture, and as of today there is no such problem of excreta disposal. Regarding waste from processing units of chicken, some of the units have got rendering plants which properly use the blood, feathers, intestines and other waste materials. Moreover, most of the poultry units in India are located in rural areas and as such do not cause several environmental problems. But considering the future global concerns over such issue, India will have to look into these matters more objectively and make plans to sort them out.

13.5.6 Control of Insects

Houseflies and mosquitoes are the common insects which may cause health problems to both birds and human beings. The insects may act as intermediate hosts or mechanical carriers of disease producing organisms. Marek's disease virus may harbour in insects from one generation to another generation. Tapeworms require an insect (like housefly, beetle, *etc.*) for their intermediate stages of development, and birds become infected by eating these insects. Common houseflies may carry caecal worm eggs. Fowl pox virus may be transmitted from one bird to other mechanically or by insect bite. Ranikhet disease virus may be found in adult flies and larvae during an outbreak of the disease. Botulism (caused by the toxin liberated by *Clostridium botulinum*) may be transmitted by the housefly larvae which feed on decaying dead bodies having the bacteria and its toxin, and birds get this infection by eating such larvae. Some mosquitoes may suck chicken blood. Fowl pox virus may be spread by several species of mosquitoes. So insect control is important to reduce the chance of such health problems of poultry.

Manure management is the most important control measure for insect control, as poultry manure is the breeding places of most of the insects. Manure should be kept in covered manure pits or it should be kept dry as far as possible, having less than 60% moisture. **Use of insecticides** for fly control is a very common method. Recommended insecticides can be applied as sprays. Spraying around the poultry shed should be done. It should also be done during cleaning of shed after disposal of birds. It is better to do spraying early in the morning or late in the evening when most of the flies will be resting during this period. Sometimes it may be needed to apply larvicide on the manure to kill the larvae present there. Butox liquid (Deltamethrin 12.5% solution, Intervet) may used as an effective insecticide @ 2 mL/L of water as spray.

13.5.7 Control of Rodents

Rats, mice and squirrels are commonly known as rodents. They hide and breed under the heaps of rubbish and unused equipment, *etc.* in the poultry farm and its surroundings. They act as reservoirs of some diseases. They themselves frequently infected with *Salmonella sp* and may transmit this organism to the birds. They contaminate the feed and litter materials with their faeces and urine. They contaminate the feed kept in the godown for the birds. They consume large quantity of feeds meant for the birds which increases feed cost and affects the FCR. A rat can consume 15–55 g of poultry feed daily, i.e. 200 rats can consume up to 11 kg feed daily and 10 times that amount of feed is contaminated by defaecating and urinating. They may attack the birds directly, especially the chicks, if their population is more in the premises. It is very difficult to remove rodents once they get entry in the premises. So rodent control should get special importance in poultry farming.

There are three methods of controlling rodents. These are rodentproof building, sanitation and rodent killing.

Rodentproof poultry shed is practically impossible, if it is operated under deep litter system of housing. However, feed godown may be constructed as rodent-proof. **Sanitation,** i.e. cleaning up of the poultry shed and its surrounding is an effective method of controlling rodents. Rodents do not like to move around in open areas. So all the rubbish and unused equipment, *etc.* should not be kept inside the premises.

Rodent killing can be done by baiting (putting rat poison at the places where they may live) and trapping. The common rodent killing agents are warfarin (multi-dose anticoagulant), bromadialone (single dose anticoagulant) or zinc phosphide (acute single dose anticoagulant). An alternative homemade rodent killing poison recipe is as follows:

1 cup of flour, 1 cup of sugar and 1 cup of baking soda (bicarbonate of soda). These are to be mixed together and to be placed in small bowls where rodent traffic is noticed. The soda will react with stomach acid and produce carbon dioxide gas to create stomach swellings and suffocates them by squashing the lungs. Cats and dogs do not normally eat the sugar and baking soda.

Rodent killing baits should be used with much precaution. Baits should be placed in the active burrows. To identify the active burrows, first day all the burrows are to be filled with soil or newspaper and very next day all the burrows are to be re-checked; and the burrows that have been reopened are considered as active and must be baited. Rodent control programme should be in operation continuously to keep the poultry shed rodent-free.

13.5.8 Poultry Welfare and Behaviour

Nowadays poultry welfare is an important consideration. According to the Prevention of Cruelty to Animals Act 1960, Government of India, amended in 2001, emphasis is given on transport of poultry. According to this Act, animal welfare measures should be complied during production at the farm as well as during distribution in the market.

General guidelines for poultry welfare (as per DEFRA, France; FAWC, UK) are five freedoms. These are:

- Freedom from pain, injury and disease
- Freedom from hunger and thrust
- Freedom for comfort
- Freedom to express normal behaviour
- Freedom from fear and distress

13.5.9 Biosecurity Checklist

1. Keep cleaned cloth and smooth-soled rubber boots at the farm, and wear them in production areas.
2. Park your vehicle at least 100 ft away from the poultry production house. Use removable vehicle floormats in your vehicle. Disinfect the floormats daily.
3. Clean and disinfect all equipments when they move between houses.
4. Take shower (if available) when you arrive at the farm; put on clean clothing and smooth-soled boots. If you leave the farm and return, shower again and put on clean clothing.
5. Change the footbath solution at each house entrance daily. Always follow the instructions of manufacturers for use of the disinfectant.
6. Clean and disinfect all equipments going into poultry houses.
7. Clean and disinfect all equipments moved between poultry houses.
8. Clean and disinfect pump houses and shower houses between flocks.
9. Follow directions to maintain effective rodent and insect control programmes.

13.6 POULTRY DRUG INDEX
(COMMONLY USED MEDICINES AND VACCINES FOR POULTRY)

This section deals with commercial medicines and vaccines available in the market and commonly used for maintenance of poultry health, along with their trade names, manufacturers, composition, indication, dose and route of administration, and pack. Medicines and vaccines are listed below as per their pharmacological groups or areas of activity.

A. List of Poultry Medicines

1. Antibiotics and other antibacterial agents (Page 254)
2. Anticoccidial drugs (Page 256)
3. Anthelmintics (dewormers) (Page 257)
4. Insecticides (ectoparasiticides) (Page 258)
5. Vitamin and mineral supplements (Page 259)

6. Liver tonics (Page 261)
7. Antistress medicines (Page 62)
8. Probiotics (Page 263)
9. Antifungal and toxin binders (Page 264)
10. Enzymes (Page 265)
11. Antibiotic growth promoters (Page 266)
12. Antioxidants (Page 267)
13. Water sanitisers (Page 268)
14. Disinfectants (Page 269)

B. List of Poultry Vaccines

1. Ranikhet disease/Newcastle disease vaccine (Page 269)
2. Gumboro/Infectious bursal disease vaccine (Page 270)
3. Marek's disease vaccine (Page 271)
4. Fowl pox vaccine (Page 271)
5. Infectious bronchitis vaccine (Page 271)

13.6.1 Antibiotics and Other Antibacterial Agents

i. **Bactrisol Powder** (Alved)

Composition: Each g powder contains 100 mg Sulphadiazine and 20 mg Trimethoprim.

Indication: It is used as a strong broad spectrum antibacterial.

Dose and Administration: 1 g/L of drinking water for consecutive 5 days; and dose may be doubled in case of severe infection.

Pack: 50 g, 250 g and 1 kg

ii. **Cosumix Plus** (Ciba)

Composition: Each 100 g powder contains 10 g Sulphachloropyridazine and 2 g Trimethoprim.

Indication: It is used as a broad spectrum antibacterial.

Dose and Administration: For broilers—1 g/L of drinking water or 1 g/1.5 kg feed during 1–4 weeks of age; and 1 g/1–1.5 L of drinking water or 1 g/2.5 kg feed during 5–8 weeks of age.

For layers—1 g/L of drinking water or 1 g/2 kg feed during 1–8 weeks of age; and 1 g/1–1.5 L of drinking water or 1 g/2.5 kg feed during 9–20 weeks of age.

Pack: 10 g, 50 g and 250 g packets

iii. **Enrocin oral 10%** (Ranbaxy)

Enrodac-10 (Sarabhai zydus)

Enrovet liquid (Vets Farma)

Meriquin liquid (Wockhardt)

Quin intas liquid (Intas)

Composition: Each mL liquid contains 100 mg Enrofloxacin or 10% Enrofloxacin.

Indication: It is used as a broad spectrum antibiotic. It is effective against CRD, colibacillosis, infectious coryza, pasteurellosis, fowl typhoid, fowl paratyphoid and other bacterial infections.

Dose and Administration: Preventive dose—1 g/2 L of drinking water for consecutive 3–5 days.

Therapeutic dose—1 g/L of drinking water for consecutive 3–5 days

Pack: 100 mL, 500 mL, 1 L and 5 L

iv. **Gentamycin injection** (Alembic/Wockhardt)

Composition: Each mL injection contains 40 mg Gentamycin.

Indication: It is used to reduce the chick mortality. In some hatcheries this injection is given to the chicks before sending them to the market.

Dose and Administration: 0.2–0.4 mg I/M injection/day-old chick. After dissolving 1 mL Gentamycin injection in 495 mL of injectable water (distilled water), 0.5 mL reconstituted injection to each chick through intramuscular route.

Pack: 30 mL and 100 mL

v. **Neodox Forte** (Vetcare)

Composition: Each g powder contains 100 mg Neomycin and 100 mg Doxycycline.

Indication: It is used as a broad spectrum antibiotic. It is very effective against Salmonella, E coli, coryza, fowl cholera, CRD, etc.

Dose and Administration: Preventive dose—1 g/10 L of drinking water for consecutive 3–4 days (for 200 chicks); after 4 weeks it is to be repeated. It is used to reduce the chick mortality.

Therapeutic dose—1 g/3–5 L of drinking water for consecutive 4–5 days

Pack: 50 g

vi. **Tetracycline HCl water-soluble powder** (Intervet)

Composition: 100 g powder contains 5 g tetracycline hydrochloride.

Indication: Broad spectrum antibiotic

Dose and Administration: Preventive dose—2.5 g per 4.5 L of drinking water. Therapeutic dose—5 g per 4.5 L of drinking water. Medicated water is to be continued till 24 hours after disappearance of symptoms.

Pack: 100 g packet.

vii. **Vendox-vet DS** (Venky's)

Composition: 2.50% Doxycycline hydrochloride, water-soluble powder

Indication: Broad spectrum antibiotic, effective against most of the gram-positive and gram-negative bacteria, mycoplasma, Rickettsia, large virus, some protozoa and fungi.

Dose and Administration: Preventive dose—1st day: 1 g/L of drinking water, 2nd and 3rd days: ½ g/L of drinking water.

Therapeutic dose—dose is doubled than the preventive dose.

Pack: 100 g and 500 g

13.6.2 Anticoccidial Drugs

These drugs are used for treatment of coccidiosis, a dreadful protozoan disease of poultry. The drugs may be used routinely to prevent the disease.

   i. **Amprolium-soluble powder** (Merind)

      Composition: Each g contains 200 mg amprolium hydrochloride

      Indication: Prevention and treatment of coccidiosis

      Dose and Administration: Preventive dose—600 mg/L of drinking water for 5–7 days (only medicated water)

      Therapeutic dose—1.2–2.4 g/L of drinking water

      Pack: 30 g and 150 g packets

  ii. **Codrinal** (Intervet)

      Composition: Each g contains 0.55 g toluene-sulphonyl beta-methoxy ethyl urethane sodium, 0.05 g tetracycline hydrochloride, 0.375 g crystalline lactose and 0.025 g dried sodium bisulphite.

      Indication: Intestinal and caecal coccidiosis; it is also effective against fowl cholera, infectious coryza, pullorum disease and secondary bacterial infections associated with viral diseases.

      Dose and Administration: Preventive dose—1 g/L of drinking water

      Therapeutic dose—4 g/L of drinking water for consecutive 3–4 days.

      Pack: 20 g and 100 g packets

 iii. **Cocciwin** (Sarabhai zydus)

      Composition: Dinitro-O-toluamide 25%

      Indication: A potent anticoccidial drug. It also enhances general condition and growth, weight gain and feed conversion.

      Dose and Administration: Layer—1 g/2–3 kg feed up to 8 weeks of age and 1 g/3–6 kg feed 9–14 weeks of age

      Broiler—1 g/2 kg of feed

      Pack: 1 kg cartons (250 g × 4)

  iv. **Esb$_3$** (Novartis)

      Composition: Each 100 g powder contains 30 g sulphachlorpyridazine sodium.

      Indication: It is effective against coccidiosis, fowl typhoid, fowl cholera, *etc.*

      Dose and Administration: Preventive dose—1 g/L of drinking water for consecutive 3 days. In case of layer birds, it is used in 3rd and 5th weeks of age and few days before egg laying starts.

      Therapeutic dose—2 g/L of drinking water for consecutive 4–5 days

      Pack: 50 g and 100 g packets

   v. **Sulphadimidine 16% Solution** (Pfizer/Ar-Ex)

      Composition: Sulphadimidine 16%

      Indication: It is used against coccidiosis and other bacterial infections.

      Dose and Administration: 7.5 mL/L of drinking water for consecutive 4 days.

      Pack: 100 mL

13.6.3   Anthelmintics (Dewormers)

i. **Albomar suspension 2.5% w/v** (Glaxo)
Composition: 2.5% solution of albendazole, a benzimidazole anthelmintic
Indication: Control and treatment of gastrointestinal and pulmonary nematodes, cestodes and trematodes. Commonly used in adult birds.
Dose and Administration: 30–45 mL in drinking water for 100 birds, only one dose
Pack: 30 mL, 60 mL and 500 mL

ii. **Almizol powder** (Alembic)
Helmonil powder (Alved)
Lemasol-P powder (Ranbaxy)
Composition: Levamisole hydrochloride 30% w/w, i.e. each g powder contains 300 mg Levamisole HCl, an imidothiazole anthelmintic.
Indication: Broad spectrum anthelmintic. Used for deworming as well as immunistimulation. It is active against benzimidazole resistant species also.
Dose and Administration: As anthelmintic—1 g in drinking water for 20 layers or 30 growers or 60 chicks, only one dose. Dose may be doubled in severe and multispecies infestation.
As immunostimulant—¼ th of the therapeutic dose, i.e. 1 g in drinking water for 80 layers or 120 growers or 240 chicks, for consecutive 3 days, then again for 3 days after a gap of 3 days.
Pack: 5 g, 100 g and 500 g

iii. **Niclex dispersible powder** (Alved)
Composition: Each g powder contains 750 mg Niclosamide, a salicylanilide anthelmintic.
Indication: Primarily used against tapeworms; also effective against amphistomes
Dose and Administration: 175 mg Niclosamide per kg body weight of bird. In general, 1 g powder per kg feed
Pack: 50 g

iv. **Panacur powder 250 mg/g** (Intervet)
Composition: Each g powder contains 250 mg Fenbendazole, a benzimidazole anthelmintic.
Indication: Broad spectrum anthelmintic; very effective against roundworms
Dose and Administration: 0.5 mL reconstituted solution (6 g powder in 100 mL drinking water) per 1.2 kg body weight, only one dose
Pack: 6 g, 60 g and 120 g

v. **Piperazine hexahydrate solution** (Merind)
Piperazine hexahydrate solution (Wockhardt)
Composition: Each 100 mL contains 46 g Piperazine hexahydrate which is equivalent to 18 g Piperazine base.
Indication: Control and treatment of gastrointestinal nematodes (roundworms). Commonly used in chicks.

Dose and Administration: 300–400 mg piperazine per kg body weight of bird, orally

Below 6 weeks—30 mL/3–5 L of drinking water for 100 birds

Above 6 weeks—60 mL/5–10 L of drinking water for 100 birds

Medicated water is to be used only for one day. It may be repeated once in a month.

Pack: 100 mL, 500 mL and 1 L

vi. **Zodex powder** (Concept)

Composition: Each 5 g powder contains 500 mg Mebendazole, a benzimidazole anthelmintic.

Indication: Effective against various gastrointestinal worms

Dose and Administration: 10 g per 50–75 birds, in drinking water or mixed with feed

Pack: 20 g, 100 g and 500 g

13.6.4 Insecticides (Ectoparasiticides)

i. **Almethrin** (Alved)—50 mL and 1 L

Butox (Intervet)—15 mL and 50 mL

Composition: Deltamethrin 12.5% solution

Indication: Ectoparasiticide, i.e. control and treatment of ectoparasites like lice, ticks, flies and mites

Dose and Administration: 1 mL/L of water for birds and 2 mL/L of water for houses and surrounding areas as spray

ii. **Flycid powder 1% w/w** (Glaxo)—10 kg

Larvadex powder (Novartis)—10 kg

Composition: Cyromazine (feed grade) 1% and inert ingredients 99%

Indication: Feed premix for control of fly in layer and breeder farms. It actually inhibits the moulting of fly larvae (maggots), retards growth and prevents pupation leading to larval death. It is ineffective against adult flies.

Dose and Administration: 500 g per tonne of feed for 4–6 weeks

iii. **Clinar liquid** (Glaxo)—5 mL, 15 mL, 50 mL and 1 L

Cyperin 100 EC (Wockhardt)—15 mL and 50 mL

Indocard (Vets Farma)—15 mL and 50 mL

Tikkil (Indian Immunologicals)—15 mL and 50 mL

Tikout (Alembic)—15 mL, 50 mL and 1 L

Composition: Cypermethrin 10% w/v, i.e. each 100 mL liquid contains 100 g Cypermethrin

Indication: Ectoparasiticide, i.e. control and treatment of ectoparasites like lice, ticks, flies and mites

Dose and Administration: 1 mL/L of water for spray; 60 L of spray mixture per 1,000 birds

13.6.5 Vitamin and Mineral Supplements

Poultry birds get vitamins and minerals from various energy-rich and protein-rich feed ingredients. Limestone, dicalcium phosphate (DCP), defluorinated rock phosphate, common salt, oyster shell, *etc.* are regarded as source of minerals for poultry. However, vitamin and mineral mixtures are mixed in concentrate feed of poultry. Besides, the vitamin and mineral mixtures may be used as such in feed or water as and when needed for continuously 5–7 days. These are used to prevent deficiency diseases, and to promote growth and production. Some trade names of vitamins and minerals along with dose, and administration are presented below.

i. **Avivita** (Cadila)
   Composition: Vitamins A, B_2, D_3 and K
   Dose and Administration: 10 g per quintal feed
   Pack: 100 g, 500 g and 1 kg

ii. **B-care Plus** (Vetcare)
   Composition: Vitamins B complex and E and folic acid
   Dose and Administration: 20–40 g per quintal feed
   Pack: 1 kg

iii. **Rovimix AB_2D_3 Feed Supplement** (Roche)
   Composition: Vitamins A, B_2 and D_3
   Dose and Administration: 20–25 g per quintal feed
   Pack: 1 kg

iv. **Meriplex Feed Supplement** (Merind)
   Composition: Vitamins B complex and E
   Dose and Administration: 20 g per quintal feed
   Pack: 1 kg

v. **Recovit** (Brihans)
   Composition: Vitamins A, D, E, C and B_{12}
   Dose and Administration: Chicks—1–2 mL, grower and broiler—2–3 mL and layer—4–5 mL per 100 birds
   Pack: 30 mL, 120 mL, 500 mL and 1 L

vi. **Biostress Soluble Powder** (Alved)
   Composition: Vitamin C, electrolytes and dextrose
   Dose and Administration: 1 g/L of water
   Pack: 250 g

vii. **Choline 500 Feed Supplement** (Vetcare)
   Composition: Choline chloride
   Dose and Administration: 100 g per quintal feed
   Pack: 1 kg

viii. **Bivinal liquid** (Alembic)
   Composition: Vitamin B complex, methionine and lysine
   Dose and Administration: 10–20 mL per 100 birds in drinking water
   Pack: 500 mL and 5 L

ix. **Aries Mineral Mixture without salt** (Aries)
Composition: Mineral feed supplement for poultry
Dose and Administration: 2 kg per quintal feed or 2.8 g per 100 birds daily
Pack: 50 kg

x. **Farmcare—M M Feed Supplement** (Farmcare)
Composition: Mineral feed supplement (without salt) for poultry
Dose and Administration: 2 kg per quintal feed
Pack: 1 kg

xi. **Farmcare—T M Feed Supplement** (Farmcare)
Composition: Trace mineral feed supplement for poultry
Dose and Administration: 50–100 g per quintal feed
Pack: 1 kg

xii. **Eggmax Mineral Mixture** (Ethicare)
Composition: Mineral mixture with salt for poultry
Dose and Administration: 2 kg per quintal feed
Pack: 1 kg and 10 kg

xiii. **Vets Mineral Mixture** (Vets Farma)
Composition: Mineral mixture without salt for poultry
Dose and Administration: 2–3 kg per quintal feed
Pack: 25 kg and 50 kg

xiv. **Vets Trace Minerals** (Vets Farma)
Composition: Trace mineral mixture for poultry
Dose and Administration: 50 g per quintal feed
Pack: 1 kg and 25 kg

xv. **Poultrymin Feed Supplement** (Aries)
Composition: Calcium, phosphorus and trace minerals
Dose and Administration: 2 kg per quintal feed
Pack: 1 kg and 50 kg

xvi. **Supplemin Mineral Concentrates** (Sarabhai)
Composition: Calcium, phosphorus, salt and trace mineral mixture
Dose and Administration: 2 kg per quintal feed
Pack: 25 kg

xvii. **Supplevite-M** (Sarabhai)
Composition: Vitamins A, B complex, D_3, E and K and minerals
Dose and Administration: 250–500 g per quintal feed
Pack: 250 g, 1 kg and 2.5 kg

xviii. **Merimix Concentrates** (Merind)
Composition: Vitamins A, B complex, D_3, E and minerals
Dose and Administration: 250–500 g per quintal feed
Pack: 2.5 kg

xix. **Concimin Feed Supplement** (Concept)
Composition: Vitamins A, B_2, D_3, E and K and minerals
Dose and Administration: 200–500 g per quintal feed
Pack: 250 g, 1 kg and 5 kg

xx. **Vitamix-M Feed Supplement** (Pfizer)
Composition: Vitamins A, B_2 and D_3 and trace minerals
Dose and Administration: 250–500 g per quintal feed
Pack: 5 kg

xxi. **Vetmix-M Feed Supplement** (Vets Farma)
Composition: Vitamins A, B_2 and D_3 and trace minerals
Dose and Administration: 250–500 g per quintal feed
Pack: 5 kg

xxii. **Vetmix Forte Feed Supplement** (Vets Farma)
Composition: Vitamins A, B complex, D_3, E and K and minerals
Dose and Administration: 250–500 g per quintal feed
Pack: 250 g and 2.5 kg

xxiii. **Cal-D-Rubra** (Cadila)
Composition: Calcium, vitamins D_3 and B_{12}
Dose and Administration: 10–20 mL per 100 broiler birds daily for consecutive 10 days
Pack: 100 mL, 250 mL, 500 mL and 5 L

xxiv. **Ossopan Vet Granules** (TTK)
Composition: Calcium and phosphorus
Dose and Administration: For 100 broiler birds aged 2–4 weeks—10–25 g and for 100 broiler birds aged 5–8 weeks—15–20 g
Pack: 100 g

13.6.6   Liver Tonics

i. **Brotone** (Agrivet)
Composition: Fresh liver extract, yeast extract, and vitamins (B_{12}, cyano-cobalamine, thiamine, nicotinic acid)
Indication: Liver tonic; it acts as supportive treatment in loss of appetite, any liver problem, aflatoxicosis, fatty liver syndrome, *etc*. It improves digestion, and enhances growth, FCR and productivity.
Dose and Administration: Broilers—5–10 mL per 100 birds daily at least for 10 days. Grower and layer—20 mL per 100 birds daily at least for 10 days. Good result is obtained, if it is used at 3 months interval in layer birds.
Pack: 120 mL and 500 mL

ii. **Liv-52 Protec Liquid** (Himalaya Drugs)
Composition: Herbal liver tonic
Indication: Liver tonic; it acts as supportive treatment in loss of appetite, any liver problem, aflatoxicosis, fatty liver syndrome, ascities, *etc*. It may be used during deworming medication.

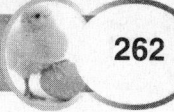
Dose and Administration: For 100 birds daily in drinking water, chicks—5 mL, grower—10 mL and layer and broiler finishers—20 mL.
Pack: 110 mL, 220 mL, 1 L and 5 L

iii. **Livol powder** (Indian Herbs)
Composition: Herbal liver tonic
Indication: Liver tonic; it acts as supportive treatment in loss of appetite, any liver problem, aflatoxicosis, fatty liver syndrome, ascities, *etc.* It may be used during deworming medication.
Dose and Administration: 5 g per kg feed for consecutive 10 days
Pack: 100 g and 1 kg

iv. **Upliv-Forte** (Venky's)
Composition: Fresh liver extract, yeast extract, and vitamin B complex, manganese, zinc, lysine and methionine.
Indication: Liver tonic; it acts as supportive treatment in loss of appetite, any liver problem. It improves digestion, and enhances growth, FCR and productivity.
Dose and Administration: 15–20 mL daily per 100 birds in drinking water
Pack: 1 L and 5 L

v. **Zigbir** (Natural Remedies)
Composition: Herbal liver tonic
Indication: Liver tonic; it acts as supportive treatment in loss of appetite, and improves digestion, enhances growth, FCR and productivity.
Dose and Administration: 25 g per 100 kg feed. It can be used for lifelong for broilers as well as layers.
Pack: 1 kg and 10 kg

13.6.7 Antistress Medicines

Transfer of birds from one farm to another, vaccination, debeaking, deworming, hot or cold weather, *etc.* may produce stress to birds. Diarrhoea and enteritis lead to dehydration and stress. Use of antistress medicines in such conditions is beneficial. It is also beneficial to improve general and specific immune status and to enhance overall health and productivity.

i. **Agrilyte** (Agrivet)
Composition: Electrolytes and vitamin C
Dose and Administration: 100 g for 1,000 chicks or 500 growers or 250 layers in drinking water
Pack: 100 g and 500 g

ii. **Stresroak** (Dabur)
Composition: Herbal antistress and performance enhancer
Dose and Administration: 5 mL per 100 chicks, 7.5 mL per 100 growers and 10 mL per 100 broiler finishers or layers. It is used in drinking water once daily.
Pack: 500 mL and 2 L

iii. **Stresvel** (Venky's)
   Composition: Vitamins A, D_3, E and C
   Dose and Administration: 1–2 mL per 100 chicks and 3–5 mL per 100 broilers or layers. It is used in drinking water once daily for 5–7 days.
   Pack: 100 mL, 500 mL and 1 L

iv. **Strexia** (Wockhardt)
   Composition: Electrolytes, dextrose, vitamin B complex and vitamin C.
   Dose and Administration: In general, 5 g in 4 L of drinking water for severe stress and 5 g in 8 L of drinking water for mild stress.
   Pack: 100 g

v. **Venlyte** (Venky's)
   Composition: Electrolytes, vitamin C and dextrose
   Dose and Administration: 1–2 g/L of water for 5 days or 200 g per tonne of feed
   Pack: 250 g and 1 kg

vi. **Zeetress** (Natural Remedies/Indian Herbs)
   Composition: Herbal antistress powder
   Dose and Administration: 0.5 g per 100 birds (broiler or layer) up to 4 weeks of age and 1 g per 100 birds aged 5 weeks and more. It is used in drinking water once daily for 10 days.
   Pack: 10 g and 50 g

13.6.8 Probiotics

Probiotics increase the efficiency of digestive system and ultimately help in weight gain, FCR and egg production of birds. Such medicines give good results, if used in diarrhoea and indigestion. Probiotics also prevent bacterial infections, drug resistance and stress.

i. **Bioboost powder** (Lyka)
   Composition: Live yeast culture, live *Lactobacillus sporogenes* culture, amino acids and liver extract
   Dose and Administration: 1–1.5 kg per tonne of feed
   Pack: 100 g and 1 kg

ii. **Biovet-YC Feed Supplement** (Wockhardt)
   Composition: Each kg contains *Lactobacillus sporogenes* 7500 million CFU, *Lactobacillus acidophilus* 30,000 million CFU, live yeast culture *Saccharomyces cerevisiae* (SC-47) 1,25,000 million CFU, α-amylase 5 g, seaweed extract 100 g, excipients qs.
   Dose and Administration: Chicks, growers and broilers—50 g per 100 kg feed Layers and breeders—100 g per 100 kg feed
   Pack: 500 g and 1 kg

iii. **G-Probiotic powder** (Vetcare)
   Composition: Live yeast culture, *Lactobacillus acidophilus*, *Streptococcus faecium*, β-gluconase enzyme and liver extract.

Dose and Administration: Chicks, growers and broilers—50 g per 100 kg feed
Layers—100 g per 100 kg feed
Breeders—150 g per 100 kg feed
Pack: 500 g

iv. **Prosol Water-soluble Powder** (Intervet)

Composition: *Lactobacillus acidophilus, L casei, Bifidus, Streptococcus faecium* and vitamin C

Dose and Administration: 10 g per 500 birds. Use in first drinking water for minimum 7 days gives good result.
Pack: 100 g

v. **Protexin Soluble Powder** (Novartis)

Composition: Multistrain probiotics containing *Lactobacillus acidophilus, L plantarum, L bulgaricus, L casei, Streptococcus faecium, S thermophilus, Bifidobacterium bifidum, Torulopsis spp* and *Aspergillus oryzae.*

Dose and Administration: Chicks—1 g/L of drinking water for 5–7 days
Adults—1 g per 4 L of water for 5 days
Use in first drinking water in chicks for 5–7 days gives good result.
Pack: 100 g and 10 kg

13.6.9 Antifungal and Toxin Binders

These medicines are used to prevent the damages caused by fungi and their toxins (like aflatoxins) liberated in feed. Such medicines contain organic salts, charcoal, organic acids and some herbal materials.

i. **Toxorid Powder** (Wockhardt)

Composition: Hydrated sodium calcium aluminium silicates, activated charcoal, organic acids, herbal ingredients

Indication: Mold inhibitor and toxin binder; for better FCR and increased productivity (weight gain, eggs)

Dose and Administration: 100 g per quintal feed, if feed contains less than 15% moisture.
200 g per quintal feed, if feed contains more than 15% moisture.
Pack: 5 kg

ii. **Ban-Tox Powder** (Venky's)

Composition: Propionic acid, acetic acid, citric acid, 3-p-cymenol, potassium sorbate, propylene glycol, silicon dioxide, essential oil extracts, zeolites

Indication: Mold inhibitor and toxin binder; for better FCR and increased productivity (weight gain, eggs)

Dose and Administration: Like Toxorid Powder (given at Sl No. i above)
Pack: 5 kg and 25 kg

iii. **Check-O-Tox Powder** (Ranbaxy)

Composition: Organic acids, salts like propionates, benzoates, sorbates and acetates together with specially treated aluminosilicates.

Indication: Mold inhibitor and toxin binder; for better FCR and increased productivity (weight gain, eggs)

Dose and Administration: Like Toxorid Powder (given at Sl no. i above)

Pack: 1 kg and 25 kg

iv. **Toximar Powder** (Glaxo)

Composition: Natural hydrated sodium calcium aluminium silicates.

Indication: Mold inhibitor and toxin binder; for better FCR and increased productivity (weight gain, eggs)

Dose and Administration: Like Toxorid Powder (given at Sl no. i above)

Pack: 1 kg and 5 kg

v. **Toxiroak Powder** (Dabur)

Composition: A herbomineral toxin binder and neutraliser

Indication: Mold inhibitor and toxin binder for control of Mycotoxin in feed; for better FCR and increased productivity (weight gain, more eggs)

Dose and Administration: For prevention—125 g per quintal of feed. For treatment—250 g per quintal of feed. Dose may be doubled in severe cases.

Pack: 2.5 kg, 10 kg and 25 kg

vi. **UTTP-5 Powder** (Vetcare)

Composition: Buffered organic acids and specially treated hydrated sodium calcium aluminium silicates.

Indication: Mold inhibitor and toxin binder

Dose and Administration: 2.5 kg per tonne of feed, if moisture content of feed up to 15%, and 5 kg per tonne of feed if moisture content is more than 15%. It may be used up to 10 kg per tonne of feed, if needed.

Pack: 5 kg

13.6.10 Enzymes

i. **Alvizyme** (Alembic)

Composition: Each g contains cellulase 400 IU, hemicellulase 300 IU, amylase 2000 IU, protease 2000 IU, pectinase 350 IU, xylanase 2000 IU and phytase 450 IU.

Indication: It improves energy utilisation of feedstuffs, improves absorption, decreases gut viscosity, improves quality of litter and reduces wet dropping and bad odour, and reduces faecal loss of phosphorus.

Dose and Administration: 500 g per tonne of feed

ii. **Anizyme Powder** (Zeus)

Composition: Endotryptase, maltase, zymase, invertase, lipase and Lactobacilli cultures

Indication: It improves digestibility and increases nutrient utilisation, improves quality of litter and reduces wet dropping and bad odour, improves FCR, egg production and egg quality, and helps in maximum assimilation of calcium and phosphorus.

Dose and Administration: Layers—300 g per tonne of feed
Broilers and Breeders—500 g per tonne of feed
Pack: 1 kg pouch and 15 kg jerry can

iii. **Caplix powder** (Wockhardt)
Composition: Cellulase, amylase, protease, pectinase, xylanase, phytase, arabinase, lipase, α-galactosidase and β-glucosidase.
Indication: It improves nutrient utilisation of feedstuffs, improves quality of litter and reduces wet dropping and bad odour, reduces faecal loss of phosphorus, reduces the undesirable effects of non-starch polysaccharides.
Dose and Administration: 500 g per tonne of feed
Pack: 5 kg

iv. **Natuzyme powder** (Novartis)
Composition: Cellulase, α-amylase, protease, pectinase, xylanase, phytase, β-glucosidase, hemicellulase, amyloglycosidase, pentosanase and phyton activities
Indication: It improves digestibility and increases nutrient availability, improves quality of litter and reduces wet dropping and bad odour, reduces faecal loss of phosphorus, decreases fat storage in broilers, inactivates mycotoxins in feed, *etc.*
Dose and Administration: 500 g per tonne of feed
Pack: 20 kg

v. **Nutrizyme-P powder** (Vetcare)
Composition: Phytase enzyme derived from *Aspergillus spp*, phytase complexes of minerals, proteins and amino acids.
Indication: It releases phytate-bound minerals, proteins, amino acids and starch, replaces effectively dicalcium phosphate, and improves FCR, laying performance and egg quality.
Dose and Administration: 1 kg per tonne of feed
Pack: 1 kg

13.6.11 Antibiotic Growth Promoters

i. **Albac 15% Granulated Powder** (Ranbaxy)
Composition: Each kg contains Bacitracin 150 g and Zinc 7.5 g.
Indication: It improves absorption of feed nutrients, improves FCR in broilers and egg production in layers.
Dose and Administration: 333 g per tonne of feed
Pack: 25 kg

ii. **Althrocin FS Powder** (Alembic)
Composition: Each g contains Erythromycin thiocyanate equivalent to 20 mg erythromycin base, excipients qs.
Indication: Growth promoter. It improves absorption of feed nutrients, improves FCR in broilers and egg production in layers. It also acts as an antistress agent.

Dose and Administration: In high challenge area—1 kg per tonne of poultry feed; week a month programme (WAMP)—500 g per tonne of poultry feed; routine inclusion level (RIL)—250 g per tonne of poultry feed. As antistress agent—1–2 kg per tonne of feed.

Pack: 1 kg Lim bag × 25 units in HDPE drum

iii. **Furazolidone powder 22.4% w/w** (Venky's)—1 kg and 5 kg

Furazolidone powder 20% w/w (Wockhardt)—25 kg

Composition: Furazolidone

Indication: It is a gut acting antimicrobial growth promoter. It also reduces chick mortality and stress.

Dose and Administration: 250–500 g per tonne of feed

iv. **Laybro Mix powder** (Glaxo)

Composition: Each kg contains colistin sulphate 1g and doxycycline 10 g.

Indication: It improves weight gain, FCR and egg production.

Dose and Administration: Broiler and layers—0.5–1 kg per tonne of feed

Breeders—2 kg per tonne of feed for 7 days

Pack: 1 kg and 5 kg

v. **TM-100 Feed Supplement** (Pfizer)

Composition: Each kg contains oxytetracycline 100 g.

Indication: It improves growth rate, FCR and egg production.

Dose and Administration: Chicks—1 kg per tonne of feed. Broiler—500 mg per tonne of feed. Pullets (up to the onset of egg production)—100–500 g per tonne. Pullets (after the onset of egg production up to 1 month)—500 g–1 kg per tonne of feed. Layers—100–500 g per tonne of feed.

Pack: 5 kg

13.6.12 Antioxidants

These additives prevent oxidative rancidity of feed, thereby reduce the loss of fat-soluble vitamins and pigments in finished feeds, and also protect the same during feed mixing and storage.

i. **Ethoxicare** (Vetcare)

Composition: Santoquin having 66.6% technical ethoxiquin

Indication: Antioxidant

Dose and Administration: 188 g per tonne of feed

Pack: 1 kg, 5 kg and 20 kg

ii. **Proviguard** (Vetcare)

Composition: Ethoxiquin, butylated hydroxyanisole (BHA), citric acid and phosphoric acid

Indication: Antioxidant and metal chelator to prevent the oxidation of feed ingredients, premixes and finished feed.

Dose and Administration: 75 g per tonne of feed

Pack: 1 kg

13.6.13 Water Sanitisers

Water sanitiser is used to reduce the bacterial load of drinking water. During rainy season water quality is generally deteriorated, and demands the use of water sanitiser. Water sanitisers should not be used 24 hours before and after vaccination, if the vaccine is used through drinking water; as sanitisers reduce the efficacy of vaccine, sometimes making it completely ineffective.

i. **Aquatreat** (Harshvardhan's Lab)

   Composition: Lactic acid, citric acid, propionic acid and ammonium salt

   Indication: Water sanitiser + water acidifier. It ceases bacterial proliferation in water, such as E coli and Salmonella; stimulates activity of digestive enzymes and improves absorption of nutrients from the gut; and ultimately improves growth and feed conversion efficiency.

   Dose and Administration: 1–4 mL/10 L of drinking water

ii. **Avitech** (Avians)

   Composition: Chlorine dioxide

   Indication: It is a broad spectrum antibacterial. It exerts quick action and is effective at very low dose level. It is effective in a wide pH range.

   Dose and Administration: 1 mL in 10 L of drinking water. It can be used for disinfection of pipelines in 2% concentration for 15–30 minutes.

iii. **Bio-quat 20** (Venky's)

   Composition: Alkyl dimethyl benzyl ammonium chloride 20%

   Indication: It is an odourless disinfectant of high germicidal and bacteriostatic potency. It is recommended for disinfecting general poultry and farm premises, vehicles, coops, crates, utensils and tools. Used for sanitising eggshells and food-contact surfaces. It can be used as a substitute of chlorine for water sanitation.

   Dose and Administration: 1 mL in 40 L of drinking water as water sanitiser. Other uses are: Surface disinfection—4 mL/L of water; eggshell sanitising—1 mL/L of water, and food surface sanitising—1 mL/L of water.

iv. **Disclor** (Polchem)

   Composition: Sodium hypochlorite having more than 5% available chlorine

   Indication: Water sanitation

   Dose and Administration: 1 mL/10 L of drinking water

   Pack: 500 mL, 1 L and 5 L

v. **Sanodrink** (Fort Dodge)

   Composition: Various forms of ammonium chloride

   Indication: Water sanitation. It prevents growth of bacteria and algae in waterers and water lines. It is effective even in presence of organic matters. It reduces the cross contamination in water.

   Dose and Administration: 1 mL/10 L of drinking water

vi. **Sokrena-WS liquid** (Glaxo)

   Composition: Didecyl dimethyl ammonium chloride 7 g/100 mL

Indication: Water sanitiser. It prevents waterborne diseases of bacterial, viral and fungal origin.

Dose and Administration: 1 mL/10 L of drinking water

Pack: 100 mL, 500 mL and 5 L

vii. **Vigorox** (Malati Fine Chemicals)

Composition: Peracetic acid, acetic acid and hydrogen peroxide

Indication: Water sanitation, and cleaning of water pipelines and poultry shed.

Dose and Administration: For drinking water sanitation—1 mL/10 L of drinking water; for flushing of water pipelines—20 mL/L of water; and for cleaning of shed—10 mL/L of water.

13.6.14 Disinfectants

These medicines are used for disinfection (killing germs) of poultry farm and its surroundings, incubator and other equipment of the farm, office and store rooms, *etc.*

i. **Kohrsolin liquid** (Glaxo)

Composition: Gluteraldehyde, hexane and polymethyl urea derivative

Dose and Administration: It is used as spray.

Hatching eggs, incubator, hatcher and other equipment—5 mL/L of water

Poultry shed and surrounding areas—10 mL/L of water

Prevention of bacterial and fungal infection—30 mL/L of water

Pack: 100 mL, 500 mL and 5 L

ii. **Aldepol-AH** (Wockhardt)

Composition: Benzalkonium chloride, gluteraldehyde and formaldehyde

Dose and Administration: Like Kohrsolin liquid (given at Sl no. i above)

Pack: 1 L and 5 L

iii. **Protekt** (Venky's)

Composition: Benzalkonium chloride and gluteraldehyde

Dose and Administration: Like Kohrsolin liquid (given at Sl no. i above)

Pack: 5 L

13.6.15 Ranikhet Disease/Newcastle Disease Vaccine

i. **Ranikhet F Strain Vaccine** (Indovax)—100, 200, 500, 1,000 and 2,000 doses

NDV-F (Intervet)—100, 500, 1,000 and 2,000 doses

Dose and Administration: It is used at the age of 4–7 days of chicks. Dose is 1 drop in eye or nostril of each bird.

ii. **Ranikhet LaSota Strain Vaccine** (Indovax)—100, 200, 500, 1,000, 2,000 and 5,000 doses

NDV-LaSota (Intervet)—100, 500, 1,000, 2,000 and 5,000 doses

Dose and Administration:

Primary vaccination—

4–7 days—1 drop in eye or nostril

Booster dose—

21–28 days—in drinking water (100 doses in 2 L)

5–6 weeks—in drinking water (100 doses in 2 L)

8–10 weeks—in drinking water (100 doses in 3 L)

Good result will be obtained, if 3–4 g of skim milk is added into drinking water before mixing vaccine.

iii. **Ranikhet Mukteshwar Strain / R_2B Vaccine** (Indovax)—100, 400 and 1,000 doses

NDV-R_2B (Intervet)—100, 500, 1,000 doses

Newcastle disease vaccine living R_2B (Ventri)—200, 400 and 1,000 doses.

Dose and Administration: 0.5 mL per bird through S/C injection given at the wing web. It may be given through I/M route. This vaccine is generally given in layer and breeder birds.

Primary vaccine—8–10 weeks of age

Booster dose—16–18 weeks of age

iv. **Newcastle disease killed vaccine** (Ventri)—200, 400 and 1,000 doses

NDV-Killed (Intervet)—100 and 1,000 doses

Dose and Administration: 0.5 mL per bird through S/C or I/M injection. This vaccine is generally given in layer and breeder birds at the age of 16–18 weeks.

13.6.16 Gumboro/Infectious Bursal Disease Vaccine

i. **Gumboro vaccine Nobilis strain D-78** (Intervet)—1,000 and 2,500 doses

Dose and Administration: Primary vaccine at 14–21 days through nasal or ocular drop or in drinking water

ii. **Gumboro / IBD intermediate vaccine** (Intervet)—100, 500 and 1,000 doses

Dose and Administration:

Primary vaccine—0–3 days, 1 drop in eye or nostril

Booster dose—at 14–21 days of age in drinking water; 3–4 g skim milk is to be added per litre of water.

iii. **IBD vaccine MB intermediate strain** (Sarabhai zydus)—250, 500, 1,000, 2,000 and 5,000 doses

Dose and Administration: In case of broiler chicks first vaccine is given at 10–12 days of age, or at 4 days and then booster dose at 17–18 days. This vaccine is used through drinking water. 5 g skim milk or 50 mL liquid milk is to be added per litre of water (for 1,000 birds) for better result. It may be given by ocular drop method.

4 days of age—1,000 doses in 8 L of water + milk

10–12 days of age—1,000 doses in 10 L of water + milk

17–18 days of age—1,000 doses in 20 L of water + milk

iv. **IBDV Killed** (Intervet)—1,000 doses

Dose and Administration:

Chick—0.3 mL S/C or I/M injection

Layer—0.5 mL S/C or I/M injection

Primary vaccine (0.3 mL per bird) is given at 14 days of age and booster dose (0.5 mL per bird) at 16–18 weeks of age.

13.6.17 Marek's Disease Vaccine

i. **Marek's disease vaccine** (Intervet)—500 and 1,000 doses
   Marek's disease vaccine (Sarabhai zydus)—1000 and 2,000 doses
   Lyomarex (Glaxo)—1,000 doses
   These are cell culture vaccines, prepared with HVT-FC 126 strain.
   Dose and Administration: 0.2 mL per chick at the age of day 1, by S/C or I/M injection.

13.6.18 Fowl Pox Vaccine

i. **Fowl Pox vaccine** (Intervet)—200 and 500 doses
   Dose and Administration: 0.2 mL per chick by I/M injection
   Primary vaccine—6–8 weeks of age
   Booster dose—13 weeks of age

ii. **Fowl Pox vaccine** (Sarabhai zydus)—1,000 doses
   Dose and Administration: Chicks at the age of day 1—each dose with the help of needle applicator in the abdominal skin between two legs.
   18–20 weeks of age—each dose with the help of needle applicator at the wing web

13.6.19 Infectious Bronchitis Vaccine

i. **Avian Infectious Bronchitis Mass type vaccine, live** (Intervet)—200 doses
   Dose and Administration:
   Primary vaccine—at 21 days of age, 1 drop in eye or nostril
   Booster dose—at 6 weeks and 14 weeks of age, in drinking water

ii. **Bioral H 120 IB FL vaccine, live** (Glaxo)—200 doses
   Dose and Administration: This vaccine may be given to layer and breeder birds.
   Primary vaccine—at 28 days of age, 1 drop in eye or nostril per bird
   1st booster dose—at 9–10 weeks of age, in drinking water or spray method
   2nd booster dose (in breeders)—at 15–16 weeks of age, in drinking water or spray method

iii. **Infectious Bronchitis vaccine, live** (Sarabhai zydus)—1,000 and 2,000 doses
   This vaccine may be given to broiler, layer and breeder birds.
   Dose and Administration:
   Primary vaccine—at 1 day of age, 1 drop in eye or nostril
   Booster dose—at 10–18 days of age, in drinking water
   Revaccination—layers at 18–20 weeks of age and breeders at 4–5 weeks of age, in drinking water.
   5 g skim milk or 50 mL liquid milk is to be added per litre of water (for 1,000 birds) for better result. It may be used as spray in the poultry shed, if primary vaccination is already done.

EXERCISE

A. Objective Questions

i. **Indicate the correct answer by putting tick (√) mark (multiple choice).**

1. Pullorum disease of poultry is caused by
   - (a) Bacteria
   - (b) Virus
   - (c) Protozoa
   - (d) Fungi

2. Marek's disease of poultry is caused by
   - (a) Bacteria
   - (b) Virus
   - (c) Protozoa
   - (d) Fungi

3. Gumboro disease of poultry is caused by
   - (a) Bacteria
   - (b) Virus
   - (c) Protozoa
   - (d) Fungi

4. Marek's disease vaccine should be given at the age of
   - (a) 3 days
   - (b) 3 weeks
   - (c) 3 months
   - (d) 13 weeks

5. The vaccine commonly given to chicken at the age of 4–7 days is
   - (a) RDF_1
   - (b) RDR_2B
   - (c) Fowl pox
   - (d) IB

6. Broiler birds are commonly vaccinated against
   - (a) Marek's disease, Ranikhet disease and Gumboro disease.
   - (b) Ranikhet disease, Pullorum disease and Gumboro disease.
   - (c) Ranikhet disease, coccidiosis and fowl pox.
   - (d) Pullorum disease, infectious bursal disease and infectious bronchitis.

7. The first vaccine against Ranikhet Disease (RDF_1 type) should be given at the age of
   - (a) 1 week
   - (b) 3 weeks
   - (c) 5 weeks
   - (d) none of these

8. Star gazing appearance is caused due to deficiency of
   - (a) Vitamin D
   - (b) Vitamin E
   - (c) Vitamin B_1
   - (d) Vitamin B_2

9. Characteristic goose stepping appearance in chicken is due to the deficiency of
   - (a) Phosphorus
   - (b) Zinc
   - (c) Manganese
   - (d) Copper

10. Which of the following is essential for prevention of Perosis?
    - (a) Choline
    - (b) Manganese
    - (c) Biotin
    - (d) Both a and b

11. Which of the following is responsible for Crazy Chick Disease?
    - (a) Vitamin B_1
    - (b) Vitamin B_2
    - (c) Vitamin D_3
    - (d) Vitamin E

12. Use of anthelmintic drugs against endoparasitic infestation is known as
   - (a) Brooding
   - (b) Deworming
   - (c) Incubation
   - (d) Culling

13. Usually break of flock immunity occurs under which of the following conditions?
   - (a) High ambient temperature
   - (b) Average nutritional status of the flock
   - (c) Administration of booster dose of vaccine
   - (d) Worm infestation

14. Caecal Coccidiosis is caused by
   - (a) *E acervulina*
   - (b) *E necatrix*
   - (c) *E tenella*
   - (d) *E maxima*

15. *Argas persicuss,* an ectoparasite which affects poultry, is actually a
   - (a) Mite
   - (b) Tick
   - (c) Louse
   - (d) Flea

16. Coccidiosis is a dreadful poultry disease caused by
   - (a) Bacteria
   - (b) Virus
   - (c) Protozoa
   - (d) Fungi

17. Ethoxyquin is a/an
   - (a) Antioxidant
   - (b) Antibiotic
   - (c) Probiotic
   - (d) None of these

18. *Lactobacillus sporogenes* is used as a/an
   - (a) Antioxidant
   - (b) Antibiotic
   - (c) Probiotic
   - (d) Coccidiostat

19. Which of the following diseases are caused due to the deficiency of vitamin?
   1. Aflatoxicosis
   2. Star gazing appearance
   3. Chronic respiratory disease
   4. Curled toe paralysis

   Select the correct answer from the code below:
   - Code (a) 1 and 2 are correct
   - (b) 3 and 4 are correct
   - (c) 2 and 4 are correct
   - (d) 1 and 3 are correct

20. Which of the following diseases are caused by bacteria?
   1. Fowl typhoid
   2. Infectious bronchitis
   3. Pullorum disease
   4. Aflatoxicosis

   Select the correct answer from the code below:
   - Code (a) 1 and 2 are correct
   - (b) 1 and 4 are correct
   - (c) 1 and 3 are correct
   - (d) 2 and 3 are correct

21. Vaccination must be done within 1st week of age of poultry against which of the following diseases?
    1. Ranikhet disease
    2. Fowl pox
    3. Infectious bronchitis
    4. Marek's disease

    Select the correct answer from the code below:

    Code (a) 1 and 2 are correct
    (b) 1 and 3 are correct
    (c) 1 and 4 are correct
    (d) 2 and 3 are correct

22. Broiler birds are not generally vaccinated against
    1. Ranikhet disease
    2. Coccidiosis
    3. Gumboro disease
    4. Fowl pox

    Select the correct answer from the code below:

    Code (a) 2 and 3 are correct
    (b) 1 and 3 are correct
    (c) 2 and 4 are correct
    (d) 1 and 4 are correct

23. Match List I with List II and select the correct answer using the code given below the lists.

List I (Name of medicine)	List II (Used for)
A. Piperazine liquid	1. Worm infestation
B. Tetracycline HCl powder	2. Coccidiosis
C. Codrinal	3. Liver tonic
D. Brotone	4. Bacterial infection

    Code (a)

A	B	C	D
3	1	2	4

    (b)

A	B	C	D
2	4	1	3

    (c)

A	B	C	D
1	4	2	3

    (d)

A	B	C	D
1	2	4	3

24. Consider the following statements in relation to the diseases of poultry.
    1. Ranikhet disease is the most devastating disease of poultry in India.
    2. Coccidiosis is also known as bacillary white diarrhoea.
    3. Gumboro disease is an infectious disease caused by bacteria.
    4. Fowl pox vaccine must be given to the broiler chickens.

    Select the correct answer from the code below:

    Code (a) 1, 2, 3 and 4 are correct
    (b) 2, 3 and 4 are correct
    (c) 2, 3 and 4 are wrong
    (d) 1 and 4 are correct

25. Which of the following diseases are caused by virus?
    1. Newcastle disease
    2. Infectious bursal disease
    3. Bacillary white diarrhoea
    4. Star gazing disease

    Select the correct answer from the code below:

    Code (a) 1 and 2 are correct
    (b) 1, 2 and 4 are correct
    (c) 1, 2 and 3 are correct
    (d) 2 and 3 are correct

ii. Fill in the blanks.

1. Thin, shelled egg is due to the deficiency of _____ (vitamin).
2. Thin, shelled egg is due to the deficiency of mainly _____ (mineral).
3. 'Crazy chick disease' (Nutritional encephalomalacia) is due to the deficiency of _____.
4. 'Curled toe paralysis' is due to the deficiency of _____.
5. 'Star gazing appearance' is due to the deficiency of _____.
6. Slipped tendon (perosis) is due to the deficiency of _____ (vitamin).
7. Slipped tendon (perosis) is due to the deficiency of _____ (mineral).
8. _____ (disease) in chicken is caused due to the deficiency of Manganese in the diet.
9. Coccidiosis is a dreadful _____ disease of poultry (as per etiology).
10. Infectious bronchitis is a _____ disease of poultry (as per etiology).
11. *Aspergillus fumigatus* causes _____ in poultry.
12. Ranikhet disease is a _____ disease of poultry (as per etiology).
13. Marek's disease is a _____ disease of poultry (as per etiology).
14. BWD is a _____ disease of poultry (as per etiology).
15. CRD is caused by _____ (name the organism).
16. Pullorum disease is caused by _____ (name the organism).
17. Fowl typhoid is caused by _____ (name the organism).
18. Gumboro disease (IBD) is a _____ disease of poultry (as per etiology).
19. *Eimeria sp* causes _____ in poultry.
20. Pullorum disease is also called _____.
21. Gumboro disease is also called _____ (organism).
22. Fowl cholera is caused by _____ (name the organism).
23. Aspergillosis in poultry is also called _____.
24. *Aspergillus flavus* causes _____ in poultry.
25. First vaccination against Ranikhet disease is done at the age of _____ week(s).
26. Type of Ranikhet disease vaccine given at 1st week of age is _____.
27. Type of Ranikhet disease vaccine given at 8th week of age is _____.
28. Marek's disease vaccine is generally given at the age of _____.
29. Diets slightly deficient in _____ (vitamin) may cause a metabolic disorder of poultry known as 'fatty liver and kidney syndrome'.
30. The parasite _____ is the most common of all roundworms in poultry.
31. Ranikhet disease of poultry was first reported from _____ town in England by Doyle in the year 1926.

32. Ranikhet disease of poultry was first reported from _____ area in India by Edward in the year 1927.

33. In India, bird flu was recorded first time in the year _____ at _____ village under Nandurbar district of Maharashtra.

34. Marek's disease was first described by the Hungarian veterinarian _____ in 1907.

35. Gumboro disease was first reported from _____ district in Delaware state of USA, in 1962.

iii. Write True (T) or False (F) against each statement.

1. Coccidiosis is a dreadful viral disease of poultry.
2. Crazy chick disease (nutritional encephalomalacia) is due to the deficiency of vitamin B_1.
3. Curled toe paralysis is due to the deficiency of vitamin B_1.
4. Star gazing appearance is due to the deficiency of vitamin E.
5. Slipped tendon (Perosis) is due to the deficiency of vitamin D.
6. Thin-shelled egg is mainly due to the deficiency of protein in feed.
7. Gumboro disease (IBD) is a dreadful bacterial disease of poultry.
8. 'All-in all-out' system is helpful to prevent poultry diseases efficiently.
9. Bird flu is caused by the Avian Influenza virus subtype H_5N_1.
10. Formalin is available commercially as 40% solution of formaldehyde in water.

B. Subjective Questions

1. Classify poultry diseases with suitable examples. Name a disease of poultry which may be transmitted through the egg from the hen to the chick?

2. What are the symptoms of Ranikhet disease? Describe briefly the preventive measures.

3. Outline a programme for maintaining a healthy poultry flock in your farm.

4. Explain various measures you would adopt for prevention and control of parasitic infestations in poultry.

5. Name any two common bacterial diseases of poultry. Mention the causative agent in each case, their incubation period, age of affected birds, mode of transmission, symptoms and control measures.

6. Name any two common viral diseases of poultry. Mention the causative agent in each case, their incubation period, age of affected birds, mode of transmission, symptoms and control measures.

7. Write the vaccination schedule for broiler chickens. What precautions should be taken during vaccination of poultry?

8. Outline in chronological order, in a tabular form, the vaccination programme to be followed from 1-day of age to the end of laying in an egg type commercial poultry farm giving name of vaccine, the target disease, age at which vaccine is given, dose and mode of administration.

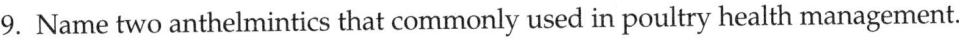

9. Name two anthelmintics that commonly used in poultry health management.

10. Name two coccidiostats.

11. Write the disease or symptoms associated with vitamin B_1 deficiency in poultry.

12. Write the disease or symptoms associated with manganese deficiency in poultry.

13. What do you mean by biosecurity? Discuss the biosecurity measures to be adopted in a commercial poultry farm for maintenance of flock health.

14. Write the cause, symptoms, and treatment and control of the following poultry diseases (any two).
    i. RD
    ii. BWD
    iii. Coccidiosis
    iv. Aflatoxicosis
    v. Bird flu

15. Write short notes on the following.
    (a) Factors that govern vaccination schedule in poultry
    (b) Pre- and post-vaccination cares in poultry
    (c) Administering medication through water and feed
    (d) Biosecurity in poultry farm

Answer of the Objective Questions

i. Multiple choice

1. (a) Bacteria   2. (b) Virus   3. (b) Virus

4. (a) 3 days   5. (a) RDF_1

6. (a) Marek's disease, Ranikhet disease and Gumboro disease

7. (a) 1 week   8. (c) Vitamin B_1 9. (b) Zinc

10. (d) Both a and b   11. (d) Vitamin E   12. (b) Deworming

13. (d) Worm infestation 14. (c) *E tenella*   15. (b) Tick

16. (c) Protozoa   17. (a) Antioxidant   18. (c) Probiotic

19. (c) 2 and 4 are correct   20. (c) 1 and 3 are correct

21. (c) 1 and 4 are correct   22. (c) 2 and 4 are correct

23. (c)   24. (c) 2, 3 and 4 are wrong

25. (a) 1 and 2 are correct

ii. Fill in the blanks

1. vitamin D   2. calcium/Ca   3. vitamin E

4. vitamin B_2/riboflavin 5. vitamin B_1/thiamin   6. choline

7. Manganese/Mn   8. Perosis/Slipped tendon

9. protozoan   10. viral

11. Brooder Pneumonia/Aspergillosis   12. viral

13. viral   14. bacterial   15. *Mycoplasma gallisepticum*

16. *Salmonella pullorum*   17. *Salmonella gallinarum*

18. viral   19. Coccidiosis

20. Bacillary white diarrhoea (BWD)

21. Infectious bursal disease (IBD)   22. *Pasteurella multocida*

23. Brooder pneumonia 24. Aflatoxicosis/Mycotoxicosis

25. first/one   26. F_1/LaSota strain   27. R_2B/Mukteswar strain

28. 0–3 days   29. Vitamin H/biotin   30. *Ascaridia galli*

31. Newcastle   32. Ranikhet   33. 2006, Navapur

34. Dr J Marek   35. Gumboro

iii. True or False

1. F   2. F   3. F   4. F   5. F

6. F   7. F   8. T   9. T   10. T

14

Hatchery Practices

14.1 INTRODUCTION

Nowadays hatching of eggs (i.e. production of baby chicks from fertile eggs) is taken as a business, and it is known as hatchery enterprise. The whole venture of hatchery enterprise includes procurement of fertile eggs, their hatching and finally selling of chicks to the poultry farmers.

14.2 FACTORS AFFECTING FERTILITY AND HATCHABILITY

Fertility and hatchability are mostly used synonymously and are expressed as the percentage of eggs that hatch from total number of eggs set. Sometimes hatchability is expressed as percentage in relation to number of fertile eggs set. (*See Chapter 4, Section 4.1.5*)

14.3 PRINCIPLES OF INCUBATION

The most important conditions for successful incubation or hatching of eggs are maintenance of optimum temperature and humidity, proper ventilation and turning of eggs. These conditions vary from one species of poultry to other.

i. Temperature

Temperature is extremely important during incubation. Variation of more than one degree from the optimum temperature will adversely affect the number of eggs that will successfully hatch. In case of hatching of chicken eggs the optimum temperature should be 37.5–37.7 °C.

ii. Humidity

Eggs lose water during the incubation period, and the rate of loss depends on the relative humidity maintained within the hatching chamber. Metabolic balance must be maintained throughout the incubation period. Thus deviation from optimum humidity will affect the number of successfully hatched eggs. Most of the poultry species including chicken require a relative humidity of 60 per cent until the eggs begin to pip, after which the relative humidity should be raised to 70 per cent.

Table 14.1: Relative humidity (%) for selected temperature readings

Wet bulb thermometer reading (°F)	Dry bulb thermometer reading (°F)			
	98	99	100	101
90	72	70	68	65
89	70	67	65	63
88	67	65	63	60
87	65	62	60	57
86	61	59	57	54
85	58	56	54	51
84	55	53	51	49
83	53	51	48	46
82	50	48	46	44
81	48	45	43	41
80	45	43	41	39

iii. Positioning and Turning of eggs

Eggs should be placed in the incubator with large end up for best results. However, a fairly good hatch can be obtained, if the eggs are placed on their sides. An extremely poor hatch will occur, if the eggs are placed in the incubator with small end up.

Turning of eggs is must for proper hatching. The yolk is less dense than the egg white. Therefore, the yolk floats to the top of the egg. Turning repositions the yolk and egg white, thereby keeping the yolk and the embryo from pressing against, and the embryo will not stick to the eggshell. Eggs should be turned at least 8 times during each 24-hour period. In large commercial incubator turning is mechanically done, controlled by automatic turning device, usually once in an hour. Turning should be continued until three days prior to hatching and or until the eggs have 'pipped'. After that turning has no effect on hatching.

iv. Ventilation

Developing embryo receives oxygen from the atmosphere and releases carbon dioxide. So the ventilation arrangement must be incorporated in the incubator. The more eggs in the incubator and the older the embryo, the more oxygen is required. The incubator should be placed in an area where fresh air containing 21% oxygen is available.

The operating details of the optimum conditions for artificial hatching of eggs of various poultry species, viz. chicken, duck and quail are depicted in Tables 14.2, 14.3 and 14.4.

Table 14.2: Optimum conditions for hatching of chicken eggs

Parameters	Conditions
	Hatching eggs
Weight	50–55 g
Storage	1–3 days (20–25 °C/68–77 °F), 4–7 days (15–17 °C/59–62.6 °F), 7–10 days (14–16 °C/57.2–60.8 °F), >10 days (10–12 °C/ 50–53.6 °F); RH 75–80%; positioning—air cell upwards.
	Setter conditions
Temperature	37.5–37.7 °C (99.5–99.8 °F) prevent fluctuation of temperature.
Humidity	28.3–30 °C (83–86 °F) wet bulb thermometer; maximum weight loss during incubation 12.6% from initial weight of egg.
Ventilation	Maximum CO_2 level 0.5%, fresh air supply 60–180 m³ per 1,000 eggs per hour.
Turning	45° *vice versa*. Common practice is once in every hour.
Candling	At day 7 and/or at transfer
Transfer	At day 18
	Hatcher conditions
Temperature	37.2–36.9 °C (99–98.5 °F)
Humidity	30–33.3 °C (86–92 °F) wet bulb thermometer; humidity is to be increased gradually when piping starts.
Turning	Not required
Hatching	21 days + hours to dry
Chick treatment	To keep the susceptible chicks free from drying out, cooling down and draught.

Table 14.3: Optimum conditions for hatching of duck eggs

Parameters	Conditions
	Hatching Eggs
Weight	65–70 g
Storage	1–3 days (20–25 °C/68–77 °F), 4–7 days (15–17 °C/59–62.6 °F), 7–10 days (14–16 °C/57.2–60.8 °F), >10 days (10–12 °C/50–53.6 °F); RH 75–80%; positioning—air cell upwards.
	Setter conditions
Temperature	37.2–37.5 °C (99.0–99.5 °F) prevent fluctuation of temperature.
Humidity	30.3–31 °C (86–88 °F) wet bulb thermometer; maximum weight loss during incubation 12.6% from initial weight of egg.
Ventilation	Maximum CO_2 level 0.5%, fresh air supply 60–180 m³ per 1,000 eggs per hour.
Turning	45° *vice versa*. Common practice is once in every hour.
Candling	At day 7 and/or at transfer
Transfer	At day 25

Contd.

Table 14.3: Optimum conditions for hatching of duck eggs *(Contd.)*

Parameters	Conditions
	Hatcher conditions
Temperature	37.0–37.2 °C (98.6–99.0 °F)
Humidity	31–35 °C (88–95 °F) wet bulb thermometer; humidity is to be increased gradually when piping starts.
Turning	Not required
Hatching	28 days + hours to dry
Duckling treatment	Keep the susceptible ducklings free from drying out, cooling down and draught. Keep them at 30 °C during the first day of their lives after taking out from the hatcher, and antistress medicines (glucose and electrolyte powder) may be provided in the drinking water.

Table 14.4: Optimum conditions for hatching of quail eggs

Parameters	Conditions
	Hatching eggs
Weight	10 g
Storage	1–10 days at 13–15 °C; RH 75%; positioning—air cell upwards.
	Setter conditions
Temperature	37.5–37.8 °C (99.5–100 °F) prevent fluctuation of temperature.
Humidity	30.3–31°C (86–88 °F) wet bulb thermometer; maximum weight loss during incubation 21.5% from initial weight of egg.
Ventilation	Maximum CO_2 level 0.5%, fresh air supply 60–180 m³ per 10,000 eggs per hour.
Turning	45° *vice versa*. Common practice is once in every hour, but once in every 3 hours is enough.
Candling	At day 7 and/or at transfer (but not done in practice)
Transfer	At day 14
	Hatcher conditions
Temperature	37.0–37.4 °C (98.6–99.3 °F)
Humidity	30–33.3 °C (86–92 °F) wet bulb thermometer
Turning	Not required
Hatching	17–18 days
Quail treatment	Keep the susceptible quails free from drying out, cooling down and draught. Keep them at 34–40 °C during the first 3 days of their lives after taking out from the hatcher, and decrease it then slowly to 24 °C at the end of second week. Antistress medicines (glucose and electrolyte powder) may be provided in the drinking water.

14.4 HATCHERY PRACTICES

The various activities of a hatchery right from the selection of hatching eggs to packing of chicks for marketing are detailed in this section.

14.4.1 Hatchery Equipment

The important hatchery equipments are incubator, egg trays, tray carts and racks, egg candler, table for traying eggs and chick boxes.

i. Incubator

Artificial incubation is done with the help of a machine called incubator (Fig. 6.3). Nowadays the incubator machine is available in two parts, viz. setter and hatcher. There are several types and models of incubating and hatching equipments available in the market today. The egg incubator may be operated by kerosene or electricity. However, presently kerosene incubator is not in use. The four basic functions of an incubator are:

a. Temperature control
b. Humidity control
c. Good ventilation, i.e. good airflow and circulation
d. Turning or rotating mechanism (hatchers do not have the turning/rotating mechanism)

There is a substantial investment in hatchery operation. So before purchasing the equipment, one has to view different models and their activities, and to get feedback on performance of the machines and after sale service of the company.

ii. Egg trays, tray carts and racks

These are used for handling of eggs for the hatching purposes.

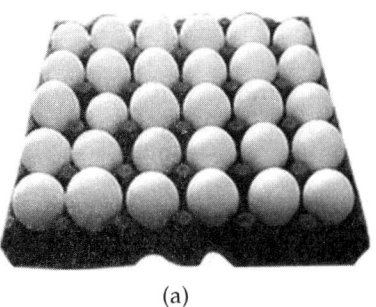 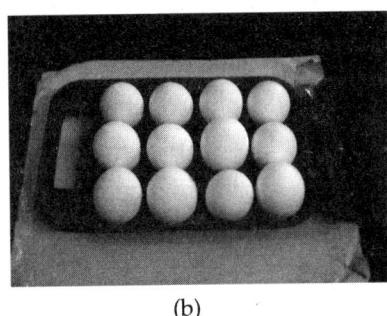

(a)   (b)

Fig. 14.1: Common egg trays
(a) 30 eggs capacity, (b) 12 eggs capacity

iii. Egg candler

It is used for candling (testing) of eggs during incubation to discard the infertile eggs and/or dead in shell, if any.

Egg candler is a wooden or metal box closed from all sides, but having an aperture of 2.5–3.0 cm in diameter, and one electric bulb is fitted inside the box.

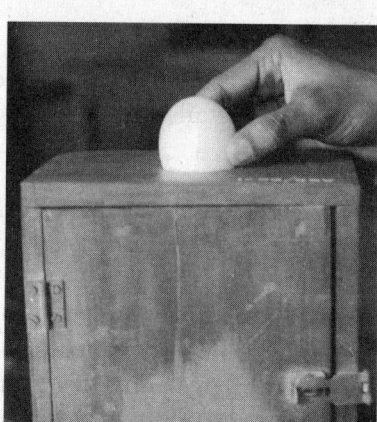

Fig. 14.2: Candler for testing of eggs

The egg is held in front of beam of light near the aperture of the candler for proper viewing of eggshell and egg contents. Porosity of eggshell, shape and size of air cell, shadow of yolk, soundness of shell, *etc.* are observed by candling of eggs. Fertile and/or infertile eggs can also be detected, if incubated eggs are candled properly on 5th to 7th days of incubation.

It is desirable to candle the eggs in darkroom.

iv. **Chick boxes** are used for packing of chicks for delivering the same to the poultry farmers.

14.4.2 Selection of Hatching Eggs

The following points are to be considered for selection of hatching eggs:

i. **Egg size:** Medium size eggs are preferred over too small or too large eggs for hatching purpose as they (later type) may create problems in setting in egg trays of the incubator and do not hatch properly.

Egg size depends on the species of poultry birds and accordingly the optimum size of hatching eggs of different poultry species may be different (Table 14.5).

Table 14.5: Optimum size of hatching eggs

Species of poultry	Egg size / Egg weight
Chicken	50–55 g
Duck	60–70 g
Quail	10 g
Turkey	80–85 g

The egg size is measured with the help of egg weighing balance. In poultry science, the terms egg size and egg weight are synonymous.

ii. **Egg shape:** The shape of hatching egg should be oval in case of chicken. Duck and turkey eggs may be less oval than chicken eggs.

Egg shape is generally known with the help of egg shape index.

$$\text{Egg shape Index} = \frac{\text{Width of egg (mm)}}{\text{Length of egg (mm)}} \times 100$$

Width and length of egg are measured with the help of slide caliper (Fig. 3.3). The optimum egg shape index of chicken egg is 74, duck egg 72 and quail egg 78.

iii. **Shell quality:** Eggshell should be clean, sound and unbroken for optimum hatchability.

Cleanliness of shell is very important. Soiled eggs should not be used for hatching purpose. The eggs with small dirt may be used after cleaning with the help of a sandpaper or rubbing with a cloth, but not with water. Because washing with water opens up the pores leading to more evaporation and poor hatching.

Egg with cracked shell is not suitable for hatching because they may be rotten during incubation. The soundness of egg shall be judged by tapping two eggs together. If there is resonant sound, the eggs will be sound. If there is a dull sound, one or both the eggs may be cracked. The cracked eggs are easily detected by candling also (Fig. 14.2).

Shell should be thick. Thin-shelled eggs are not suitable for hatching and should be discarded.

iv. **Shell colour:** The colour of eggshell is very characteristic to the species and breed of poultry birds. Chicken of Mediterranean class (e.g. White Leghorn, Minorca) always lays white-coloured egg, while chicken of other classes (e.g. Rhode Island Red, New Hampshire, Australorp, *etc.*) lay brown-shelled eggs. If the white-shelled eggs are used for hatching, they should be free from any tints. In case of brown-shelled eggs medium and dark brown colour is better than light brown.

v. **Interior quality of eggs:** Hatching eggs should have good quality albumin and yolk. Albumin should be clean and reasonably firm. Yolk should be fairly well-centred. Albumen and yolk should be free from blood and meat spots or any other defect.

vi. **Age of eggs:** Fresh eggs are best for optimizing hatchability. However, eggs of 3 days in hot weather and up to 7 days in cold weather may be used for hatching. In these cases eggs are to be stored properly.

vii. **Conditions of parent stock or breeding flock:** Parent stock should be well-nourished, disease free and healthy. Parent stock (both male breeder and layer) should be provided balanced ration; otherwise eggs produced for hatching purpose may be infertile and deficient in nutrients.

Parent stock should be disease free and healthy; otherwise eggs produced by them may spread disease. Eggborne diseases like chronic respiratory disease (CRD), PPLO (pleuropneumonia-like organism), *etc.* may spread from breeders to chicks through eggs. So hatching eggs should be collected from disease free stock.

Fertile eggs are must for hatching; and to obtain fertile eggs males should be kept with female birds. Usually one male for 10–12 females for broiler chicken is optimum for good fertility.

14.4.3 Handling and Care of Hatching Eggs

Careful and proper handling of hatching eggs is important to obtain maximum hatchability with viable and strong chicks.

i. **Collection of eggs**: Eggs are to be collected as frequently as possible from the poultry shed. In winter months eggs are to be collected at least three times a day and in summer months at least five times a day to avoid undue effect of weather on eggs, particularly on embryos within the eggs. Just after collection of eggs, these are to be set in incubator or stored properly.

ii. **Storage of eggs**: Prolonged storage of eggs leads to lower hatchability, longer incubation period and poorer chicks' quality. However, from practical point of view some storage is always necessary.

Hatching eggs may be stored for a maximum period of 7 days before incubation. However, storing of eggs for 3 days gives best result. If eggs are to be kept for 3 days, they may be stored in 18–30 °C temperature. Eggs may be stored in 16–17 °C temperature (below the physiological zero level) when they are to be kept for a period of 7 days. In some unavoidable circumstances, if the eggs are to be stored for more than 7 days, 10 °C (55 °F) storage temperature is suggested. Storage room should have a relative humidity of 75–80% and proper ventilation.

iii. **Positioning of eggs/placement of eggs**: Normally hatching eggs are kept in narrow end down position, *i.e.* broad end having air cell upwards position. This position probably helps to maintain the air cell in normal position and provides highest rate of hatchability.

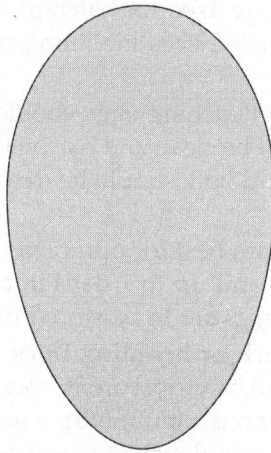

Fig. 14.3: Right position of egg with narrow end down

iv. **Turning of eggs**: There is no need of turning of eggs before incubation, if stored for a period of 7 days or less. Turning is must during incubation and, if stored for more than 7 days at the rate of at least 4 times a day.

v. **Transportation of eggs**: During transportation hatching eggs may be shaken or jarred. These eggs should be allowed to settle for about 24 hours before setting in incubator.

14.4.4 Management of Incubator

The following steps are to be followed properly for successful hatching of eggs.

i. **Cleaning and disinfection of incubator**

The incubator is to be cleaned thoroughly. The interior of the machine is to be washed with 4% solution of washing soda followed by disinfection with phenyl or lysol. Loose fittings of the machine are to be removed, and washed and disinfected separately, and be fitted at their respective places.

ii. **Fumigation**

The incubator is to be fumigated with formaldehyde gas [40% formalin on potassium permanganate $(KMnO_4)$].

Quantity required: 20 g $KMnO_4$ and 40 mL formalin for 100 ft³ area (1 × concentration) for 3–4 hours.

$KMnO_4$ crystals are to be taken in an enamel bowl and kept at the bottom of the incubator; then formalin is to be poured over it to liberate formaldehyde gas. The enamel bowl should have sufficient volumetric capacity to avoid overflowing during reaction.

Before fumigation thermometers are to be removed as during fumigation excessive heat generation may damage these sensitive parts of the incubators. Air inlet and outlet are to be closed properly to conserve the fumigated gas inside the incubator. However, it is to be ventilated properly before setting of eggs to remove traces of poisonous gas. Birds or humans to prevent fatal effects should not inhale the formaldehyde gas.

iii. **Testing of incubator**

Before actual setting of eggs, the incubator machine is to be tested for its various functions like maintaining desired temperature and humidity, turning of eggs and ventilation mechanism. The incubator is to be on for at least 24 hours to make sure that it is all right.

iv. **Actual management of the incubator**

- Adjusting the incubator for all functions according to the manufacturer's instructions and as per the requirements to a specific species of bird—like temperature, humidity (dry bulb and wet bulb thermometers), turning mechanism and ventilation.
- Placing of eggs: The selected eggs are to be placed in upright position, i.e. with broad end up position.
- All the principles are maintained automatically; so strong vigil is to be kept for mechanical fault, if any.
- After adjusting the incubator and setting of eggs, the machine should not be opened frequently to avoid interference in maintaining temperature and humidity in it.
- For maintaining humidity quantity of water in the respective containers is to be checked daily, and if needed, water is to be poured in the respective containers.

14.4.5 Testing of Incubated Eggs

Incubated eggs are tested by means of candling at two different times during incubation, viz. on 5–7th day of incubation (to discard the infertile egg, if any) and again on 18th day of incubation (to discard the dead-in-shell, if any and to maintain the business liaison in case of commercial hatchery).

On 5–7th day of incubation, spider-like red radiating lines can be seen in fertile eggs and movement of developing embryos is quite visible. At this stage infertile eggs will be clear like fresh eggs, but they have bigger air cell.

On 18th day of incubation, about two-third of the egg will show dark in appearance and a pulsating movement will be observable at the edge of the air cell in case of fertile eggs. Infertile eggs with dead embryos at this stage will be less developed.

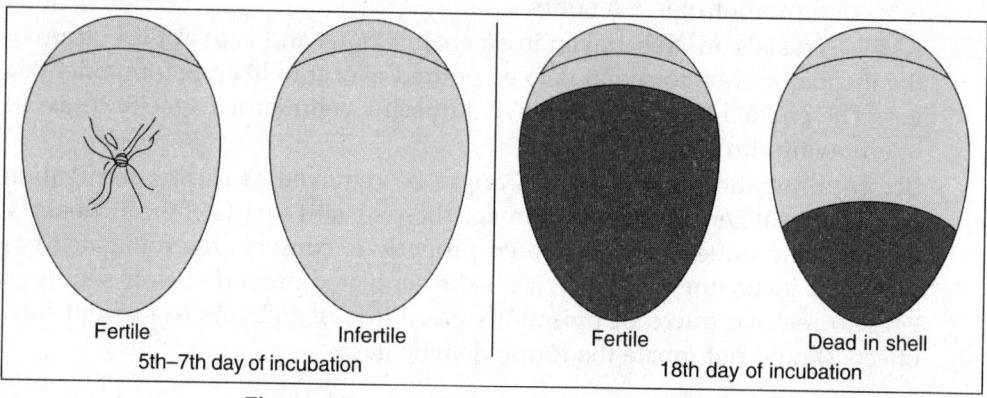

| Fertile | Infertile | | Fertile | Dead in shell |
| 5th–7th day of incubation | | | 18th day of incubation | |

Fig. 14.4: Testing of incubated eggs by candling

14.4.6 Sexing of Chicks

The method of segregation of male and female birds is called as sexing. It is a common practice and essential for breeder and layer chicks at day-old stage. The methods of chick sexing are described below.

i. Japanese method or vent method of sexing

This method was first developed in Japan and considered to be the most popular method of the recent time. The sexing is done on the basis of genital eminence of the day-old chicks.

Table 14.6: Male–female determination based on various characters

Sl no.	Characters	Male	Female
1.	Elasticity of genital eminence	More elastic	Less elastic
2.	Boundary and contour of the genital eminence	Distinct boundary and contour	No distinct boundary or contour
3.	Lusture and colour of eminence	Distinct lusture	Transparent appearance, colour does not differ from other part of cloaca.
4.	Difference in the position of eminence	Much more outside	Further inside

ii. **Proctoscope method**

Proctoscope is an optical instrument with an illuminated glass tip which is inserted into the chick's bowel through cloaca, enabling the sexer to view the testicle of the cockerel or the ovary (left) of the pullet.

iii. **Sex-linked characters**

    a. **Colour of plumage:** In this method sex-linked characters are used to identify the sexes of chicks. For example, when a Rhode Island Red male is mated to Barred Plymouth Rock female, all the female progenies will be black and male progenies barred.

    b. **Feather growth:** Slow-feathering and rapid-feathering genes are used in breeding programmes so that the sex of day-old chicks can be easily determined. Feather sexing is common in layer and broiler parent stocks.

14.4.7 Care of Newly Hatched Chicks, Their Grading, Packing and Dispatch

Care of newly hatched chicks

Chicks are required to be handled before they are delivered to the customers for sexing and grading, vaccination and packing (for proper transportation). These operations should be performed in hygienic and comfortable atmosphere having about 26 °C room temperature.

Properly hatched chicks do not require feed and water for first 72 hours as they have enough yolk in their abdominal cavity to take care of. However, to avoid risk and to give them a good start, efforts must be made to put them on feed and water as early as possible. Glucose and electrolyte water may be given to the chicks during this period.

The favourable temperature of the holding room for chicks should be 25 °C along with 70% relative humidity.

Grade standards for day-old chicks should be as follows:

Eggs should be obtained from flock certified free from Pullorum disease. Chicks should be free from all physical deformities. Physical defects or deformities means crossed beak, curled toes, lameness, having one or both eyes blind, *etc.* Chicks should be vigorous and healthy. The appropriate grade designation mark shall be labeled or stenciled on each chick box, carte or carton by the grading staff at each packing centre.

Packing of chicks

Chicks are commonly packed in chick boxes for sending them to the market. Chicks shall be packed in clean, dry and well-ventilated boxes of cardboard or any other suitable commercial packages. Boxes of cardboard used once shall not be used again for packing purposes. Plastic chick boxes are also coming in the market. These are to be washed and fumigated before reuse.

The size of chick box should be 60 cm × 45 cm × 12 cm for 80 chicks (as per Transport of Animals Amendment Rules, 2001, in Chapter VII: Transport of Poultry by Rail, Road and Air). The chick box is generally partitioned into four compartments. Season, distance to be traveled by chicks and mode of transportation should be considered for packing of chicks in the chick boxes.

Dispatch and transportation of chicks

This is the final stage of hatchery operation. Transporting birds is stressful for them. So every effort should be made to protect birds from the adverse effects of direct sunlight, radiant and reflected heat, wind and rain. The most common problem at this stage is overheating and lack of oxygen. To ensure the quality of chicks, they should not be overpacked, and sufficient holes should be there in the chick boxes. Vehicles carrying chicks should not be stopped under direct sunlight for an extended period. Air-conditioned vehicle is always preferable for transporting the chicks. Unnecessary transport of chicks must be avoided, and it is always desirable to use shortest possible route. Any transport that is required should be carried out safely and in a manner that minimises stress, pain and suffering.

As per the 'Transport of Animals (Amendment) Rules, 2001', the following points should be considered while transporting day-old chicks and poults by rail, road and air.

- Chicks and poults shall be packed and dispatched immediately after hatching and shall not be stored in boxes for any length of time before dispatch.
- Chicks and poults shall not be fed or watered before and during transportation.
- Every effort shall be made to ensure that chicks and poults arrive as quickly as possible at the dispatching site. The consignee shall be informed about the train, flight or road vehicles and its approximate time of arrival well in advance. Seventy-two hours shall be normally regarded as the maximum period to be taken from incubator to brooder in winter and 48 hours in summer.
- Personal attention shall be given by the forwarding agent or the consignor to ensure that all consignments are kept out of direct sunlight, heat and rain.
- Care shall be taken to carry the boxes at a leveled position so that chicks are not in danger of falling over onto their backs, and putting up of other merchandise over and around chick boxes shall be avoided. The boxes should be properly secured to avoid pilferage.
- Chicks shall not be transported continuously for more than 6 hours and whole batch shall be inspected on every 6 hours interval. The transportation shall not remain stationery for more than 30 minutes.
- All precautions against fire shall be taken and there shall be provision of fire extinguishers in transport.
- 'Care in Transit' words shall be tagged or printed on the chick boxes.

14.5   TROUBLESHOOTING HATCH FAILURE

Eggs can fail to hatch for many reasons. Among these are inadequate diet of the hen, incorrect environment within the incubator, and malposition of the embryo within the egg, *etc.* The probable causes and corrective measures of common problems encountered during artificial hatching are presented here.

Table 14.7: Common hatching problems, their causes and corrective measures

Sl no.	Problem	Probable causes	Corrective measures
1.	Early embryonic death (blood rings seen on candling)	Incubation temperature too high or too low	To check temperature and humidity control devices. To ensure proper electric supply in the incubator.
		Improper storage of eggs	Recommended egg storage conditions should be followed.
		Improper breeder nutrition	Balanced diet should be offered to the breeder stock.
		Improper fumigation	Fumigation recommendations should be followed.
2.	Many 'dead-in-shell'	Poor ventilation	To check the fresh air circulation in the incubator and hatchery room.
		Faulty turning of eggs	To maintain the turning schedule of eggs properly and seriously.
		Infection, e.g. BWD, *etc.* Ill-health of breeder stock including poor nutrition.	To maintain the hatchery hygiene. To maintain the disease free and well-nourished breeder stock.
3.	Chicks fully formed, but failing to hatch (pipped)	Low level of moisture in the incubator	To maintain the humidity requirement inside the machine.
		Improper setting of eggs causing malpositioned embryos	Set eggs with small end down. Turn eggs properly, but avoid turning within 3 days of hatching.
		Improper ventilation in incubator	Increase ventilation rate in incubator and/or room, but avoid drafts.
4.	Malformed chicks	Faulty setting of eggs	To set eggs properly with broad end up position.
		Faulty turning of eggs	To turn eggs properly as per schedule.
		Faulty incubation temperature (usually too high)	To check thermometer.
		Improper hatching trays	Use trays with wire floors
		Improper nutrition of breeder flock	Provide a well-balanced nutritional diet to the breeders.

Contd.

Table 14.7:   Common hatching problems, their causes and corrective measures
(Contd.)

Sl no.	Problem	Probable causes	Corrective measures
5.	Clear eggs with no embryonic development (infertile eggs)	Males undernourished	Recommended feeding programme should be followed to provide adequate nutrition. Underweight males should be replaced with vigorous ones.
		Too few males	Increase the number of males in the flock.
		Seasonal decline in fertility	Young cockerels, more resistant to environmental stress, should be used.
		Diseased flock	Conduct an approved disease control programme.
		Old males	Replace with younger males.
		Male sterility	Replace males in the pen/house.
		Crowded breeders	Provide recommended floor space, at least 3 ft²/bird.
		Eggs damaged by environment	Gather eggs frequently (at least once daily).
		Eggs stored too long or incorrectly	Store eggs at proper environmental conditions. Incubate eggs within 7 days of lay.
		Respiratory disease of breeder flock	Health status of breeder flock should be assured. A thorough clean up and disinfection of incubator and hatching facilities are needed.
6.	Early hatching	Improper storage of eggs	Proper egg storage conditions should be followed.
		High incubation temperature	Follow recommended incubation temperature. Check equipment for proper functions.
7.	Late hatching or not hatching uniformly	Low incubation temperature	Follow recommended incubation temperature.
		Old or improperly stored eggs	Collect eggs frequently, cool immediately and store eggs properly. Do not store for longer than 7 days in such cases.

Contd.

Table 14.7: Common hatching problems, their causes and corrective measures (Contd.)

Sl no.	Problem	Probable causes	Corrective measures
8.	Embryos sticking or adhering to shell	Low humidity (especially during the later part of hatching)	Increase incubation humidity by increasing water evaporation.
		Excessive ventilation rate	Reduce ventilation rate, but maintain minimum air exchange to prevent suffocation of embryos.
9.	Large, soft-bodied mushy chicks; dead on trays; bad odour	Low average incubation temperature	Follow recommended incubation temperature.
		Poor ventilation	Increase ventilation rate in incubator and/or room, but avoid drafts.
		Navel infection (omphalitis)	Incubator unit should be cleaned and disinfected between settings of eggs. Hatching trays to be kept dry. Storage and fumigation of eggs should be proper.
10.	Chicks with laboured breathing	Excessive fumigation	Follow recommended fumigation procedure.

14.6   DISPOSAL OF HATCHERY WASTE

The common hatchery wastes are infertile eggs, dead embryos, eggshells and dead chicks, *etc.* These are the primary sources of contamination in a hatchery. So these should be removed as early as possible after the hatch is finished. During handling of hatchery wastes, care should be taken to avoid spread of infection. To overcome the strong objectionable odour from these wastes, chemical treatments may be required. Gaseous sterilents like methyl bromide and ethylene oxide are commonly used chemicals for this purpose.

The hatchery wastes can be effectively converted into hatchery by-product meal. This hatchery by-product meal can be used as protein-rich feed item of poultry.

14.7   HATCHERY RECORDS

All the happenings in the hatchery should be recorded. In addition, all other information regarding egg source, hatchability, comments on unusual happenings, *etc.* should be recorded for technical study. The business records are also important for economic analysis of the hatchery business. The most common hatchery record format is given below.

Hatchery Record Format

Incubator	Date of setting eggs:	Date of candling 1st: 2nd:					Date of hatching
Sl no.	No. of eggs set and source	Infertile eggs	Dead in Shell	No. of chicks hatched	Hatchability (%)		Remarks
					On total eggs set	On fertile eggs set	

14.8   BIOSECURITY IN THE HATCHERY

The following biosecurity measures should be strictly followed at all times to prevent the introduction of infection to a hatchery site or transfer from one building to another.

Hatchery hygiene

Hatchery hygiene is very much essential. Thorough cleaning followed by disinfection of hatchery and its surroundings can reduce the microbial load in the hatchery. There is no substitute of this activity to prevent the occurrence of any disease. Mode of using disinfectants for various components of a hatchery is inscribed in Table 14.8.

Table 14.8:   Disinfectants for various components/operations in a hatchery

Sl no.	Components of hatchery to be disinfected	Types of disinfectant and mode of use	When to use
1.	Hatching eggs	Formaldehyde gas by fumigation	Before setting in incubator
2.	Storage and traying room (wall and floor)	Detergent—sanitiser and formalin—water aerosol	Weekly
3.	Setting room (wall and floor)	Detergent—sanitiser and formalin—water aerosol	Weekly
4.	Hatcher room (wall and floor)	Detergent—sanitiser and formalin—water aerosol	Weekly
5.	Dispatch room (wall and floor)	Detergent—sanitiser and formalin—water aerosol	Weekly

Contd.

Table 14.8: Disinfectants for various components/operations in a hatchery
(Contd.)

Sl no.	Components of hatchery to be disinfected	Types of disinfectant and mode of use	When to use
6.	Egg boxes and trays (plastic-made and reusable), egg graders	Detergent—sanitiser	Before and after use
7.	Setter (1st part of incubator)	Fog with iodophor	Before each setting
8.	Hatcher (2nd part of incubator)	Detergent—sanitiser and washing followed by formaldehyde fumigation	After each hatch
9.	Hatching trays	Detergent—sanitiser and washing with the help of power house clean	After each hatch
10.	Trolley and van	Detergent—sanitisers washing	Before use
11.	Operators	Should use apron, clean hand towel, medicated soap, hot water, footbath for shoes	As and when required, without any negligence.

NB: The details of disinfectants, their concentrations and recommended procedures are discussed in Chapter 13.

Use of disinfectant pits

All personnel and visitors must use disinfectant pits (footbaths), containing a broad spectrum disinfectant solution, on entering hatchery. The disinfectant solution should be changed daily.

Disinfection of vehicle and mobile equipment

Any vehicle entering the hatchery site must pass through a disinfectant vehicle spray using an appropriate disinfectant solution. The vehicle spray should be topped-up regularly to avoid dilution or contamination. Mobile equipment brought on to the site from other units must be washed and disinfected before being allowed to enter in the hatchery.

Handwashing

Dirty hands may transfer infection. All visitors must be required to wash their hands before entering. It is to be ensured that all staffs wash their hands when entering and leaving the production area, and before chick and egg handling operations (like traying up, setting, transfer, candling, take-off, sexing, vaccinating and packing).

Personnel and visitors

Care should be taken to ensure that all staffs and visitors follow the biosecurity measures, a 'shower-in, shower-out' policy should be put into place wherever possible, and suitable protective equipment and clothing should be issued to both personnel and visitors where appropriate.

Insect and rodent control

Insects and rodents may be responsible for the spread of a number of diseases, including Salmonella infection. It is to be ensured that an effective control programme is put in place against the insects and rodents in the hatchery.

14.9   ECONOMICS OF HATCHERY BUSINESS

Economics of any business is visualised through calculation of benefit-cost ratio and breakeven point. Benefit-cost ratio is the ratio between total gross receipts and total recurring expenditure for a specified period.

$$\text{Benefit-cost ratio} = \frac{\text{Gross receipts}}{\text{Total recurring expenditure}}$$

A value of less than 1 indicates that the enterprise has incurred losses, a value of 1 indicates no loss no profit, and a value higher than 1 indicates net profits, during that specified period. A sound enterprise should maintain a value of benefit-cost ratio of 1.2 and above. The breakeven point is the minimum level of output at which the business revenue is sufficient to cover its cost of production, otherwise a no profit no loss state.

Nowadays hatchery business is recognised as a profitable business. Hatchery may be of two types, viz.

i. Hatchery with parent stock where breeder birds are reared for production of hatching eggs (fertile eggs). It may be again of two types—broiler hatchery and layer hatchery.

ii. Hatchery without parent stock where breeder birds are not reared and eggs are procured from outside sources.

Technical specification of broiler hatchery

Technical details of broiler hatchery is depicted below, based on which economics of the hatchery can be calculated or project report can be prepared on the basis of local price of inputs and outputs.

- Types of parent stock—Hubbard, Vencob, Anak-2000, Pearl-bro Samrat, Starbro, Keggbro, *etc.* as per the local demand.
- Culling age—70 weeks.
- Batch interval—may be 26 weeks, i.e. 2 batches per year.
- Housing system—may be deep litter for chicks and growers, and cages for breeders.
- Chick-cum-grower house space—2 sq ft per bird under deep litter system.
- Breeder house space (including cages)—2 sq ft per bird.
- Breeder cage floor space for hen—135 sq inches per bird.
- Breeder cage floor space for cock—189 sq inches per bird.
- Mating technique—artificial insemination, freshly harvested undiluted semen will be used once in 5 days to get optimum fertility.

- Feed consumption per bird up to 24 weeks—12 kg per bird.
- Feed consumption during laying period (25–70 weeks)—58 kg per bird (180 g/bird/day).
- Mortality and culling during chick-cum-growing period (0–24 weeks)—10%.
- Mortality and culling during laying period (25–70 weeks)—12%.
- Total eggs per hen housed—190.
- Hatching eggs per hen housed—180.
- Saleable chicks per hen housed—150.
- Average manure produced per bird housed—50 kg.
- Empty feed bags for sale—1 saleable bag per 70 kg feed, and 70 kg feed required per bird.
- Depreciation of building and equipment—5% and 10% respectively.

For preparation of economics of broiler hatchery the following statements are to be made as per the above technical specification and local price of the inputs and output.

Statement I: Cost of land development, construction of building and other civil works. It includes land development, fencing, roads, brooder-cum-grower house, breeder house, feed mill (in case of large establishment for the production of own feeds), hatchery building, office and quarters for the farm and hatchery staffs (in case of large establishment).

Statement II: Cost of equipment. It includes chick-cum-grower house equipment, feeders and waterers, breeder cages, feed mill equipment, setter and hatcher, generator, chick delivery van, and office equipment, *etc.*

Statement III: Working capital. It includes cost of parent stock, feed cost, management cost including medicines, insurance, *etc.*, office and hatchery expenditure, *etc.*

Statement IV: Total project cost. It includes the cost of above three items.

Statement V: Annual recurring expenditure. It includes chick cost, feed cost, miscellaneous farm expenses, hatchery expenses, and office and marketing expenses.

Statement VI: Gross return, net profit and benefit-cost ratio. Receipts are coming from sale of chicks, sale of culled birds, sale of eggs unfit for hatching, sale of manure, and sale of feed bags. Based on the receipts yearly returns and profits can be calculated.

Statement VII: Bank loan repayment schedule. If the project is implemented by taking bank loan, it is also to be prepared.

14.10 COMPUTER APPLICATIONS FOR HATCHERY MANAGEMENT

Nowadays application of computer in various hatchery related activities is must, especially for large establishments. In breeder farm section of a hatchery, computer can be used for keeping records of individual stock for selection of next generation, least cost feed formulation by using unconventional feedstuff for the breeder stock, *etc.* In the hatchery section, computer helps to keep the records of eggs and chicks, hatchability, and all business records in relation to receiving of hatching eggs and selling of day-old chicks, *etc.* Besides, one can maintain a good business liaison with the help of a computer. Computer helps to save time and labour. Processing of hatching related data is easier with the help of computer for better interpretation and future planning.

14.11 COMMERCIAL HATCHERIES AND THEIR ROLES IN POULTRY DEVELOPMENT

Commercial hatcheries are engaged in hatching of eggs and supplying of chicks to the poultry farmers. They directly supply the chicks to the poultry farmers through their agents.

The important roles of commercial hatcheries in poultry development are:

  i.   Supply of high quality hybrid chicks
  ii. Providing technical service after sales to the poultry farmers
  iii. Providing laboratory disease diagnosis and feed analysis
  iv. Training of personnel
  v.   Marketing support

14.11.1 Supply of High Quality Hybrid Chicks

A lot of commercial hatcheries are doing researches for evolving high yielding broiler and layer varieties, as a result nowadays we have many such high yielding varieties of poultry (Table 14.9). They supply these high yielding varieties to the poultry farmers through their authorised agents. Starting of poultry farm with high quality birds is possible due to the constant efforts made by many of these commercial hatcheries.

Table 14.9: Few commercial hatcheries and their hybrid varieties in India

Sl no.	Hybrid chicks	Parent stock (foundation stock)
i.	BV-300 (white egg layer)	Venkateshwara Hatcheries Ltd, Pune (India)
	BV-380 (brown egg layer)	Do
ii.	Vencob*	Venco Research and Breeding Farms Ltd, Pune (India)
iii.	Starcross-288 (layer)	Ranishaver Hatcheries Ltd, New Delhi (India)
	Starbro*	Do
iv.	Keggbro*	Kegg Farms, New Delhi (India)
v.	Hyline layer	Hi-bred India Pvt Ltd, Karnal (USA)
	Indian River*	Do
vi.	H & N (layer)	Asian-Agro, Talegaon, Dist Pune (India)
vii.	Lohmann (brown egg layer)	BLV Hatcheries Ltd, Hyderabad (India)
	Lohmann broiler*	Do
viii.	Hubbard*	Kasila Farms (P) Ltd, Hyderabad (India)
ix.	Anak-2000*	Tarakeshwara Hatcheries Ltd, Nasik (India)
x.	Pearl—Rupali and Sonali, Tara-287 (layer)	Poona Pearls Hatcheries Ltd, Hadapsar, Pune (India)
	Pearl-bro Samrat*	Do

* indicates broiler type chicks.

Note: The above list is indicative, not exhaustive.

14.11.2 Providing Technical Service After Sales to the Poultry Farmers

The after sale service from the recognised hatcheries is remarkable. They provide first hand training to the poultry farmers in terms of housing, feeding, vaccination and other preventive medication as well as diagnosis of disease and treatment advice, if needed. They provide poultry management manual in local language also. The hatcheries recruit experts/veterinarians for providing these technical services to the poultry farmers.

14.11.3 Providing Facilities of Disease Diagnosis and Feed Analysis

Many commercial hatcheries have established disease diagnosis and feed analytical laboratories. Poultry farmers may take these helps from the concerned hatcheries as and when required. The services are either free of cost or a nominal charge may be taken from the customers/poultry farmers.

14.11.4 Training of Personnel

Many hatcheries have their own training institutes where trainings of various capacities are being offered, like training for technicians (debeaking, vaccination), farm supervisors, farm managers, besides training for the poultry farmers.

14.11.5 Marketing Support

National Egg Coordination Committee (NECC) was established by the initiates of commercial hatcheries. This NECC is responsible for orderly marketing of eggs by declaring egg selling rates, monitoring of egg stock from area to area by supplying surplus eggs to the deficient production places, promotion of egg consumption through advertisement, *etc.*

Few hatcheries have established egg powder plant and poultry dressing plant. The excess/surplus eggs are purchased by such hatcheries for production of egg powder and it reduces the fluctuation of egg price in the market. One such hatchery is Venkateshwara Hatcheries Ltd, Pune.

EXERCISE

A. Objective Questions

i. **Indicate the correct answer by putting tick (√) mark (multiple choice).**

1. For artificial incubation of chicken eggs are kept in the setter for
   - (a) 3 days
   - (b) 18 days
   - (c) 21 days
   - (d) 28 days
2. Hatching eggs can be preserved for 7 days at a storage temperature of
   - (a) 2–8 °C
   - (b) 16–17 °C
   - (c) 25–30 °C
   - (d) 37–38 °C
3. Optimum shape index of duck egg is
   - (a) 74
   - (b) 72
   - (c) 78
   - (d) 70

4. Optimum shape index of quail egg is
   - (a) 10
   - (b) 60
   - (c) 74
   - (d) 78

5. Optimum shape index of chicken egg is
   - (a) 60
   - (b) 72
   - (c) 74
   - (d) 78

6. Time taken for hatching of fowl eggs into chicks in the incubator is
   - (a) 16–17 days
   - (b) 20–21 days
   - (c) 27–28 days
   - (d) 34–35 days

7. To get best result hatching eggs should not be stored for more than
   - (a) 1 day
   - (b) 3 days
   - (c) 10 days
   - (d) 21 days

8. For successful hatching of chicken eggs, turning of eggs is essentially needed during
   - (a) The total incubation period
   - (b) The first 18 days of incubation
   - (c) The last 3 days of incubation
   - (d) The first 3 days of incubation

9. For successful hatching of duck eggs, turning of eggs is must during
   - (a) The total incubation period
   - (b) The first 25 days of incubation
   - (c) The last 3 days of incubation
   - (d) None of these

10. When turning of chicken eggs is not required?
    - (a) During the first 18 days of incubation
    - (b) After 18 days of incubation
    - (c) At 21st day of incubation only
    - (d) None of these

11. Optimum level of oxygen in hatcher should be
    - (a) Less than 0.5%
    - (b) 5%
    - (c) 78%
    - (d) 21%

12. Optimum level of CO_2 in the incubator should be
    - (a) Less than 0.5%
    - (b) 5%
    - (c) 78%
    - (d) 21%

13. Turning of eggs in the setter should be done at least at
    - (a) 4 hours interval
    - (b) 6 hours interval
    - (c) 8 hours interval
    - (d) 12 hours interval

14. Turning of eggs in the hatcher should be done at least
    - (a) At 4 hours interval
    - (b) At 6 hours interval
    - (c) At 8 hours interval
    - (d) No turning is needed in hatcher

15. Male-female ratio of broiler parent stock (chicken) for production of hatching eggs should be
    - (a) 1:3
    - (b) 1:10
    - (c) 1:20
    - (d) 1:50
16. Position of eggs in the incubator should be
    - (a) Broader end down
    - (b) Narrow end up
    - (c) Narrow end down
    - (d) Slanting position
17. If tapping of two eggs generates resonant sound, it indicates
    - (a) Any one egg is cracked
    - (b) Both the eggs are cracked
    - (c) Both the eggs are good
    - (d) None of these
18. Desired temperature and relative humidity for storage of hatching eggs for 7 days:
    - (a) 18–30 °C and 75–80%
    - (b) 16–17 °C and 75–80%
    - (c) 10 °C and 75–80%
    - (d) None of these
19. To know the presence of infertile eggs, candling of incubated eggs is done at
    - (a) 5–7th day
    - (b) 9–10th day
    - (c) 17–18th day
    - (d) 20th day
20. During candling of incubated eggs, if spider-like red radiating lines are seen, it indicates
    - (a) Infertile eggs
    - (b) Fertile eggs
    - (c) Dead embryo
    - (d) None of these
21. When a Rhode Island Red male is mated to Barred Plymouth Rock female
    - (a) Male progenies will be black
    - (b) Female progenies will be barred
    - (c) Both a and b
    - (d) None of these
22. For commercial purpose chick sexing is done
    - (a) At day old stage
    - (b) After 3 days of hatching
    - (c) At 5–7th day
    - (d) After 2 weeks of hatching
23. What is/are the method(s) of sexing chicks at day-old stage?
    - (a) Japanese method (vent method)
    - (b) By proctoscope
    - (c) By observing sex-linked characters
    - (d) All of these
24. Probable cause of 'pipped eggs' (i.e. chicks fully formed, but failing to hatch)
    - (a) Low level of moisture in the incubator
    - (b) Improper setting of eggs causing malpositioned embryos
    - (c) Improper ventilation in incubator
    - (d) All of these
25. If incubated egg with live embryo is placed in water at 18th day, it will
    - (a) Float in water
    - (b) Sink in water
    - (c) Wriggle in water
    - (d) None of these

ii. Fill in the blanks.

1. Properly hatched chicks do not require feed for _____ hours.
2. The eggs are placed in the incubator as _____ end up.
3. The desirable temperature for proper hatching of chicken eggs is _____°C.
4. The desirable relative humidity for proper hatching of chicken eggs is _____.
5. The incubator should be placed in an area where air should contain _____% oxygen.

iii. Write true (T) or False (F) against each statement.

1. Turning of eggs is essential during the last three days of incubation to prevent sticking of egg white to one side of eggshell.
2. Eggs should be placed in the incubator with narrow end up position.
3. Anak-2000 is a layer type high yielding hybrid chick.
4. 200 eggs/year with 58 g average egg weight should be the target for selection of layer type hybrid chicken.
5. Turing of eggs is essential in both setter and hatcher machines.
6. The egg shape index of chicken and duck eggs are 72 and 74 respectively.
7. Blood rings seen on candling of incubated eggs indicate early embryonic death.
8. Chicks fully formed, but failing to hatch is known as 'pipped eggs'.
9. Low humidity in hatcher may result embryos sticking or adhering to eggshell.
10. Faulty setting of eggs in the incubator may result malformed chicks.

B. Subjective Questions

1. What are the factors affecting fertility and hatchability?
2. Enlist the activities of a poultry hatchery.
3. Explain briefly how the following practices are being carried out in a hatchery.
   i. Selection of hatching eggs
   ii. Management of incubator
   iii. Testing of incubated eggs
   iv. Sexing of day-old chicks
   v. Care of day-old chicks before marketing
   vi. Grading, packing and dispatch of day-old chicks
4. What is incubation? Describe in detail about the artificial incubation of chicken eggs.
5. Describe the important factors based on which selection of hatching eggs is done.
6. What is the purpose of turning eggs during incubation?
7. Why and how eggs are tested during artificial incubation?
8. What do you mean by candling of eggs and how is it done?

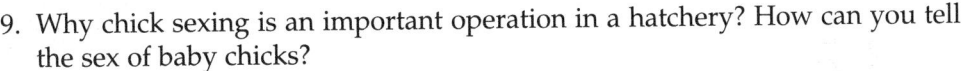
9. Why chick sexing is an important operation in a hatchery? How can you tell the sex of baby chicks?
10. What is autosexing? Explain it with example.
11. Enlist the common hatching problems, their causes and corrective measures.
12. What do you mean by 'dead-in-shell'? What measures are to be taken to reduce this case?
13. What do you mean by 'pipped eggs'? What measures are to be taken to reduce this case?
14. Write short notes on the following.
   (a) Troubleshooting hatch failure
   (b) Biosecurity in the hatchery
   (c) Computer applications for hatchery management
   (d) Principles of incubation
   (e) Factors affecting hatchability
   (f) Disposal of hatchery waste

Answers of the Objective Questions

i. Multiple choice

1. (b) 18 days
2. (b) 16–17 °C
3. (b) 72
4. (d) 78
5. (c) 74
6. (b) 20–21 days
7. (b) 3 days
8. (b) The first 18 days of incubation
9. (b) The first 25 days of incubation
10. (b) After 18 days of incubation
11. (d) 21%
12. (a) Less than 0.5%
13. (c) 8 hours interval
14. (d) No turning is needed in hatcher
15. (b) 1:10
16. (c) Narrow end down
17. (c) Both the eggs are good
18. (b) 16–17 °C and 75–80%
19. (a) 5–7th day
20. (b) Fertile eggs
21. (d) None of these
22. (a) At day-old stage
23. (d) All of these
24. (d) All of these
25. (c) wriggle in water

ii. Fill in the blanks

1. 72
2. broad/large
3. 37–38
4. 60–70%
5. 21

iii. True or False

1. F
2. F
3. F
4. F
5. F
6. F
7. T
8. T
9. T
10. T

15

Record Keeping and Economics of Poultry Farming

15.1 POULTRY FARM RECORDS

Keeping records in poultry farm is must for scientific care and management as well as for economic analysis of the farm. Records may be different for different types of poultry farming. The necessary information is to be recorded in a simple, but scientific manner, either in the form of register or record sheet.

In brooder-cum-grower house, the most important information to be kept are number of day-old chicks and their hatch dates, daily mortality and culling, average biweekly body weight and uniformity of stock, feed specification and daily feed intake, source of water and daily water intake, light on/off time, in-house temperature—maximum and minimum, vaccination, medication, debeaking, transfer of pullets from grower house to layer house. In layer house, daily information are to be recorded on mortality and culls, feed consumption and egg production in addition to other technical information including medication.

For calculation of cost of egg production in layer or breeder farming, all expenditures and incomes must be recorded. The expenditures on various heads are to be kept as they occur like cost of day-old chicks or pullets up to point of lay, mortality, feed, labour, vaccines and other medicines, consumables, maintenance cost, vehicles/repairs, depreciation of equipment and farm buildings, electricity and water, miscellaneous expenses like telephone, postage, etc. The incomes on various heads are sale of eggs, sale of manure and gunny bags, sale of culls, *etc.*

Following are some examples of formats used for different operations in poultry farm.

Rearing Records for Broilers and Pullets

Strain: Feed source:
Source:
Number received:

Date	Age	Deaths	Culled	Balance number	Vaccination/medication	Weekly weight

Monthly Laying Record Sheet

Date of transferring: Strain: Vaccination done:

The flock in layer: Layer house no.:

House:

Date	Deaths	Culled	Feed intake (kg)	Eggs collected			Observations
				1st	2nd	Total	

Egg Collection and Disposal Register

Year: Strain:

Source:

Month:

Date	Laying house no.	Eggs collected			Broken	Disposal	Balance
		1st	2nd	Total			

Mortality Register

Month: Year:

Sl no.	Strain	Sex	Date of death	Cause of death	PM report no.	Book value	Remarks

Feed Register

Month: Year:

Date	Opening balance (kg)	Received (kg)	Source	Issued (kg)	Closing balance (kg)	Composition of ration

Layer Farm Performance Record Card

Card no.:	Name of the farm:		Date:
	Address:		

Sl no.	Flock no.	Date of receiving chicks	Number of chicks (including extra)	Culling%	Mortality%	HHP%	Average HDP%	Feed consumed to produce one dozen of eggs/month (kg)	Feed cost to produce one dozen of eggs	Feed cost to egg rate ratio	Price of spent hen	Remarks	Signature

Broiler Farm Performance Record Card

Card no.:	Name of the farm:		Date:
	Address:		

Sl no.	Flock no.	Date of receiving chicks	Number of chicks (including extra)	Date of selling birds	Mortality%	FCR	PEF%	Discrepancy	Gross margin per unit floor space	Average finished weight	Remarks	Signature

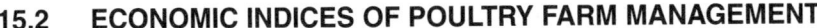

15.2 ECONOMIC INDICES OF POULTRY FARM MANAGEMENT

Various types of economic indices are used in poultry farm management. These indices are used (a) to evaluate the production performances of birds, (b) to assess the financial condition of the enterprise, (c) to suggest the correcting measures for improvement of the economic efficiency of the business, and (d) to formulate the guidelines for future improvement, planning and expansion of the farm.

Various economic indices applicable in case of different types of poultry farming (broiler farming, layer farming, breeder farming and pullet rearing, *etc.*) are depicted below.

Production Indices for Broiler Birds

1. **Average body weight at market age (6 weeks of age):** It is calculated by dividing the total body weight of a flock by the number of birds at the time of marketing.

   Ideal value becomes 1.80–2.0 kg

2. **Feed conversion ratio (FCR):** It is obtained by dividing the total amount of feed consumed by the total weight of live broilers.

   i.e. $\text{FCR} = \dfrac{\text{Total amount of feed consumed}}{\text{Total body weight}}$

   A value of less than 2.00 at 6 weeks of age is preferable. Presently, there are farms in India which attain less than 1.7 FCR in broiler.

3. **Feed cost per kg of broiler produced:** It is calculated by the multiplication of FCR with cost per kg of feed.

4. **Performance efficiency factor (PEF):** The PEF is derived by dividing the live body weight of the flock by FCR and number of chicks purchased, multiplied with 100.

   i.e. $\text{PEF} = \dfrac{\text{Total live body weight of the flock}}{\text{FCR} \times \text{no. of chicks purchased}} \times 100$

   The higher the PEF, the better will be the performance of the flock. A value of 100 or higher is desirable.

5. **Gross margin per unit floor space:** It is calculated by subtracting the total cost of raising (cost of chicks, feed, medication, *etc.*) from gross income and then dividing the result by the total area of floor space.

   i.e. Gross margin per unit floor space $= \dfrac{\text{Gross income} - \text{Total raising cost}}{\text{Total floor area (in sq ft/sq m)}}$

6. **Broiler performance efficiency score:**

   It is calculated based on the body weight, feed efficiency and livability at 6 weeks of age; giving appropriate score for each of these three traits; based on their relative economic importance.

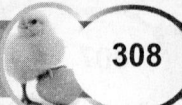
Score card to judge the broiler performance efficiency

Trait	Optimum	Range	Score
i. Average live weight at 6 weeks of age (kg)	> 1.6	1.3 to 1.8	50
ii. FCR	< 2.0	1.8 to 2.1	30
iii. Per cent livability	> 95.0	92 to 98	20

A broiler farm should try to attain a minimum score of 70.

7. Formula for calculating the cost of production/kg live broiler:

    i. Chick cost = 0.55 × Cost of one day-old chick = A

    ii. Feed cost = Feed efficiency × Cost/kg of feed = B

    iii. Miscellaneous expenditure = 12% of (A + B) = C

Hence, production cost/kg live broiler = A + B + C

8. Formula for calculating the cost of production/broiler:

    i. Chick cost = 1.05 × Cost of one day-old chick = A

    ii. Feed cost = Live weight in kg × Feed efficiency × Cost/kg of feed = B

    iii. Miscellaneous expenditure = 12% of (A+B) = C

Hence production cost/broiler = A + B + C

9. Livability% = $\dfrac{\text{Number of birds sold}}{\text{Number of chicks bought (including extra)}} \times 100$

Production indices for Layer Birds

1. Percentage of hen housed production (HHP%): It is computed as the percentage of dividing the number of eggs of the day by number of birds housed.

    i. HHP% = $\dfrac{\text{Number of eggs produced on a day}}{\text{Number of hens housed at the beginning of the laying period}} \times 100$

    (for one day)

    ii. HHP% = $\dfrac{\text{Average number of eggs produced per day during the period}}{\text{Number of birds housed at the beginning}} \times 100$

    (for a long period)

2. Percentage of hen day production (HDP%)

    i. HDP (%) = $\dfrac{\text{Number of eggs produced on the day}}{\text{Number of birds on the day}} \times 100$ (for one day)

    ii. HDP (%) = $\dfrac{\text{Total number of eggs produced over the period}}{\text{Total number of hen days}}$

    (for a long period)

NB: Total number of hen days are calculated by adding daily number of live hens over the concerned period.

3. Feed consumed to produce one dozen of eggs per month

$$= \frac{\text{Total feed consumed per month}}{\text{Total dozen of eggs per month}}$$

4. Feed consumed per hen per day

$$= \frac{\text{Total feed consumed}}{\text{Average number of birds per day} \times \text{Number of days}}$$

5. Feed cost to produce one dozen of eggs per month

$$= \frac{\text{Total feed cost per month}}{\text{Total dozen of eggs per month}}$$

6. Percentage of livability per month

$$= \frac{\text{Number of birds at the end of month}}{\text{Number of birds at the start of month}} \times 100$$

7. Performance efficiency index (PEI)

$$\text{PEI} = \frac{K\,(EW)^2\,P}{BW \times F}$$

where   K   = 30
BW = Body weight (g)
EW = Egg weight (g)
P   = Percentage hen day production
F   = Feed consumed per day per bird (g)

8. Percentage of culling

$$= \frac{\text{Total number of birds culled}}{\text{Total number of birds received}} \times 100$$

9. Stage breakeven point:

It is the stage at which the sum of prices of all inputs and outputs are same. It depends upon (1) rate of egg production, (2) prevailing egg price, (3) culled (spent) hen price, (4) daily feed intake, (5) predictable future trends in egg, feed and culled hen prices.

10. Income: Expenditure

$$= \frac{EN \times EP}{FI \times FC} \times 1.176$$

where   EN = Total number of eggs produced/day by the existing flock
EP = Selling price/egg in rupees
FI   = Daily feed intake by the flock in kg
FC   = Cost/kg of feed in rupees

The farmer can retain his/her birds as long as the value is greater than one. A week average value is to be taken into account. Normally the breakeven point should be 1.3 times the feed expenditure, i.e. suppose the feed expenditure is ` 100.00 then the receipt should be ` 130.00.

Production Indices for Breeder Birds

1. Number of settable eggs produced per dam
2. Number of saleable chicks produced per dam

Efficiency Measure of Breeding Farms

1. Percentage of fertility $= \dfrac{\text{Number of eggs fertile}}{\text{Total number of eggs}} \times 100$

2. Percentage of hatchability $= \dfrac{\text{Number of chicks hatched out}}{\text{Total number of eggs}} \times 100$

   i. on total eggs set
  ii. on fertile eggs set

Efficiency Measure of Pullet Farm

(Rate of uniformity)

Percentage of pullets within 10% of average flock weight	Uniformity rating
85% and over	Excellent
80–85%	Very good
75–85%	Satisfactory
70–75%	Fair
Less than 70%	Not satisfactory

It is done at 18 weeks of age of flock.

Efficiency Measure of Utilizations of Farm Land

Construction coefficient $= \dfrac{\text{Total constructed area}}{\text{Total farmland area}} \times 100$

For an ideal farm, it should be 25 to 35.

15.3 PREPARATION OF PROJECT REPORTS FOR VARIOUS AVIAN SPECIES

Project reports for various categories of poultry are presented here, viz. **broiler**, **layer**, **duck** (free range system), **duck** (intensive system), **Japanese quail** (broiler type), **turkey** (free range system) and **cockerel** (all-in all-out system).

The project cost may vary depending on the prices prevailing in different localities, but the method for preparation of project reports is same and the following project reports may be taken as guide.

15.3.1 Project Report for a Broiler Farm

Technical details and assumptions:

   i. House: Open-sided, tile-roofed, deep litter house.
  ii. Floor space: Half square feet per bird up to 25 days of age and one square feet per bird thereafter.
 iii. Cost of poultry house: ` 100/sq ft

iv. Other building cost: ₹ 200/sq ft

v. Equipment cost: ₹ 20/bird

vi. Cost of medicine, vaccine, insurance, labour, electricity, fuel, *etc.*: ₹ 6/bird

vii. Total number of birds in the farm: 7,000

viii. Total number of birds per batch (including extra 5%): 1,050

ix. Batch interval: 1 week

x. Down time: 1 week

xi. Saleable broilers per batch per week: 980

xii. Growing period: 42 days

xiii. Feed efficiency: 1.7 (average body weight = 2 kg)

xiv. Cost of feed (average cost of pre-starter, starter and finisher feeds): ₹ 25/kg

xv. Mortality: 7%

xvi. Manure production: 4 kg per bird

xvii. Bank holiday period: 2 months from completion date

xviii. Loan repayment period: 5 years, including holiday period

xix. Bank interest: 15%

Farm buildings

i. **Orientation of poultry house:** Houses are built east-west with long axis facing north and south, and short axis on east and west.

ii. **Construction details:** Houses are constructed with concrete pillars with brick and cement walls, and floor plastered with cement, elevated one foot above the ground level. The inside height at eaves will be about 7'; while at ridge height will be around 12'. The two long sides are provided one foot high wall with 60° inside slope at top. The partition wall specification is like that of side walls. The remaining 5' height is covered with 1'' GI 12 gauge chain link mesh throughout except at the doors. There will be 3' overhang of roofs at eaves. The doors are made up of MS angle frame and 1'' × 3'' mesh of 10 gauge thickness, with provision to lock from both sides. The two sides are made up of solid brick wall. Roof structure is built by seasoned wood and tiles.

The house is provided with 3-phase power supply.

iii. **Other buildings:** The feed room, store and workers, quarters will have brick side walls to the full height.

iv. **Specification of farm buildings for the project**

A. One shed will be 30' × 120' size outer to outer with 4 pens each of 500 sq ft area to accommodate 4 batches × 1,000 birds from 0 to 25 days of age with ½ sq ft/bird.

B. i. One 400 sq ft owner/supervision quarters

ii. 200 × 2 = 400 sq ft for two workers, quarters

iii. 600 sq ft feed room

iv. 200 sq ft office-cum-store room

C. Another shed with 30′ × 133.3′ outer size, partitioned into 4 × 1,000 sq ft rooms to rear 4 batches of broilers from 26th day onwards = 4,000 sq ft
Total area required for birds = 2,000 + 4,000 = 6,000 sq ft
Total area required for other purposes = 400 + 400 + 600 + 200 sq ft
$$= 1,600 \text{ sq ft}$$

STATEMENT I

Non-recurring expenditure	Amount (₹ in lakhs)
1. Cost of 2,000 sq ft broiler brooder + 4,000 sq ft broiler grower houses @ ₹ 100/sq ft	= 6.00
2. Cost of 1,600 sq ft feed store, supervisor and workers' quarters	= 3.20
3. Land development charges like fencing, provision of gate, farm roads, *etc.*	= 0.50
4. Cost of deep tube well, water pump, overhead tank and pipeline to all sheds	= 1.00
5. Cost of feeders, waterers, platform weighing scales, wheel-barrow, brooders, *etc.* @ ₹ 20/bird for 7,000 birds	= 1.40
Total	**12.10**

STATEMENT II

Working capital	Amount (₹ in lakhs)
1. Cost of 1,000 × 7 batches of day-old chick @ ₹ 25/each	= 1.75
2. Feed cost for 7 batches at an average of 3.4 kg/bird × ₹ 25/kg	= 5.95
3. Medicine, vaccine, insurance, labour, electricity, health coverage, *etc.* @ ₹ 6/bird	= 0.42
Total	**8.12**

STATEMENT III

Total capital investment, share of promoter (margin money), bank finance needed
Amount (₹ in lakhs)

Sl no.	Description	Total capital	Promoter/ farmer share	Bank finance required
1.	Land cost (1 acre)	2.00	2.00 (100%)	–
2.	Non-recurring expenditure (vide Statement I)	12.10	3.02 (25%)	9.08
3.	Working capital (vide Statement II)	8.22	2.03 (25%)	6.09
Total		**22.22**	**7.05**	**15.17**

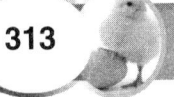

STATEMENT IV

Annual recurring expenditure	Amount (₹ in lakhs)
1. Cost of 1000 day-old chicks × 52 batches/year @ ₹ 25/each	= 13.00
2. Feed cost for 52,000 broilers × 3.4 kg/bird @ ₹ 25/kg	= 44.20
3. Other miscellaneous cost @ ₹ 6/bird	= 3.12
Total	**60.32**

STATEMENT V

Annual gross and net returns	Amount (₹ in lakhs)
1. By sale of 980 live broilers per batch × 52 batches × ₹ 70/kg live weight (2.0 kg)	71.34
2. By sale of about 2,500 empty gunny bags @ ₹ 7.50/each	0.18
3. By sale of about 200 tonnes of manure @ ₹ 500/tonne	1.00
Total	**72.52**

LESS

Annual expenditure (statement IV)	:	60.32
Net returns (before repayment of bank loan) (72.52 – 60.32)	:	12.20

STATEMENT VI
(₹ in lakhs)

Year	Gross receipts	Expenditure	Net surplus before loan repayment	OB of bank loan	Interest (15%) on loan	Total bank loan	Loan repaid loan	CB of bank loan	Net profit after loan repayment	Benefit-cost ratio
	A	C			B					(A –B)/C
1	62.80*	52.20	10.60	15.17	2.28	17.45	4.50	12.95	6.10	1.10
2	72.52	60.32	12.20	12.95	1.94	14.89	4.50	10.39	7.70	1.13
3	72.52	60.32	12.20	10.39	1.56	11.95	4.50	7.45	7.70	1.13
4	72.52	60.32	12.20	7.45	1.12	8.57	4.50	4.07	7.70	1.13
5	72.52	60.32	12.20	4.07	0.61	4.68	4.68	nil	7.52	1.12
6	72.52	60.32	12.20	nil	nil	nil	nil	nil	12.20	1.20

* The annual gross returns during first year will be ₹ 62.80 lakhs as there will be no sales during first 6–7 weeks period; only 45 batches will be sold instead of 52 batches. Therefore, the net surplus before repayment will be ₹ 10.60 lakhs.

Certificate

It is certified that this project is prepared by me taking into account the prevailing prices of various farm inputs and outputs and the latest technical and production standards. It appears that this project will be technically feasible and financially viable.

Enclosures

1. Land ownership document
2. Farm site map
3. Blue print and estimates of farm buildings

15.3.2 Project Report for a Layer Farm [(1 + 3) System]

Technical details and assumptions

The project is a layer farm, having 20,000 birds at any given time where 15,000 are layers and 5,000 are growers in (1 + 3) batches, i.e. 1 batch of grower and 3 batches of layers. Once in every 20–21 weeks, 5,400 new chicks are to be purchased and out of this 5,000 are expected to be available at pullet stage. At about 19 weeks of age, about 5,000 pullets are to be shifted to layer cages; where they will stay up to the age of 80 weeks after which they will be culled. At a point of time there will be about 14,400 (5,000 + 4,800 + 4,600) layers which will lay 11,500 eggs daily with 80% yearly average production level. There will be down time of one week for each batch of new arrival in respective house or cage. Number of culled hens at 20–21 weeks interval will be 4,500. Each pullet will consume 7 kg of feed up to 20 weeks of age and about 110 g of feed/day during laying period. As such a bird from 0 to 80 weeks of age will consume 53 kg of feed and lay 336 eggs in 420 days and produce around 40 kg of manure.

It will take minimum three months for land development and grower shed construction to receive first batch of chicks, second and third batches will arrive 20 and 40 weeks later. The third batch comes to production in 60 weeks after arrival of first batch. Therefore, a minimum of 18 months repayment holiday period is needed. The principal and interest will be repaid in 72 months after 18 months of holiday period, i.e. by 90 months.

1. House: i.   Open-sided, tile-roofed, deep litter house for grower birds.
            ii.   Raised platform cage layer house for layers.
2. Cost of grower house = ₹ 100/sq ft
3. Cost of layer house = ₹ 150/sq ft
4. Cost of other farm buildings = ₹ 200/sq ft
5. Cost of layer cages = ₹ 50/bird
6. Cost of grower equipment = ₹ 20/bird
7. Cost of medicines, vaccines, electricity, labour = ₹ 15/bird
8. Pullet chicks purchased/batch = 5,400 (excluding extra)
9. Average number of batches/year = 2.5
10. Cost of day-old chick = ₹ 20/each
11. Mortality: 0 to 20 weeks = 8%
               21 to 80 weeks = 10%
12. Cost of feed = ₹ 20/kg
    (average of starter, grower and layer)
13. Average number of saleable eggs/day = 11,500 eggs

14.	Average number of spent/culled hens	= 11,250 hens
		= (2.5 × 4,500 hens)
15.	Average egg selling price	= ₹ 3.75/egg
16.	Average manure production/year	= 500 tonnes
17.	Average selling pric e of manure	= ₹ 500/tonne
18.	Sale price of empty gunny bag	= ₹ 10/each
19.	Insurance premium	= ₹ 4/bird
20.	Average number of batches	= 2.5/year
21.	Feed/bird (0 to 80 weeks)	= 53 kg

Farm buildings

i. **Orientation:** Same as other poultry houses.

ii. **Grower house**

The deep litter' brooder-cum-grower house to accommodate 5,000–5,500 replacement pullets is of 30' width (north to south) and 167' length (east to west); total 5,010 sq ft with one sq ft/bird. The two *long sides* are provided one foot high wall with 60° inside slope. The remaining height is covered by 1" eye, 12 gauge GI chain link mesh throughout, except at the four doors. The inside height at eaves will be about 7' while at ridge the height will be 12'. The roof at eaves is provided with 3' overhang. The roof structure is supported by 9" thick concrete pillars. The inside floor is made up of cement, elevated one foot above the ground level.

The 4 doors are made up of MS angle frame and 1" × 3" weld mesh of 10 gauge thickness, with provision to lock both sides. Two rows of water pipelines are provided 7–8' above the ground level throughout the length of the shed, to connect it to automatic waterers.

iii. **Raised platform cage layer house**

The layer house is 33' wide and 292' long (total 9,636 sq ft) to accommodate 15,000 layers in 3 divided batches with 0.64 sq ft/hen. The 3 cage units, one for each batch will be separated by two 10' wide and 33' long platforms with staircase. The platforms are 6' above the ground level. Two store rooms are constructed below the two 10' × 33' platforms to store eggs, *etc*. The two sides of layer house on east and west are brick wall type, supported by 9" thick concrete pillars, with a height 15' at eaves and 23' at ridge. The lengthwise north and south sides are having concrete pillars at 20' interval. The asbestos roof will have ridge ventilation at the centre and have 5' overhang at the eaves. Three platforms, each of 2' width and 290' length will be provided in each shed, which will be supported by 5" thick 'T' shaped concrete pillars at the bottom at 5' interval.

iv. **Cages**

Two 'M' type and two 'L' type cages, each of three-tier will be fixed in between the platforms. There will be 12 'M' and 6 'L' units of cages; of which 4 'M' and 2 'L' units will be allotted to each batch of layers. Each 'M' unit will have 6 rows and 'L' unit have 3 rows of cages. The 'M' units are at the centre and the 'L' are near the pillars. Each row will have 52 cage boxes. The size of cage box

20″ length in front, 17″ to 18″ height at front, depth will be 15″ (front to back) in bottom and middle row cages to house 5 hens and depth will be 18″ in top row cages to house 6 hens with 60 sq inch cage space/hen. The middle row overlaps the bottom row cages and the top row overlaps the middle row cages by 2″. Cage floor gradient will be 7° from back to front. The cage bottom is made up of 1″ × 3″, 10 gauge weld mesh, whereas top, back and front mesh size will be 2″ × 3″, 8 gauge weld mesh. The cage partition mesh size will be 1″ × 3″, 12 gauge weld mesh. The feeders are made up of 24 gauge aluminium sheet and plastic water pipe with two nipple drinkers are there at each cage partition of top front portion. Two rows of foggers are provided over each M cage.

The poultry house is provided 3-phase power supply. Compact fluorescent lamps are used in two rows.

v. **Other buildings**

A rodent and seepage proof warehouse of 40′ × 20′ size for feed storage; supervisor quarter 30′ × 20′; 30′ × 20′ egg store with 12′ height and asbestos roof are to be built. Total = 800 + 600 + 600 = 2,000 sq ft.

STATEMENT I

Non-recurring expenditure	Amount (₹ in lakhs)
1. Cost of grower house with asbestos roof @ ₹ 100/sq ft (5,010 sq ft)	5.01
2. Cost of elevated platform, asbestos roof cage layer house @ ₹ 150/sq ft (9,636 sq ft) for 15,000 layers	14.45
3. Cost of other buildings @ ₹ 200/sq ft (2,000 sq ft)	4.00
4. Land development charges, fencing, manure pit, burial pit, farm road and other infrastructure facilities.	0.70
5. Cost of deep tube well, water pump, overhead tank and pipeline to all sheds.	1.00
6. Cost of chick and grower equipments @ ₹ 20/bird for 5,000 birds	1.00
7. Cost of layer cages @ ₹ 50/ bird for 15,000 birds	7.50
Total	**33.66**

STATEMENT II

Working capital	Amount (₹ in lakhs)
1. Cost of 5,400 day-old chicks × 3 batches @ ₹ 20/each + insurance premium @ ₹ 4/each	3.88
2. Feed cost for 3 batches up to the point of lay (20 weeks) for 5,000 pullets/batch × 3 batches × 7 kg feed/bird × ₹ 20/kg	21.00
3. Miscellaneous cost : 5,000 birds × 3 batches × ₹ 15/bird	2.25
Total	**27.13**

STATEMENT III

Sl no.	Description	Total cost	Margin money	Bank loan required
	Total project cost, margin money, bank loan required			**Amount (₹ in lakhs)**
1.	Land (3½ acre)	7.00	7.00	–
2.	Non-recurring expenditure (Statement I)	22.13	8.41 (25%)	25.25
3.	Working capital (Statement II)	27.13	6.75 (25%)	20.38
Total		**67.79**	**22.16**	**45.63**

STATEMENT IV

Period (quarter)	Purpose	Total loan/quarter
	Calendar of loan disbursement	**Amount (₹ in lakhs)**
1	Land development charges	
	Chick-cum-grower shed	
	Deep tube well, overhead tank, *etc.*	6.60
	Equipment cost	
2	First batch of chicks	
	Feed room and other buildings	
	Layer house	22.80
	Cost of layer cages	
	Feed cost	
	Miscellaneous cost	
3	Second batch of chicks	
	Cost of layer cages	8.40
	Feed cost	
	Miscellaneous cost	
4	Third batch of chicks	
	Cages for layer house	7.83
	Feed cost	
	Miscellaneous cost	
Total loan released		**45.63**

- Repayment holiday = 18 months from the time of starting of farm
- Repayment period = 72 months (after 18 months holiday period)
- Total repayment period = 72 + 18 = 90 months
- The entire loan amount along with accrued interest at the rate of 15% will be repaid after the commencement of the project or within 72 months from commencement of full egg production.

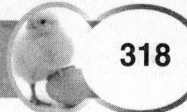

STATEMENT V

Annual recurring expenditure (Amount in ₹ in lakhs)

Year	Chick cost including insurance premium		Feed cost		Misc cost @ ₹ 15/bird/ annum	Total expenditure
	Nos.	Cost	Quantity (tonnes)	Cost		
1	16,200	(3.88)*	105 + 169	(21.0)* + 33.80	(2.25)* + 0.75	(27.13)* + 34.55
2	10,800	2.59	640	128.0	3.0	133.59
3	16,200	3.88	670	134.0	3.0	140.88
4	10,800	2.59	670	134.0	3.0	139.59
5	16,200	3.88	670	134.0	3.0	140.88
6	10,800	2.59	670	134.0	3.0	139.59
7	16,200	3.88	670	134.0	3.0	140.88
8	10,800	2.59	670	134.0	3.0	139.59
9	16,200	3.88	670	134.0	3.0	140.88

* Values in parenthesis indicate the working capital. In 1st year it is expected that two batches will cover 44 weeks of laying period.

STATEMENT VI

Annual gross and net returns (Amount in ₹ in lakhs)

Year	By sale of eggs		By sale of culled hens		By sale of manure		By sale of empty feed bags		Total gross receipts	Total expenditure	Net surplus
	Nos. (million)	Amount (₹ 3.75/ egg)	Nos.	Amount (₹ 65/ hen)	Quantity (T)	Amount	Nos. (₹ 500/ T)	Amount (₹ 10/ bag)			
1	1.30	48.75	–	–	70	0.35	2,800	0.28	49.38	34.55	14.83
2	3.90	146.25	9,000	5.85	500	2.5	8,106	0.81	155.41	133.59	21.82
3	4.19	157.12	13,500	8.77	500	2.5	8,320	0.83	169.22	140.88	28.34
4	4.19	157.12	9,000	5.85	500	2.5	8,320	0.83	166.30	139.59	26.71
5	4.19	157.12	13,500	8.77	500	2.5	8,320	0.83	169.22	140.88	28.34
6	4.19	157.12	9,000	5.85	500	2.5	8,320	0.83	166.30	139.59	26.71
7	4.19	157.12	13,500	8.77	500	2.5	8,320	0.83	169.22	140.88	28.34
8	4.19	157.12	9,000	5.85	500	2.5	8,320	0.83	166.30	139.59	26.71
9	4.19	157.12	13,500	8.77	500	2.5	8,320	0.83	169.22	140.88	28.34

STATEMENT VII

Cash flow statement, net profit and benefit-cost ratio (Amount in ₹ in lakhs)

Source of funds	At start	At the end of the year								
		1	2	3	4	5	6	7	8	9
Land cost	7.00	–	–	–	–	–	–	–	–	–
Promoter's fund	–	10.75	4.41	–	–	–	–	–	–	–
Borrowings	–	37.80	7.83	–	–	–	–	–	–	–
Increase in net profit	–	9.16	9.98	12.25	14.12	14.95	16.82	24.90	24.55	28.34
Net assets (cumulative)	7.00	64.71	86.93	99.18	113.30	128.25	145.07	169.97	194.52	222.86
Net surplus (cumulative)	–	9.16	19.14	31.39	45.51	60.46	77.28	102.18	126.73	155.07
Cash outflow										
Cost of chicks	–	–	2.59	3.88	2.59	3.88	2.59	3.88	2.59	3.88
Cost of feed	–	33.80	128.00	134.00	134.00	134.00	134.00	134.00	134.00	134.00
Misc cost	–	0.75	3.00	3.00	3.00	3.00	3.00	3.00	3.00	3.00
Repayment of loan with interest	–	5.67	11.84	16.09	12.59	13.39	9.89	3.44	2.16	–
Total cash outflow (A)	–	40.22	145.43	156.97	152.18	154.27	143.03	144.32	141.75	140.88
Cash inflow										
Sale of eggs	–	48.75	146.25	157.12	157.12	157.12	157.12	157.12	157.12	157.12
Sale of spent/culled hens	–	–	5.85	8.77	5.85	8.77	5.85	8.77	5.85	8.77
Sale of manure	–	0.35	2.50	2.50	2.50	2.50	2.50	2.50	2.50	2.50
Sale of gunny bags	–	0.28	0.81	0.83	0.83	0.83	0.83	0.83	0.83	0.83
Total cash inflow (B)	–	49.38	155.41	169.22	166.30	169.22	166.30	169.22	166.30	169.22
Net surplus	–	14.83	21.82	28.34	26.71	28.34	26.71	28.34	26.71	28.34
Benefit-cost ratio (B/A)	–	1.23	1.07	1.08	1.09	1.10	1.16	1.17	1.17	1.20

STATEMENT VIII

Bank loan repayment schedule (Amount in ₹ in lakhs)

Year	OB of loan	Borrowings	Interest (15%)	Total	Repayment Principal	Repayment Interest	Repayment Total	CB of loan
1	–	37.80	5.67	43.47	–	5.67	5.67	37.80
2	37.80	7.83	6.84	52.47	5.00	6.84	11.84	40.63
3	40.63	–	6.09	46.72	10.00	6.09	16.09	30.63
4	30.63	–	4.59	35.22	8.00	4.59	12.59	22.63
5	22.63	–	3.39	26.02	10.00	3.39	13.39	12.63
6	12.63	-	1.89	14.52	8.00	1.89	9.89	4.63
7	4.63	–	0.69	5.32	2.75	0.69	3.44	1.88
8	1.88	–	0.28	2.16	1.88	0.28	2.16	nil
9	–	–	–	–	–	–	–	–
Total	–	45.63	29.44	–	45.63	29.44	75.07	–

Certificate

Certified that this project report is prepared by taking into account the latest technical standards and prevailing market prices for various farm inputs and outputs. The report is technically feasible and economically viable.

Enclosures

1. Farm site map
2. Farm buildings blue print and estimates from civil engineer
3. Land ownership document
4. Quotation for cages, *etc.*
5. Other relevant documents

15.3.3 Project Report for a Duck Farm (Free Range System)

Technical details and assumptions:

i. Number of layer ducks = 200
ii. Number of ducklings (straight run) purchased = 450
iii. Type of duck = Khaki Campbell × Desi cross
iv. Feeds (mostly grains) will be given in first one month brooding period and during the scarcity in summer months.
v. Source of feed by foraging mainly
vi. Cost of day-old straight run ducklings = ₹ 15 each
vii. Feed required for brooding period = 1.5 kg each
viii. Cost of feed = ₹ 20/kg
ix. Feed required for dry summer season (2 months/year) = 2 kg/bird/month (part feeding)

x. Selling price of drakes at 2 months of age = ₹ 60/each

xi. Selling price of eggs = ₹ 4/each

xii. Selling price of culled ducks = ₹ 65/each

xiii. No housing, except a nylon wirenet circular enclosure for night shelter

xiv. Replacement stock: Next batch of 450 ducklings are to be purchased six months before the disposal of the old batch.

xv. Farmer will look after his own farm.

xvi. Mortality = Average 12%

STATEMENT I

Expenditure per batch (2.5 years)	(Amount in ₹)
1. Cost of feeders, waterers, fencing net, egg boxes, *etc.*	5,000
2. Cost of 450 day-old straight run chicks	6,750
3. Cost of feeding (brooding period) ($450 \times 1.5 \times 8$)	13,500
4. Cost of vaccines, medicines and misc expenditure	2,400
5. Cost of feeding during summer season ($200 \times 2 \times 4 \times 8$)	
[2 years = 4 summer months]	32,000
Total	**59,600**

Cost of replacement stock	(Amount in ₹)
1. Cost of feeders, waterers, *etc.*	3,000
2. Cost of 450 ducklings (straight run)	6,750
3. Cost of feeding them during brooding period	13,500
4. Cost of vaccination, medication, *etc.*	2,000
Total	**25,250**

STATEMENT II

Gross income per batch	(Amount in ₹)
1. By sale of 200 drakes at 8 weeks of age	12,000
2. By sale of 200 eggs in first year + 180 eggs in second year/dam ($200 \times 200 + 200 \times 180) \times 4$	3,04,000
3. By sale of 170 ducks at the end of 2½ years (170×65)	11,050
Total	**3,27,050**

Net return = (Gross income/Batch – Expenditure/Batch) – Cost of replacement stock

= ₹ (3,27,050 – 59,600 – 25,250)

= ₹ 2,42,200

Net return after 30 months (2½ years) = ₹ 2,42,200

Net return/month = ₹ 8,073

Benefit-cost ratio = 3.85

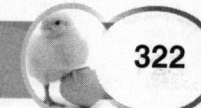

15.3.4 Project Report for a Duck Farm (Intensive System)

Technical details and assumptions:

i. Number of female ducklings purchased = 1,100
ii. Mortality = 5% up to 12 weeks of age, and 10% after that
iii. Feed consumption = 13 kg (0 to 20 weeks of age) + 47 kg (20 to 72 weeks of age)
iv. Cost of vaccines, medicines, misc cost, *etc.* = ₹ 6/bird
v. Equipment cost = ₹ 20/bird
vi. Floor space required = 2.5 sq ft/bird
vii. Cost of construction of duck house = ₹ 75/sq ft
viii. Selling price of eggs = ₹ 4/egg
ix. Selling price of spent duck = ₹ 65/each
x. Cost of feed (average) = ₹ 20/kg
xi. Selling price of empty gunny bag = ₹ 10/bag
xii. Cost of ducklings = ₹ 20/duckling

STATEMENT I

Non-recurring expenditure	Amount (₹ in lakhs)
1. Building @ ₹ 75/sq ft for 1,000 birds	1.875
2. Equipment cost @ ₹ 20/bird	0.20
Total	**2.075**

STATEMENT II

Working capital	Amount (₹ in lakhs)
1. Cost of 1,100 ducklings @ ₹ 20/each (10% extra to cover mortality)	0.22
2. Cost of feeding up to 20 weeks of age (1,100 × 13 × 20)	2.86
3. Misc cost (1,100 × 6)	0.066
Total	**3.146**

STATEMENT III

Annual recurring expenditure	Amount (₹ in lakhs)
1. Cost of feeding 1,000 ducks (1,000 × 47 × 20)	9.40
2. Misc cost (1,000 × 6)	0.06
3. Cost of raising replacement stock* (3.146 ÷ 2)	1.573
4. Depreciation 10% (buildings and equipment)	0.207
Total	**11.24**

* Ducks lay profitably during 2nd even 3rd year laying. So the replacement stock may be raised on every alternate year or half of the stock is replaced on every year.

STATEMENT IV

Gross receipt	Amount (₹ in lakhs)
1. Sale of eggs @ ₹ 4 each @ 300 eggs/year/bird (1,000 × 300 × 4)	12.00
2. Sale of 25 tonnes of manure @ ₹ 500/T	0.125
3. Sale of empty gunny bag (800 × 10)	0.080
4. Sale value of 950 spent duck	0.617
Total	**12.822**

Net receipt = Gross receipt – Recurring expenditure

= ₹ 12.822 lakhs – ₹ 11.240 lakhs

= ₹ 1.582 lakhs/annum

Benefit-cost ratio = 1.14.

15.3.5 Project Report for a Japanese Quail Farm (Broiler Type)

Technical details and assumptions:

 i. Growing period = 5 weeks
 ii. Livability = 90%
 iii. Average body weight at 5 weeks of age = 130 g
 iv. Feed conversion efficiency = 1:3
 v. Total feed consumed = 400 g/bird
    (0 to 5 weeks of age)
 vi. Cost of feed = ₹ 25/kg
 vii. Cost of empty feed bags of 75 kg capacity = ₹ 10/bag
 viii. Cost of day-old Japanese quail chick = ₹ 5/chick
 ix. Growing will be entirely in battery cages, each battery consisting of 5 tiers and each tier is of 160 cm × 80 cm dimension; this will be used for rearing of 100 quails in each tier @ ₹ 30,000.
 x. Manure production by 1,000 birds = 25 kg
 xi. Cost of manure = ₹ 500/T

STATEMENT I

Fixed capital	Amount (₹ in lakhs)
1. Cost of cage grower house to keep 6 batches of quail = 1,000 sq ft @ ₹ 200/sq ft	2.00
2. Cost of 6 cage units for 6 batches of 3,000 birds each @ ₹ 30,000/battery cage unit	1.80
3. Tube well, motor pump, pipelines, *etc.*	1.00
Total	**4.80**

Annual depreciation @ 10% = 0.48

STATEMENT II

Working capital (2 months)	Amount (₹ in lakhs)
1. Cost of quail chicks (8 batches × 3,000 chicks × ₹ 5/chick)	1.20
2. Feed cost (average 0.3 kg/bird) @ ₹ 25/kg	1.80
3. Misc expenditure @ ₹ 2/bird	0.48
Total	**3.48**

STATEMENT III

Capital investment	Amount (₹ in lakhs)
1. Fixed cost + Working capital	8.28
2. Bank loan (75%)	6.21
3. Promoter's share	2.07
Total	**16.56**

STATEMENT IV

Annual recurring expenditure	Amount (₹ in lakhs)
1. Cost of chicks (52 batches × 3,000 chicks × ₹ 5/chick)	7.80
2. Feed cost (52 × 3,000 × 0.4 × ₹ 25/kg of feed)	15.60
3. Misc expenditure @ ₹ 2/chick	3.12
Total	**26.52**

STATEMENT V

Annual returns	Amount (₹ in lakhs)
1. Returns by sale of 52 batches of 2,700 quails/batch @ ₹ 23/bird	32.292
2. By sale of manure @ ₹ 500/T	0.019
3. By sale of empty gunny bags (890 × ₹ 10)	0.089
Total	**32.400**

Annual expenditure including depreciation (10%) and interest (15%) = ₹ 27.93 lakh

Annual net profit = ₹ 32.40 lakh – ₹ 27.93 lakh = ₹ 4.47 lakh

15.3.6 Project Report for a Turkey Farm (Free Range System)

Technical details and assumptions:

  i. Requirement of land: 1 to 2 acres with good foraging capacity.
 ii. Shelter: A thatched house of 300 sq ft will be required for brooding and rearing up to one month of age.
iii. Cost of day-old poult: ₹ 60/each
 iv. Growing period: 6 months, i.e. 2 batches/year
  v. Expected body weight at 6 months: 4 kg
 vi. Feeds: Broiler starter supplemented with kitchen waste will be fed up to one month of age. Thereafter, they will be let out for foraging.

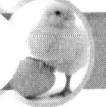

STATEMENT I

Fixed capital	Amount (₹ in lakhs)
1. Cost of 300 sq ft thatched house for brooding and night shelter	0.15
2. Cost of equipment	0.02
Total	**0.17**

STATEMENT II

Working capital	Amount (₹ in lakhs)
1. Cost of 100 day-old poultry @ ₹ 60/each	0.060
2. Broiler started feed for one month @ 1.5 kg/bird @ ₹ 25/kg	0.037
3. Feeds during scarcity (dry season) @ 10 kg/bird × ₹ 20/kg	0.200
Total	**0.297**

STATEMENT III

Annual recurring expenditure	Amount (₹ in lakhs)
1. Cost of 100 × 2 batches @ ₹ 60/each	0.120
2. Broiler starter feed (200 × 1.5 × 25)	0.075
3. Misc items include feeds in dry season (200 × 10 × 20)	0.400
Total	**0.595**

STATEMENT IV

Gross returns	Amount (₹ in lakhs)
1. By sale of 95 (5% mortality) × 2 batches at ₹ 200/ kg each weighing 4 kg.	0.912
Total	**0.912**

Net annual return = ₹ 0.912 – ₹ 0.595 = ₹ 0.317 lakhs

Benefit-cost ratio = 1.53

15.3.7 Project Report for a Cockerel Farm (All-in All-Out System)

Technical details and assumptions:

i. Cost of day-old male chicks (egg type) = ₹ 5/chick

ii. Area required per bird = ½ sq ft

iii. Equipment cost = ₹ 10/bird

iv. Feed required = 2 kg/bird

v. Cost of feed = ₹ 20/kg

vi. Body weight at 8 weeks = 650 g

vii. Age at marketing = 8 weeks

STATEMENT I

Capital investment	Amount (₹ in lakhs)
1. Thatched house for 2,000 chicks @ ½ sq ft/ bird = 1,000 sq ft @ ₹ 50/sq ft	0.50
2. Store room 200 sq ft (asbestos roof) @ ₹ 100/sq ft	0.20
3. Equipment cost	0.20
Total	**0.90**

STATEMENT II

Annual recurring expenditure	Amount (₹ in lakhs)
1. Cost of day-old male chicks 2,000 × 5 batches × ₹ 5/each	0.50
2. Feed cost for an average of 1,900 × 5 batches × 2 kg/bird × ₹ 20/kg of feed	3.80
3. Misc cost @ ₹ 5/bird for 2,000 × 5	0.50
Total	**4.80**

STATEMENT III

Annual gross and net returns	Amount (₹ in lakhs)
1. By sale of 1,850 cockerels × 5 × ₹ 58/each	5.365
2. By sale of empty bag 270 nos. × ₹ 10/each	0.027
3. By sale of 20 tonnes of manure @ ₹ 500/tonne	0.100
Total	**5.492**

Net returns/year = (₹ 5.492 – ₹ 4.80) lakhs = ₹ 0.692 lakhs

Net returns/month = ₹ 0.692 lakhs/12 = ₹ 5,766

Benefit-cost ratio = 1.14

15.4 DESIGNER MEAT AND EGG PRODUCTION

Meaning and Concept

Simply 'designer egg and meat' are those food items in which the contents have been modified from the normal products. The term 'designer egg' is more popular than 'designer meat'. These speciality products can be produced by flocks of chickens which have been fed special diets. Biotechnological intervention for genetic modification of hens for producing designer eggs was also tried with unconfirmed results. Obviously the cost of designer products will be more than normal ones. However, many consumers are ready to pay more for the products with respect to safety, healthfulness, freshness, taste, colour, *etc.*

The content modification of designer eggs is mainly inclined to increase vitamins A, E, C, carotenoids (mainly lutein), omega-3 fatty acid, selenium, iodine, *etc.* and decrease cholesterol. Vitamins E, Se and the carotenoids are important antioxidants and contribute significantly to the body's defence against free radical attack. Cooking did not alter the fatty acid composition of eggs, and functional properties of eggs are also retained. Research showed that cooking characteristics of designer omega-3 eggs including emulsification capacity, hardiness and springiness of sponge cakes prepared using these eggs are the same as in ordinary eggs. The major antioxidant constituents of the egg, vitamin E and lutein, are also stable during egg boiling.

The results of various experiments in relation to designer eggs are:

i. Designer eggs have been produced that contain higher concentrations of several **vitamins.** Two vitamins A and E, are receiving the most interest as components of designer eggs.

ii. The fatty acid profile of egg yolk lipid can easily be changed, simply by changing the type of fat used in the diet of poultry. Different feeds, such as safflower oil, marine algae, fish, fish oil and vegetable oil have been added to chicken feeds to increase the **omega-3 fatty acid** content in the egg yolk. Grass has a relatively high proportion of alpha-linolenic acid (53.4%) in total fatty acids and eggs from hens fed under free-range conditions had a higher concentration of total n-3 fatty acids than eggs from hens fed the commercial diet.

iii. It is possible to increase the content of selenium, iodine and chromium of egg through dietary supplementation of the hen. These three minerals are important in human health, however, there has been very little success in changing the calcium and phosphorus content of the albumen and yolk.

iv. Most of the carotenoids in egg yolk are hydroxy compounds called xanthophylls. Lutein and zeaxanthin are two of the most common xanthophylls found in egg yolk. Lutein and zeaxanthin are high in pigmented feed ingredients such as yellow corn, alfalfa meal, corn gluten meal, dried algae meal and marigold-petal meal. Fortunately, both lutein and zeaxanthin are efficiently transferred to the yolk when these various feed ingredients are fed to laying hens.

v. Another group of designer eggs is iodine-enriched eggs. Iodine deficiency still exists in many countries worldwide. Therefore, these eggs could be a good source of iodine in human diet. A typical egg of this type contains about 700 mg iodine.

vi. It is not possible to significantly decrease cholesterol levels in eggs without decreasing egg weight or egg production. Genetic selection of hens for lowered cholesterol has not been successful in lowering the egg cholesterol content. Chromium supplementation to laying hen diets at concentrations of less than 1 ppm have been shown to lower egg cholesterol and also improve egg interior quality. Research has also shown that the most effective way to lower egg cholesterol content is to lower the energy consumption of the hen. However, the use of drugs in lowering cholesterol is not yet approved in America for commercial use.

Commercial production of designer eggs in India and abroad

Various types of designer eggs (also called super eggs) are available in different countries. For example, in the UK there are free range eggs, organic eggs, and

Columbus eggs, *etc*. The nutritive values of these eggs are quite similar containing increased level of unsaturated linolenic acid. In some countries eggs enriched with iodine (Japan) or omega-3 fatty acid (Canada) are also produced. Pilgrim's Pride Company, a largest producer of poultry products in North America and Mexico introduced a speciality egg called EggsPlus with an increased level of vitamin E and omega-3 fatty acids. Similar eggs are produced by Gold Circle Farms, Colorado, USA; they are called Gold Circle Farms Eggs (containing 150 mg omega-3 fatty acid and 6 mg vitamin E). Omega Tech (USA) launched the sale of DHA eggs (rich in omega-3 fatty acid) in Germany, Spain, Portugal, Belgium, Norway and Andorra. They are sold under different names: OmegaDHA Eggs (Germany), BrudyEggs (Spain, Portugal and Andorra), DHA Food Products-Benelux (Belgium) and DHApluss (Norway). DHA-enriched eggs were recognised with the "Most Innovative Finished Food Product Award" in 1996 at the Annual Food Ingredients Europe Conference in Paris. A survey conducted in 5 major Texas cities with over 500 consumers indicated that 65% of consumers were willing to purchase n-3 fatty acid-enriched table eggs and, of these, 71% were willing to pay an additional price for this.

The designer eggs are gaining popularity in many countries of the world, even with higher price. However, this concept is in the virgin state in India.

15.5 EXPORT/IMPORT OF POULTRY AND POULTRY PRODUCTS

India's participation in the world trade in poultry has so far been negligible. India exports mainly day-old chicks (DOC), hatching eggs, table eggs, egg powder and frozen egg. On the other hand, India mainly imports parent stock, whole chicken fresh/chilled/frozen, and some additives such as lysine, methionine, choline chloride and vitamins.

The top export markets for India's table and hatching eggs are UAE, Kuwait, Oman, Saudi Arabia and Yemen. Similarly, for egg powders are the European Union (EU) and Japan. India also exports live poultry in the form of DOC to other South Asian countries (Table 15.1).

During 2010, the world trade (exports) in chicken meat amounted to around 11.63 million tonnes. But India's export of chicken meat was only 2.23 thousand tonnes i.e. only 0.02 per cent of the world's exports on a volume basis. Egg and egg-based products account for most of India's poultry exports. Exports of hatching and table eggs have increased dramatically due to a higher demand from the Middle East and south eastern countries (Table 15.2). In 1990 it was 1.52 thousand tonnes ($1.2 million) whereas it was more than 34.86 thousand tonnes in 2010 ($38.8 million).

India's import of poultry products is very negligible (Table 15.3) which may be due to a web of import restrictions. Only hotels and restaurants were permitted to import poultry meat under import licensing till early 2000. However, in beginning April 1, 2001, all quantitative restrictions on India's imports have been dismantled, and poultry items can be freely imported. Presently, effective from April 2001, chicken may be imported without license, but subject to an import duty of 30 per cent for whole chicken fresh/chilled/frozen and 100 per cent for cut in pieces, grandparent breeding stock can be imported without any barriers, and some additives such as lysine, methionine, choline chloride and vitamins can be freely imported.

Export of poultry products from India has tremendous potential. There are no restrictions on exports of poultry and poultry products in India. The government provides some transportation subsidies to facilitate the exports. India has competitive advantage in exporting poultry and poultry products, since the cost of poultry production is comparatively low, next only to Brazil. However, the government support is not adequate, and international price structure is another important problem to exploit the potentiality of this sector. Poultry and poultry products are subsidised in some countries like USA and EU; this factor has impeded India's export of such products not only to these countries but also to other countries where they compete with India. Improvements are also required in technology of packaging, preservation and transportation. Consumer preferences in international markets are to be kept in mind for increasing the exports of poultry from India. As for example, in Dubai, our major sales of eggs are in institutional markets like caterers, hotels and restaurants. Retail stores prefer eggs from the USA and Europe. Indian eggs are considered as of low quality and price is US $ 2–3 less per carton (360 eggs) than the eggs from the USA and Europe. With the onset of WTO agreement, strict quality and hygiene standards are being prescribed by countries intending to import poultry products. Infrastructure facilities including cold chain facilities, better veterinary inspection, disease screening and certification facilities are required to be provided at international airports.

Table 15.1: India's major markets for export of poultry and poultry products

Live poultry	Sri Lanka (50%) Bangladesh (32.5%) Nepal (8.2%)
Hatching eggs	UAE (38%) Oman (26.8%) Kuwait (5.4%)
Table eggs	UAE (72.8%) Kuwait (8.3%) Oman (8.3%)
Egg powder	Japan (16%) Poland (14.5%) UAE (8.9%) Belgium (5.5%)
Frozen eggs	UAE (83%) Oman (5%) Kuwait (3.9%)

Source: Rahman SA (2005).

Table 15.2:   India's export of poultry, 1990–2010

(Quantity in tonnes, Value in '000 USD)

Year	Chicken meat— fresh, chilled or frozen		Birds eggs— without shell dried		Birds eggs— without shell liquid		Hen eggs— with shell		Poultry total
	Quantity	Value	Quantity	Value	Quantity	Value	Quantity	Value	Value
1990	–	–	22	19	1	2	1,524	1,154	1,175
1995	70	60	305	1,249	44	97	13,175	4,238	5,644
2000	84	92	957	2,481	4,539	6,620	11,344	12,741	21,934
2005	476	602	7,699	25,544	1,500	2,423	58,744	42,841	71,410
2010	2,234	2,948	6,085	26,770	600	1,070	34,861	38,790	69,578

Source: FAOSTAT; FAO Statistics Division, 2013.

Table 15.3:   India's import of poultry, 1990–2010

(Quantity in tonnes, Value in '000 USD)

Year	Chicken meat— fresh, chilled or frozen		Birds eggs— without shell dried		Birds eggs— without shell liquid		Hen eggs— with shell		Poultry total
	Quantity	Value	Quantity	Value	Quantity	Value	Quantity	Value	Value
1990	–	–	–	–	–	–	–	–	–
1995	–	–	–	–	–	–	–	–	–
2000	–	–	–	–	–	–	23	40	40.12
2005	–	–	3	11	1	12	366	986	1,009
2010	–	–	–	–	24	116	144	576	692

Source: FAOSTAT; FAO Statistics Division, 2013—negligible.

15.6   KEY PLAYERS IN POULTRY INDUSTRY IN INDIA

Important large scale integrated players in Indian poultry industry are Venkateshwara Hatcheries (VH) group, Suguna Poultry Product Limited, Godrej Agrovet Limited, Charoen Pokphand (India) Private Limited, Arambagh Hatcheries Limited, *etc.* They have their own grandparent and parent breeding farms, hatcheries, feed mills, in-house veterinary services, and marketing set up. They have also moved into vertical integration by setting up retail chains, processing, branding and aggressively marketing their products under frozen/chilled and ready-to-cook categories. They are also engaged in poultry production through contract farming model which is spread across the country. The farm sizes under this contract farming model are typically ranging from 2,000–10,000 of DOCs, though there are few larger farms also. The strong growth in Indian poultry industry is attributed to the successful implementation of this large scale contract poultry farming model. In this model, integrators provide farmers with DOCs, feed, medicines, necessary training and standard growing fee, while farmer needs to provide farm space, labour and power. The growing fee is usually a minimum guaranteed fee plus bonus based on gain body weight of the birds with typical per kg growing fee of ₹ 3.5/kg. Poultry farming provides a healthy source of alternative income for large rural population of the country and has been growing strongly across the country especially in Southern India, and in the states of Maharashtra, Haryana and Punjab.

EXERCISE

A. Objective Questions

i. **Indicate the correct answer by putting tick (√) mark (multiple choice).**

1. Average weight of a good quality broiler chicken at the age of marketing is expected to be
   (a) 1.0 kg   (b) 2.0 kg
   (c) 2.8 kg   (d) 3.5 kg

2. The content modification of designer eggs is mainly inclined
   (a) To increase omega-3 fatty acid
   (b) To decrease cholesterol
   (c) To increase vitamin A
   (d) All of these

3. Which of the following feed item(s) has/have been added to chicken feed to increase the omega-3 fatty acid content in the egg yolk?
   (a) Marine algae   (b) Safflower oil
   (c) Fish oil   (d) All of these

4. India's major market for export of live poultry is
   (a) Bangladesh   (b) Nepal
   (c) Sri Lanka   (d) None of these

5. India's major market for export of table eggs is
   (a) Kuwait   (b) Oman
   (c) Sri Lanka   (d) UAE

6. India's major market for export of frozen eggs is
   (a) Kuwait   (b) Oman
   (c) UAE   (d) None of these

7. Cost of which of the following inputs in poultry farm is maximum?
   (a) Housing   (b) Nutrition
   (c) Brooding   (d) Medicine

8. Which of the following poultry related enterprises is most profitable?
   (a) Broiler farming
   (b) Layer farming
   (c) Poultry hatchery
   (d) All are equally profitable

9. India exports mainly
   (a) Day-old chicks   (b) Hatching eggs
   (c) Table eggs   (d) All of these

10. Match List I with List II and select the correct answer using the code given below the lists.

List I (Term)

A. Cull bird

B. Broiler

C. Layer

D. Day-old chick

List II (Meaning)

1. Egg type chicken generally kept in the farm for 72 weeks for economic egg production.
2. Meat type chicken marketed at 5–6 weeks of age.
3. Egg type chicken used as meat purpose after completion of laying.
4. A chicken just after hatching.

Code (a) A B C D
         3 1 2 4

(b) A B C D
    3 4 1 2

(c) A B C D
    1 3 4 2

(d) A B C D
    3 2 1 4

ii. Fill in the blanks.

1. Two vitamins, viz. _____ and _____ are receiving the most interest as components of designer eggs.
2. Most of the carotenoids in egg yolk are hydroxy compounds called _____.
3. India exports frozen eggs mainly to _____, Oman and Kuwait.
4. India exports day-old chicks mainly to _____, Bangladesh and Nepal.
5. Feed cost per kg of broiler produced is calculated by the multiplication of _____ with cost per kg of feed.

iii. Write True (T) or False (F) against each statement.

1. The top export markets for India's table and hatching eggs are UAE, Kuwait, Oman, *etc.*
2. The fatty acid profile of egg yolk can easily be changed, simply by changing the type of fat used in the diet of poultry.
3. Eggs from hens fed under free-range conditions had a higher concentration of total n-3 fatty acids than eggs from hens fed commercial diets.
4. The concept of producing the designer eggs is to decrease the omega-3 fatty acid content in the egg yolk.
5. Sri Lanka is the major export market of India for live poultry especially in terms of day-old chicks.

B. Subjective Questions

1. Enlist the important poultry farm records. What are the advantages of keeping records in poultry farms? Prepare the formats of records related to feeds and feeding, and broiler rearing and its performance.
2. Discuss the factors affecting costs and returns in poultry farming.

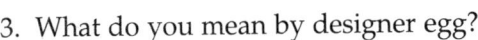

3. What do you mean by designer egg?

4. What technical assumptions should be made for preparation of a project for establishment of a layer/broiler farm?

5. Which will be the most profitable on your farm, rearing of broilers or layers? Justify your answer.

6. Prepare a model scheme for establishment of a commercial broiler chicken farm in your locality with 1,000 birds/lot/month capacity.

7. Prepare a project report for rearing of 10,000 layer chickens.

8. Calculate the mortality percentage and FCR of a commercial broiler farm from the following information.

Number of birds housed: 1,200, total feed intake up to 6 weeks: 3,904 kg, total no. of birds died: 25, and total live weight up to 6 weeks: 2,058 kg.

9. Calculate the mortality percentage and hen housed egg production in a year of a commercial poultry farm from the following information.

Number of birds at the onset of production: 2,000, total egg production: 5,60,000, and total no. of birds died: 76.

10. Write short notes on the following.
   (a) Hen housed egg production
   (b) Hen day egg production
   (c) Calculation of FCR in broiler
   (d) Designer egg
   (e) Export–import of poultry and poultry products

Answers of the Objective Questions

i. Multiple choice

1. (b) 2.0 kg   2. (d) All of these   3. (d) All of these
4. (c) Sri Lanka   5. (d) UAE   6. (c) UAE
7. (b) Nutrition   8. (c) Poultry hatchery 9. (d) All of these
10. (d)

ii. Fill in the blanks

1. vitamin A, vitamin E   2. xanthophylls   3. UAE
4. Sri Lanka   5. FCR

iii. True or False

1. T   2. T   3. T   4. F   5. T

Appendices

Appendix 1
VCI Syllabus

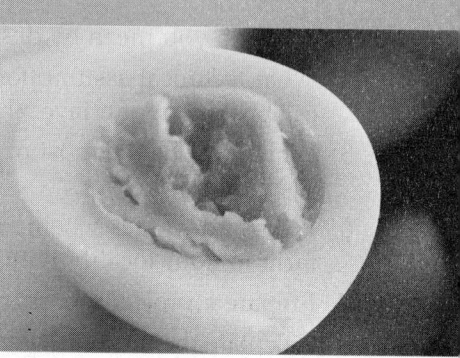

Course Name: AVIAN PRODUCTION MANAGEMENT

[LPM-211, Credit hours 1 + 1 = 2, Semester III]

THEORY

Indian Poultry Industry — brief outline of the different segments, poultry statistics. Classification of poultry, common breeds of poultry including duck, quail, turkey and Guinea fowl and their descriptions. Description of indigenous fowls. Reproduction in fowl, male and female reproduction systems, formation of eggs and structure of eggs. Important economic traits of poultry, egg production, egg weight, egg quality, growth, feed consumption and feed efficiency, fertility and hatchability, plumage characteristics and comb types. Scavenging system of management: Raising of chicks, scavenger feed base of village. Low input technology; backyard and semi-intensive unit of various sizes; their descriptions, management and economic achievements. New coloured feathered birds developed in public and private sectors for meat and egg production for rural poultry; their acceptability and assimilation in rural ecosystem. Mixed farming and poultry raising. Concept of self-local market unit. Brooding and rearing practices used for chicken, duck, quail, turkey and Guinea fowl. Economic production of chicken, and other classes of poultry. Hatching and feeding norms for different species of poultry. Marketing of poultry and poultry products. Setting of farms for different classes of poultry. Organic and hill farming.

PRACTICAL

Morphological description of common exotic poultry breeds like White Leghorn (WLH), Rhode Island Red (RIR), Plymouth Rock, Cornish and New Hampshire. Diagrammatic illustration of body parts of chicken, duck, quail, Guinea fowl and turkey. Descriptive specialities of indigenous birds, listing of its advantageous value in rural areas. Diagrammatic representation of scavenging, backyard and semi-intensive units; with habitats, feed base and shelter. Conservation of indigenous germplasm; listing of conservation techniques. Demonstration of newly developed breeds in rural environment. Housing, equipments, nesting and brooding requirements. Vaccination, medication and incubation requirements. Preparation of projects for rural people on poultry and other species (duck, quail, Guinea fowl and turkey).

Course Name: COMMERCIAL POULTRY PRODUCTION AND HATCHERY MANAGEMENT

[LPM-221, Credit hours 1 + 1 = 2, Semester IV]

THEORY

HOUSING: Location of poultry. Types of poultry house. Different types of rearing — advantages and disadvantages. Space requirement for different age groups under different rearing systems. Environmentally controlled housing.

BROODING MANAGEMENT: Brooding, types of brooder, preparation of shed to receive chicks and importance of environment (temperature, humidity and ventilation). Feeding and vaccination in early stages of chicks.

REARING AND MANAGEMENT: Care and management of growing, laying/broiler birds of both breeders and commercial categories of poultry. Battery cage management: Different types and sizes. Poultry judging.

LITTER MANAGEMENT: Litter materials, litterborne diseases and control; potential for poultry litter used as fertilisers; recycling for livestock feeding and power generation. Special management care in adverse weather conditions/stress; summer management; modification of housing, light reflectors, insulators, sprinklers, foggers and other methods; dietary modification to minimise heat stress; special management during rainy and winter seasons; other stress management — vice in poultry and its remedial measures.

WATER MANAGEMENT: Standard for drinking water in terms of total solids, pH, mineral levels, sanitisers and water sanitations, disease spread through water contamination — prevention.

BIOSECURITY: Proactive measures to minimise entry of infections in farm premises — farm fencing, disinfectant pits, personnel management, restriction of movement, *etc*. Poultry welfare and behaviour.

FEEDING: Digestive system and digestion in chicken. Classification, selection of common feed ingredients and their nutrient compositions. Nutrient requirement for different age groups. Feed formulation, economics of feed formulation — cost/unit nutrient. Feeding systems and feeding management, economisation of poultry feeding. Feed restriction — separate male feeding, non-nutrient feed additives including herbal bioenhancers. Antinutritional factors and toxins.

HEALTHCARE: Common poultry diseases: Bacterial, viral, fungal, parasitic and nutritional deficiencies. Vaccination schedule for commercial layers and broilers: Factors that govern vaccination schedule; vaccination principles type, methods, pre- and post-vaccination cares. Medication: Types of administration — general principles and precautions with emphasis on administering medication through water and feed; commonly used drugs in poultry diseases. Disinfection: Types of disinfectant, mode of action, recommended procedure, precaution and handling.

ECONOMICS: Economics of layer and broiler production; project reports of layer in different systems of rearing. Project reports for broilers: Feasibility studies on poultry rearing in context of small units and their profitability. Designer meat and egg production. Export/import of poultry and poultry products.

BREEDER FLOCK MANAGEMENT: Layer and broiler breeder flock managements, housing and space requirements. Different stages of management during life cycle; light management during growing and laying periods. Artificial insemination. Feeding: Feed restriction, separate male feeding. Nutrient requirement of layer and broiler breeders of different age groups. Health care: Vaccination of breeder flock, difference between vaccination schedule of broilers and commercial birds. Common diseases of breeders (infectious and metabolic disorders) — prevention. Fertility disorder — etiology, diagnosis and corrective measures. Selection and culling of breeder flocks. Economic parameters on returns from breeders — for example, saleable chicks/hen/production cycle, *etc.*

HATCHERY PRACTICES: Management: Principles of incubation. Factors affecting fertility and hatchability. Disposal of hatchery waste; sexing, grading, packing and dispatch of day-old chicks. Economics of hatchery business; trouble-shooting hatch failure: Importance of hatchery records, breakeven analysis of unhatched eggs. Biosecurity in the hatchery. Computer applications for hatchery management.

PRACTICAL

Male and female reproductive systems, artificial insemination. Selection of breeder flock.

Working of hatchery, incubation requirement; incubators' working, care. Hatchery layout and equipment. Handling of eggs prior and during incubation. Candling. Fumigation. Project reports of setting up a hatchery. Hatchery records and maintenance.

Exposure to commercial broiler and layer farms — different systems of housing. Demonstration of litter and cage rearing systems. Feed equipment and maintenance; hammer mill, mixture, pellet mill types, principle of working, comparison of different types, premix preparations, quality control of raw materials. Feed mill operation. Demonstration of different types of feeders, waterers, foggers, sprinklers, *etc.* Maintenance of farm records.

Medication — demonstration of routinely employed methods of administration. Vaccination practice in general and demonstration of different routes of administration in particular.

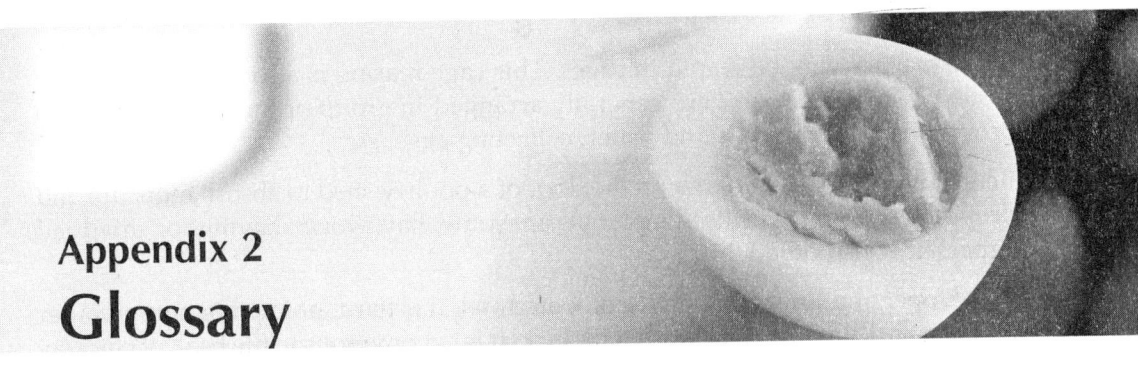

Appendix 2
Glossary

A

Abdominal capacity: It is the capacity of abdomen of a bird, measured by placing fingers between two pubic bones. If the abdominal capacity is more, it will be a good layer. In case of good layers the distance between two pubic bones should be at least three fingers.

Air cell: The air space between the two shell membranes, usually present at the large end of an egg, which can be simply seen when the egg is candled. It indicates the age of an egg, larger air cell means more age of egg.

Albumen: The white portion of an egg. It is about 58% of the total weight of a chicken egg. In liquid form, the albumen is composed of water and proteins. In dry form, it is composed of proteins.

Ambient temperature: The prevailing temperature or surrounding temperature.

Animal protein factor: APF. Vitamin B_{12} is called animal protein factor. It is present to some extent in the built up deep litter.

Anthelmintic: An antiworm drug, e.g. Piperazine, Fenbendazole, Albendazole, Levamisole, Niclosamide, *etc.*

Antibiotic: A soluble chemical produced by a microorganism or fungus and used to destroy or inhibit the growth of bacteria and other microorganisms, e.g. Tetracycline, Gentamycin, Enrofloxacin, *etc.*

Autosexing: Determination of sex on the basis of sex-linked morphological characters. It is one of the methods of sexing of poultry.

Avian: The term is related to all species of birds including domestic fowl. Zoologically they are under the class Aves.

Aviculture: The science of raising avian species. It is specially related to keeping birds.

Avidin: It is a specific protein component of egg albumin. It is present in the raw egg. If raw egg (uncooked) is eaten, it interacts with biotin (a vitamin of B complex group) to render it unavailable leading to the syndrome called egg white injury. Avidin is denatured by heat and thereby inactivated.

B

Battery: Birds may be reared in cages. This cage rearing is also known as battery system of rearing. Cages are generally arranged in group or multiple decks with provision of giving feeds and water, collecting eggs, *etc.*

Bedding: Materials scattered on the floor of a poultry shed to absorb moisture and droppings. Commonly used materials are straw, hay, wood shavings or shredded paper, *etc.* Also called 'litter'.

Bill: Upper and lower mandibles of waterfowl. It is hard, pointed or curved outer part of a bird's mouth. It is present in duck. It is synonymous to the beak of chicken.

Biosecurity: Disease Prevention Management. A management system to minimise the disease exposure in flocks. In poultry health management biosecurity measures are of great importance.

Blood spot: It is a defect of egg. Sometimes reddish spot is seen in the egg white (albumen) portion of an egg. This spot is called blood spot. It is generally due to nutritional and management faults including low level of vitamin A. Eggs with blood spot are not suitable for hatching purpose.

Blastoderm: The site of fertilisation on the egg yolk in fertile eggs. Also a fertilised true egg.

Blastodisc: The site of fertilisation on the egg yolk. Also a true egg that was not fertilised.

Booster: Vaccination other than the first one in a series.

Bran: The seed coat of wheat and other cereal grains. It is obtained during the processing of the cereal grains as by-product. For example, wheat bran is obtained during preparation of the wheat flour. The bran is used as poultry feed ingredient.

Breast: The forward part of the body between the neck and the keel bone in poultry.

Broiler: Broiler is a young chicken of either sex, which has tender meat with smooth textured skin and soft and pliable breast bone, weighing about 1.5–2.0 kg at the age of 6 weeks and consuming 1.7–1.8 kg feed per kg live weight.

Brooder: It is the device which provides heat to the birds at their early part of lives generally up to 4–6 weeks of age or until they are well-feathered. There are various types of brooders, e.g. bamboo basket, hover or canopy (round, conical or angular shaped structure usually made up of galvanised iron sheets fitted with bulbs), infrared lamps (electricity), infrared brooder (gas), radient brooder (gas), cage or battery brooder, *etc.* Choice of brooder depends on the system of keeping poultry, economy and number of chicks to be reared, source of fuel, *etc.*

Broody hen: The hen used for natural hatching of eggs is called broody hen. A broody hen should be light in weight, well-feathered and good sitter. *Deshi* hens are ideal broody hens.

Bursa of fabricius: Cloacal bursa.

C

Calciferol: Vitamin D_2 is commonly known as calciferol.

Calorie (cal): The amount of heat required to raise the temperature of 1 g water from 14.5 to 15.5 °C is called calorie. It is equivalent to 4.185 J. **Kilocalorie (Kcal)** is the equivalent of 1,000 small calories.

Candler: The light device used to examine the contents on an intact egg. It is a wooden or metal box closed from all sides except an egg-sized aperture (2.5 cm diameter) on one side and has an electric bulb fitted inside the box. Commonly known as egg candler.

Candling: Testing of eggs with the help of a light source is popularly known as candling. Testing of egg is done by viewing through egg by holding it in front of a source of light in a darkroom. Initially candle was used as a source of light, so the name is candling. Presently, it is done with the help of an egg candler. Observation is taken while viewing through and twirling the egg before the aperture of the candler.

Cannibalism: It is a vice or bad habit of some fowls like plucking of feathers, pecking of vent, wings, toes and head, breaking or eating of eggs, *etc.* The probable causes of cannibalism are overcrowding, mineral (salt) deficiency, high temperature and brighter light, overgrown beak and very low fibre in the diet. As it is due to faulty management, cannibalism can be prevented by proper stocking density, timely debeaking, proper feeds having required salt and fibre percentage, toe clipping in case of breeder birds, *etc.*

Cape: It is a narrow feather, only present in male fowl between chicken's neck and back.

Capon: Castrated male chickens (that have had their reproductive organs/testes surgically removed) are called capon. They lose some of their male sex characteristics. Usually accompanied by underdeveloped comb and wattles and longer hackle, saddle and tail feathers than a normal male. The sex libido is lost.

Caponettes: Male chickens that have had their reproductive organs made useless by injection of an estrogenic hormone (like stilbestrol).

Caponisation: The process of surgical removal of reproductive organs (testes) of male chickens.

CARI: Central Avian Research Institute of India is located at Izatnagar near Bareilly of Uttar Pradesh state. It is one of the India's most modern research infrastructures in the field of poultry science with all its interdisciplines. It was established in 1979 under the administrative control of Indian Council of Agricultural Research (ICAR), New Delhi.

Celsius: The temperature expressed in degrees, where 0° C and 100° C are the freezing and boiling temperatures respectively, of water at sea level. It is a centigrade temperature scale. It can be converted to fahrenheit by using formula [(°C × 9/5) + 32 = °F].

Chalazae: The two whitish cords on opposite sides of the yolk that hold the yolk in the centre of the albumen and serve as a rotating axis to keep the germ cell on the top side of the yolk and next to the heat of the hen's body. Singular — chalaza.

Chalaziferous layer: Thin layer of thick white surrounding the yolk, continuous with the chalazae.

Chick: Newborn fowl or chicken is called chick. It may be of either sex. The term is also used to denote the baby quail. In case of layer farming (chicken) the term 'chick' is used up to the age of eight weeks and during this period 'chick ration' is offered to the birds.

Chicken: The term is synonymous to fowl. It is the major species of poultry. Its scientific name is *Gallus domesticus* (domestic chicken) or *Gallus gallus* (wild chicken). Chickens have been domesticated for thousands of years and have been developed into many different breeds and varieties by man. They are an efficient source of protein, producing both meat and eggs. They are one of the most prevalent forms of livestock bred around the world today. The meat of fowl/chicken is commonly known as chicken. In India, the term poultry is used synonymously to chicken, as chicken accounts for more than 90% of the poultry population. Indian poultry industry is chicken oriented.

CLFMA: The Compound Livestock Feed Manufacturers' Association. CLFMA was formed in June 1967 as an association of feed manufacturers and associated industries such as ingredient suppliers, importers, feed additive manufacturers, consultants, hatcheries and milk cooperatives and feed machinery manufacturers. The objectives of CLFMA are to promote the concept of nutritionally balanced compound feed; to assist and coordinate scientific research in the field of animal nutrition; to conduct, sponsor or cosponsor surveys and studies; to collect, classify and circulate information related to animal feed to its members and government; to offer suggestions to government in formulating policies; and to impart training to livestock farmers, feed mill personnel, veterinarians, students and others. The office-bearers of CLFMA are elected and operate for a maximum of two years at one level. Over the years, CLFMA has been able to solve many problems of the animal feed industry.

Cloaca: The chamber just inside the vent in birds at which the digestive, excretory, and reproductive tracts open.

Clutch size: The number of eggs laid on consecutive days without gap in an egg laying sequence is known as clutch size. Clutch size is more in good layer birds than in *deshi* birds.

Clutch: The eggs laid by a hen on consecutive days before she skips a day and begins a new laying cycle. Also a batch of eggs that is incubated and hatched together, either in an incubator or in a nest under a hen.

Coccidiosis: A parasitic protozoal infection, usually occurring in damp and unclean housing.

Coccidiostat: A drug used to prevent coccidiosis, e.g. Amprolium.

Cock: A mature male chicken (or fowl) usually above one year of age is called cock. Its skin is coarse; meat is toughened and darkened along with hard chest bone. It is also known as rooster.

Cockerel: A young male chicken/fowl usually below one year of age. Its meat is comparatively better than cock in respect of its texture, tenderness, chest bone structure, *etc.*

Comb: A piece of red flesh (tissue) present on the head of chicken. It may be of various shapes like pea comb, single comb, rose comb, *etc.*

Coop: The house in which a chicken lives.

CPBF: Central Poultry Breeding Farm. These farms are under the overall supervision and control of Department of Animal Husbandry, Dairying and Fisheries, Ministry of Agriculture, Govt of India. CPBFs are located at Bengaluru, Mumbai, Gurgaon and Bhubaneswar.

Crop: A pouch at the base of a chicken's neck that bulges after the bird has eaten. It stores and softens feed for digestion.

Crude fibre (CF): It is the least digestible part of a feed. This portion of feedstuffs is composed of cellulose, hemicellulose, lignin, *etc.* It is high in forages and less in cereal grains. Ruminants (cattle, buffalo, sheep and goat) can digest large quantity of crude fibre, but poultry and non-ruminants (pig) can digest little quantity of crude fibre. As per BIS specification, CF content (in per cent, maximum) of chick, grower and layer mash should be 4, 7 and 6, and of broiler starter and broiler finisher mash should be 3.5 and 4.

Crude protein (CP): This is the total protein of a feedstuff. In calculating the crude protein percentage of a feedstuff, first the nitrogen content is chemically analysed, and then it is multiplied by 6.25 to give the CP percentage; since on average, the nitrogen content of natural protein is approximately 16 per cent ($100 \div 16 = 6.25$). As per BIS specification, CP content (in per cent, minimum) of chick, grower and layer mash should be 20, 16 and 18, and of broiler starter and broiler finisher mash should be 22 and 19–20.

Crumble: It is the rough mixture of poultry feed, not as fine as mash. Its consistency is coarser than mash, looks like broken pellets (small cylindrical-shaped feed). These are generally offered to the starting chicken.

Cull bird: The laying birds (chicken) after one year of economic laying (i.e. after 72 weeks of age) are sold in the market for meat purpose. These birds are generally known as cull birds. In broader sense, all the undesirable birds which are removed from the flock are called cull birds.

Culling: Removal of undesirable birds from the flock is called culling. It is an important and continuous process in commercial poultry farming as it improves the economics of poultry farming by culling unproductive or less productive birds at appropriate time. It also reduces the chance of spreading disease from unhealthy birds to the apparently healthy birds of the flock.

D

Dead-in-shell: Late embryonic death during incubation is known as 'dead-in-shell'. Causes may be poor ventilation, faulty turning of eggs, infection (like BWD), and ill-health of breeder stock including poor nutrition. It is commonly detected by testing of incubated eggs on 18th day of incubation in commercial hatcheries.

Debeaking: Removal of a portion of bird's top beak. In poultry farming ½ to 1/3rd portion of upper beak is removed and lower beak is trimmed to some extent at an early age manually or by electrical debeaker machine. Debeaking is done to reduce feed wastage and to prevent cannibalism in poultry.

Deep litter: This is the bedding of poultry under deep litter system of management. The floor of the house is covered with dry materials like rice husk, sawdust, wood shavings, chopped straw, dried leaves, groundnut shells, *etc.* as per the cost and availability. The depth of deep litter is 3 inches in broiler and 6 inches in layer house.

Depigmentation: Depigmentation is used as a tool for judging layer birds. Depigmentation or bleaching acts as an index in assessing the persistency of egg production. The pigment, xanthophylls is derived from the feed (principally from yellow maize) and stored in different parts of the body. The bird looses this pigment as the laying age progresses. At the last stage, i.e. in the last 20 weeks of egg productions, when the production is less the pigments reappear in the same order.

Designer eggs: Speciality eggs in which contents are modified. Generally vitamins A and E, carotenoids, selenium, iodine, omega-3 fatty acids are increased in the designer eggs by offering special diets to the birds.

Dewlap: The single flap of skin below the beak of turkeys and some geese.

DHA: Docosahexaenoic acid, commonly known as DHA. It is an omega-3 essential fatty acid. In chemical structure, DHA is a carboxylic acid with a 22-carbon chain and six *cis* double bonds; the first double bond is located at the third carbon from the omega end. Fish oils are rich in DHA. It is also commercially manufactured from microalgae. Most animals make very little DHA through metabolism. However, small amounts are manufactured internally through the consumption of α-linolenic acid, an omega-3 fatty acid found in plants, animals and milk. DHA is metabolised to form the docosanoids—several families of potent hormones. It is a major fatty acid in sperm and brain phospholipids, and especially in the retina. Dietary DHA may reduce the risk of heart disease by reducing the level of blood triglycerides in humans. Presently, there is an approach to produce designer eggs, rich in DHA. In many countries of the world DHA-rich eggs are available in the markets.

Disinfectant: Anything used to destroy disease-causing organisms.

Double yolker: Egg containing two yolks.

Drake: Adult male ducks are called drake. They are capable of breeding.

Drakelet: Male day-old duckling.

Droppings: The excreta of bird is known as droppings. It is the mixture of faeces and urine passed through the vent of birds. It is very rich in fertiliser value (NPK), can be used as biofertiliser in agri-horti fields and also in the pond for aquaculture. It can be fed in the biogas plant for production of biogas.

Drumstick: Thigh portion of meat type bird used for table purpose.

Dry bulb thermometer: Thermometer that expresses air temperature reading in number of degrees fahrenheit (F) or centigrade/celsius (C).

Dubbing: Surgical removal or trimming of comb and wattle of poultry.

Duck: It is used as a common term which indicates the species of duck (*Anas platyrhynchos*) under the family *Anatidae*. Specifically adult female ducks are called duck.

Duckling: Newborn and young ones of duck are called duckling. They are of either sex.

Dust bath: The habit of chicken, thrashing around in soft soil to clean their feathers and discourage body parasites.

E

Earlobes: The fleshy skin below the ears, varying in size, shape and colour. The colour may be red, white, blue or purple, according to the breed.

Ectoparasites: External parasites like lice, ticks, flies, mites, *etc.*

Edema: Accumulation of excessive fluid in swollen or damaged tissues.

Egg size: The egg weight and egg size are synonymous. Standard egg sizes of various species of poultry are chicken egg—58 g, duck egg—70 g, quail egg—10 g, *etc.*

Egg: The microscopic germ cell of the female animal or bird. It is also a common term to denote the shelled egg, which is used as a nutritious and palatable food item.

Embryo: The developing chick within the egg.

Endoparasite: Internal parasite, commonly known as worm.

Etiology: The study of causes of disease.

F

Feed conversion efficiency: The units of feed consumed per unit of weight gain. Sometimes it is also called **FCR** (feed conversion ratio) or simply **feed efficiency**. In case of broiler chicken farming the **FCE** should be 2 or less.

Fertile egg: An egg that is fertilised; the capability of an egg to develop into a chick.

Fertilisation: The act or process of making or becoming fertile; the union of a male cell with a female cell. It takes place in the infundibulum or funnel part of oviduct in hen, generally within 18 minutes after ovulation.

Flight feathers: Primary feathers of the wings, sometimes used to denote the primaries and secondaries.

Flock: A group of birds living together.

Fluff: Downy feathers around the vent of a fowl, abdominal feathers of fowl. These are very soft feathers. Initial hairy covering of baby chicken or turkey is also called fluff or **down**.

Fowl: It is a species of poultry, also known as chicken. Its scientific name is *Gallus domesticus* (domestic fowl) or *Gallus gallus* (wild fowl).

Frizzle: Feathers that curl rather than lay flat; also a chicken with such feathers.

Fryer: Fryer and broiler are synonymous. *See broiler.*

G

Gallus domesticus: The domestic chicken or fowl.

Gallus gallus: The red jungle fowl. It is considered as the origin of all current chicken breeds.

Game birds: Any of several species including pheasant, quail and partridge that have traditionally been hunted for food and sport. Game birds may be raised in captivity, but are not domestic in the senses that chickens are. The term can also be used for wild turkey and some species of wild waterfowl.

Gander: A mature male goose.

Germinal disc: Site of fertilisation on the egg yolk; blastodisc.

Giblets: Edible viscera (internal organ) of a fowl used as food. The term used to describe the portion of poultry carcasses that consist of heart, gizzard and liver.

Gizzard: An internal organ of birds specifically the muscular stomach. It has thick muscular wall and a tough lining. It crushes and grinds feed by muscular action and with grits. It is an edible part of the digestive system of poultry.

Goose: A mature female goose.

Gosling: A young goose of either sex.

Growers: Growing birds of egg type chicken aged between 9 to 20 weeks or point of lay; pullets between 9 weeks to point of lay.

Guinea fowl: Guinea fowl are referred by various local names as *Chittra* in Western region, *Titri* in Northern plains, and *China Murgi* (*Cheena Murgi*) in southern peninsular and Eastern parts of India. Scientific name of Guinea fowl is *Numida meleagris*. A pheasant like bird from Africa raised for ornamental qualities, meat, feathers or vermin control. They are gregarious, and very interesting. They are watchful and territorial, making them good natural alarms. They can be noisy, tend to be only partially domesticated, and if allowed to roam will cover a fairly wide range.

H

Hackles: Erectile hairs on the back of certain animals. Neck feathers of fowl are commonly known as hackles. These feathers are present both in male and female fowls. The ends are usually pointed in males and rounded in females.

Hairline crack: Hair like fine cracks may be present in the eggshell which cannot be seen by naked eye, but can be identified with the help of candling.

Hatchery: A place where eggs are incubated and hatched, or a place having facility for hatching of eggs. Nowadays hatching of eggs is taken as a business, and it is known as hatchery enterprise. The whole venture of hatchery enterprise includes procurement of fertile eggs, their hatching and finally selling of chicks/ducklings to the poultry farmers. Fertilised eggs are placed into an incubator, a hatching machine that maintains conditions favourable for hatching. Chicken eggs will hatch 21 days after they are set and duck eggs after 28 days.

Hatching egg: A fertilised egg used to hatch; fertile egg.

Hatching: Hatching means production of baby chicks from fertile eggs. The term 'hatching' is also known as incubation. The hatching of eggs may be of two types, viz. natural hatching (with the help of broody hen) and artificial hatching (with the help of machine/incubator). In commercial poultry production hatching is done by the artificial method. The optimum conditions are to be maintained for successful hatching of eggs, viz. optimum temperature (37.2–37.7 °C in case of chicken), relative humidity (60–70% in case of chicken), proper ventilation (to provide 21% oxygen in air) and turning of eggs (at least 4 times a day during first 18 days of incubation in case of chicken).

Hen: The female of all classes of poultry, except goose, whose age can vary considerably depending on the class of poultry. A female chicken over 1 year of age is commonly called hen. Sometimes the term pullet is used to denote the female hen up to one year of age.

Hock: The knee joint of a chicken's leg, between the lower thigh and the shank.

Hover: Canopy used on brooder stoves to hold heat near the floor when brooding young stock.

I

Incubation period: The period between setting of eggs and hatching is known as incubation period. It varies from one species of bird to other. The incubation period of chicken is 21 days, duck, turkey, Guinea fowl and geese 28 days, Japanese quail 18 days, and Muscovy duck 35 days.

Incubation: *See hatching*

Incubator: It is a machine used for production of chicks from fertile eggs. All the favourable environments are created and maintained in this machine artificially. Nowadays two types of incubators are in use, viz. combined incubator (setter-cum-hatcher) where chicken eggs are kept for 21 days, and setter and hatcher where chicken eggs are kept for 18 days in setter and remaining 3 days in hatcher.

IU: International unit. It is a unit of measurement of biologicals (like vitamins, hormones, antibiotics, *etc.*) as defined and adopted by the International Conference for Unification of Formulas. The potency depends on the bioassay that produces a specific biological effect agreed on internationally. For example, as per BIS specification, vitamin A requirement for broiler mash is 6500 IU/kg of feed.

K

Keet: A Guinea fowl chick.

L

Layer: The adult female birds reared for production of eggs — most commonly chickens and ducks. In case of high yielding hybrid chicken, layer birds are generally kept in the farm up to 72–80 weeks of age. These chickens are usually at least 18–20 weeks of age and may include the breeder hen that produces broiler type or egg type hatching eggs.

Laying period: This is the period when birds are in egg laying stage. Poultry (chicken or duck) starts to lay egg at the age of 18–20 weeks and continued till death. However, one year laying period in chicken and 2–3 years in duck are economical.

Laying: Act of giving eggs in chicken or duck. Also called oviposition.

Litter: Absorbent bedding materials used to cover the floor in poultry houses.

M

ME: Metabolisable energy. It is generally expressed as Kcal/kg of feed.

Meat spot: It is a defect of egg. Sometimes blackish spot is seen in the egg white (albumen) portion of an egg. It is generally due to nutritional and management faults including low level of vitamin A. This spot is called meat spot. Eggs with meat spot are not suitable for hatching purpose.

Milking: Collection of semen from poultry by applying gentle massage to sex organ of cock.

Morbidity: Percentage of birds in a flock affected by a disease.

Mortality: Percentage of birds in a flock died by a disease.

Moulting: It is the shedding of feathers of birds. It provides some indication about the laying capacity of birds. Poor layers moult early, take more time to complete the moulting process and generally do not lay eggs during this period. On the other hand, good layers moult late, complete the moulting period quickly and sometimes continue to lay eggs even during moulting period.

N

NECC: National Egg Coordination Committee. A farmers' cooperative for promotion of poultry industry in India.

Nest: A secluded place where a hen feels she may safely lay her eggs; also the act of brooding.

O

Oesophagus: Tube-like structure of digestive system that moves feed from the throat to the stomach. Also called gullet.

Offal: The non-edible viscera and trimmings (feet, head) of a slaughtered animal or bird removed in dressing.

Ornithology: The study of the science of birds. Salim Ali is a renowned ornithologist, sometimes called as the father of ornithology.

Oviposition: The laying (expelling) of a fully formed egg from the reproductive system of poultry.

Ovulation: Release of ovum from the ovary. The ovary of a hen contains a series of ova, size of which may vary from microscopic to a large size looks just like a yolk of an egg. With the help of gonadotropic hormones like FSH and LH, mature ovum (i.e. yolk) is released from the ovary in laying hens.

Ovum: The round female germ cells attached to the ovary; plural form is ova. They are releases and drop into the oviduct and become the egg yolk.

P

Pause size: Number of consecutive days without egg in an egg laying cycle is known as pause size. It is more in *deshi* birds and less in good layer.

Pellet: Pellets are small cylindrical-shaped feeds, made up of dry mash under high pressure. Generally, pellets are offered to the chicken/fowl.

Perch: It is also called roost. Pole of wood placed on a higher level of poultry house for perching/sitting of birds on it.

Pheasant: A species of game bird that comes in many breeds and varieties. They are primarily raised for meat, and also for feathers and ornamental value.

Pin bones: Pubic bones. Two sharp, slender bones that end in front of the vent.

Pip: To break through or peck holes in the shell by the chick; the hole a newly formed chick makes in its shell.

Plumage: The total set of feathers covering a chicken or other fowl.

Poult: After hatching, a young turkey of either sex that is between one day and a couple weeks old. Sometimes the term 'poultry' is abbreviated as 'poult' in some journals.

Poultry: The domesticated species of birds which are reared for production of meat and/or eggs for the benefit of human beings are called poultry. It is a broad term, and it includes number of avian species, viz. fowl/chicken, duck, quail, turkey, Guinea fowl, goose, *etc.*

Poultry science: That branch of Animal Science which deals with study of poultry (birds). In includes scientific breeding, feeding, housing and management, and health control measures of poultry birds (viz. chicken, duck, quail, turkey, *etc.*) for production of meat and/or eggs.

Pullet: Young female chicken less than a year old.

R

Ratite: The family of birds including Ostrich and Emu.

Ready-to-cook: Processed young poultry and its parts which are ready to be cooked with very little additional preparation.

Roost (Perch): Resting place of fowl. Wooden slats or GI pipes (5 cm², round at top and flat at bottom) placed horizontally at lengthwise in the poultry house at a distance of 35–40 cm apart giving 20–25 cm space per bird are regarded as roost or perch. It satisfies the natural instinct of birds to sit at higher places like branches of a tree.

Rooster: A male chicken usually kept for breeding. *See cock.*

S

Saddle: It is a feather, only present in male fowl.

Setter: Incubator used during the first 18 days of incubation in case of chicken egg hatching.

Sexing: Determination of sex, i.e. separation of male and female. Sexing can be done by vent method or Japanese method at day-old stage of birds (by observing male sex organ at the fold of cloaca through the vent) or by autosexing method (by observing some sex-linked characters). In case of broiler farming (birds of either sex are reared), sexing of birds is not needed. But in layer farming (only female birds are reared for production of eggs), sexing of birds is essentially needed.

Sex-link character: A genetic trait that creates a difference (usually in colour) between males and females. Most often this is used to refer to traits that make chicks of different genders visibly distinct for ease of sexing. The term may apply to the gene or characteristic, or is often applied to hybrid crosses that display this characteristic such as the Golden Sex-link.

Shell membranes: Two thin membranes next to the shell and surrounding the albumen and yolk; known as inner and outer shell membranes; they are one of the egg's chief defenses against bacterial invasion.

Shell: The hard outer surface of an egg made up largely of calcium carbonate; the shell has pores allowing loss of carbon dioxide and moisture from the egg. It is about 11% of the total weight of a chicken egg.

Sickle feather: It is a sickle shaped feather, only present in the tail region of male fowl.

Spent hen: A breeder or commercial egg type hen after completion of economic production life is known as spent hen. In case of layer farming birds are generally kept for 1st laying year, i.e. up to 72–80 weeks of age, after this period they are disposed of as spent hen.

Spur: The sharp horny protrusion from the inside rears of a bird's shanks, usually a cock or rooster has spur, but absent in its female counter part.

Squab: Baby pigeon, either male or female, also called squeaker.

Sternum: Breastbone or keel bone in poultry.

Straight run chicks: Day-old chicks that have not been separated according to sexes, i.e. a flock of straight run chicks is composed of both male and female. Generally, broiler chicks are of such type.

Stress: Any physical or mental tension that reduces resistance to disease.

Subcutaneous: Just beneath the skin.

Swan: A large elegant species of waterfowl. Some breeds are raised for their ornamental qualities, adding a stately grace to ponds and waterways.

Symptom: Detectable evidence of a disease.

Syndrome: A group of symptoms that occur in combination in a particular disease.

T

Tom: A male turkey.

Turkey: A large game bird native to the America reared primarily for meat. Males are called toms, females called hens and chicks are known as poults.

V

Vaccine: Product made from disease-causing organisms and used to produce immunity.

Vent: The common external opening of the cloaca in birds through which the intestinal, urinary and reproductive tracts empty.

Vitelline membrane: Thin membrane that encloses the yolk of an egg.

W

Wattles: The fleshy, red growths that hang from the side and base of the chicken's beak.

Web: A piece of skin that joins the toes of some birds and animals like duck. It helps them to swim in water.

Wet bulb thermometer: A thermometer used to measure the amount of moisture or water vapour in the air.

WPSA: World Poultry Science Association.

Y

Yolk: The yellow portion of the egg composed of water, protein and fat. The yolk contains practically all of the known vitamins except vitamin C. It is about 31% of the total weight of a chicken egg.

Appendix 3

ICAR and Private Institutions in the Field of poultry Science in India

1. **Central Avian Research Institute**
   CARI, Izatnagar, Pin: 243122, Uttar Pradesh, India
   Tel: EPABX Lines
   91-581-2301220; 2301320
   91-581-2303223; 2300204
   Fax: 91-581-2301321.
   E-mail: cari_director@rediffmail.com
   Website: http://www.icar.org.in/cari/index.html

2. **Central Poultry Development Organisation**
   (Southern region)
   Hessarghatta, Bangalore 560088
   Karnataka, India
   Tel: 080-28466236/28466226.
   Fax: 080-28466444.
   E-mail: cpdosr@yahoo.com
   Website: http://www.cpdosrbng.kar.nic.in

3. **Central Poultry Development Organisation (CPDO),** Western Region, Aarey
   Milk Colony, Mumbai 400065
   Tel: 022-29272497
   Fax: 022-29272488
   E-mail: cpdo_mum@yahoo.com
   Wedsite: http://www.cpdomumbai.gov.in

4. **Central Poultry Development Organisation (CPDO),** Eastern Region,
   Nayapalli, Bhubaneswar 751012
   Tel: 0674-2420175
   Fax: 0674-2420635
   E-mail: cpdo_er@rediffmail.com
   Website: http://www.cpdobbser.gov.in

5. **Central Poultry Development Organisation (CPDO),** Northern Region,
   Phase-I, Industrial area, Chandigarh 160001
   Tel: 0172-2655460

E-mail: cpdonr-chd@nic.in

Website: http://www.cpdonrchd.gov.in

6. **Project Directorate on Poultry**, Hyderabad 500030, Andhra Pradesh.

7. **Indian Veterinary Research Institute** (IVRI), Izatnagar 243122, Uttar Pradesh.

8. **Central Poultry Performance Testing Centre, Gurgaon,** Begumpur, Khatok Narsingpur, Gurgaon, Haryana

   Fax: 0124-2215194

   E-mail: cpptcggn@gmail.com

9. **High Security Animal Disease Laboratory**, Bhopal, Madhya Pradesh.

10. **Centre of Advanced Studies in Poultry Science**

    a. **Veterinary College and Research Institute**

       Namakkal 637002, Tamil Nadu.

       Phone: Direct (04286) 266494

       PBX (04286) 266491, 266492, 266493

       EXT 402

       Fax: (04286) 266494

       (04286) 266484

       (04286) 228693

       E-mail: caspsc@rediffmail.com

    b. **College of Veterinary and Animal Sciences,** Kerala Agricultural University, Mannuthy, Kerala.

11. **Poultry Diagnostic Research Centre (PDRC),** Division of Venkateshwara Hatcharies (P) Ltd, Pune, Solapur Road, Lonikolbhor, Pune, Maharashtra 412201 [Private Institute]

    Tel: 020-26913315, 26913416

    Fax: 020-26913417

    E-mail: pdrcpune@bsnl.in

    Website: http://www.venkys.com

12. **Dr BV Roa Institute of Poultry Management & Technology (IPMT),** Tilekarwadi, PO Urulikanchan 412202, Pune, Maharashtra 412202 [Private Institute]

Universities Awarding Postgraduate Degree in Poultry Science

THE LIST OF INDIAN UNIVERSITIES OFFERING PG DEGREE IN POULTRY SCIENCE

(This list may be considered as indicative, not exhaustive.)

ANDHRA PRADESH

College of Veterinary Science, Rajendra Nagar, **Acharya NG Ranga Agricultural University**, Hyderabad.

College of Veterinary Science, Tirupati.

ASSAM

Faculty of Veterinary Science, Khanapara Campus, **Assam Agricultural University**, Guwahati.

GUJARAT

College of Veterinary Science & Animal Husbandry, **Gujarat Agricultural University (GAU)**, Anand.

College of Veterinary Science & Animal Husbandry, **Gujarat Agricultural University (GAU)**, Sardar Krushi Nagar.

KARNATAKA

Karnataka Veterinary, Animal & Fisheries Sciences University (KVAFSU), Bidar. College of Veterinary Science, Bangalore.

KERALA

College of Veterinary & Animal Sciences, **Kerala Agricultural University**, Mannuthy, Thrissur.

MADHYA PRADESH

College of Veterinary Science & Animal Husbandry, **Jawaharlal Nehru Krishi Vishwavidyalaya (JNKV)**, Jabalpur.

College of Veterinary Science & Animal Husbandry, **JNKV**, Mohow.

MAHARASHTRA

Nagpur Veterinary College, **Maharashtra Animal & Fishery Sciences University (MAFSU)**, Nagpur.

College of Vetreianry & Anmal Sciences, **MAFSU**, Parbhani.

Bombay Veterinary College, **MAFSU**, Mumbai.

Postgraduate Institute of Veterinary & Animal Science, **MAFSU**, Akola.

ODISHA

College of Veterinary Science & Animal Husbandry, **Orissa University of Agriculture & Technology**, Bhubaneshwar.

PONDICHERRY

Rajiv Gandhi College of Veterinary & Animal Sciences, **Pondicherry University**, Pondicherry.

TAMIL NADU

Madras Veterinary College, **Tamil Nadu University of Veterinary & Animal Science (TNUVAS),** Chennai.

Veterinary College and Research Institute, **TNUVAS**, Namakkal.

UTTAR PRADESH

College of Veterinary Science & Animal Husbandry, **Uttar Pradesh Pandit Deen Dayal Upadhyaya Pashu Chikitsa Vigyan Vishwavidyalaya Evam Go Anusandhan Sanstha**, Mathura, UP.

Indian Veterinary Research Institute (Deemed University), Izatnagar, UP.

Appendix 5
List of Poultry Journals and Magazines

INDIAN JOURNAL OF POULTRY SCIENCE

(Print ISSN: 0019-5529, Online ISSN: 0974-8180). Established in 1965, Indian Journal of Poultry Science (IJPS), a leading peer-reviewed Indian journal in the field is an official publication of the Indian Poultry Science Association (IPSA), Izatnagar 243122 (UP). The publication is aimed at providing access to academicians, researchers and industry professionals from across the globe to publish their work on all aspects of poultry science through research papers, short communications and review articles. The journal is published three times in a year as one volume in April, August, and December and circulated to IPSA members free of cost. The editorial board of IJPS welcomes the submission of manuscripts within the aim and scope of the journal for publication.

Address: Central Avian Research Institute, Izatnagar 243122, Uttar Pradesh, India; **Phone:** +91-0581-2303223, 2300204 Extn. 3060; **Fax:** +91-0581-2301321; **E-mail:** ijpseditor@gmail.com; **Website:** www.ipsa-cari.org.in.

INDIAN POULTRY REVIEW

Address: 57B, Townshend Road, Kolkata 700025; **Phone:** 033-24740549/24192487/24750838; **E-mail:** pouljag@vsnl.net, pouljag_vsnl@bsnl.in.

POULTRY ADVISER

Address: 97, St. John's Church Road, Bengaluru 560005.

POULTRY FLAME

This is an English newspaper, published every week. It contains an article and important national and international news. The total number of pages is eight. It is published every Thursday and posted on Friday. This newspaper is very popular because of its updated information. The wide circulation in India, SAARC, Gulf and Middle East countries, make it an instant hit with the readers.

Address: Poultry Punch Publications (I) Pvt Ltd, 25, Thyag Raj Nagar Market, New Delhi 110003.

POULTRY GUIDE

Address: 20, Thyag Raj Nagar Market, New Delhi 110003.

POULTRY INTERNATIONAL

It is a leading international publication serving the commercial poultry industry for many years. Poultry International serves commercial broiler, turkey, duck and egg producers, in addition to poultry and egg processing and further processing plants, hatcheries, feed manufacturers, and others allied to the integrated poultry supply chain.

Address: Watt Publishing Co, 18, Chapel Street, Petersfield, Hampshire GU 32, 3DZ, England; **Website:** www.wattagnet.com.

POULTRY JAGAT

A Bengali poultry magazine.

Address: M/S Salmali Publications, 57B, Townshend Road, PS-Bhawanipur, Kolkata 700025; **Phone:** 033-24740549/24192487/24750838; **E-mail:** pouljag@vsnl.net, pouljag_vsnl@bsnl.in.

POULTRY PUNCH

It is an English magazine, published every month. It encompasses a wide range of popular updated articles from experts on the topic. The news content comprises the latest national and international events in poultry. This magazine is published and posted on the last date of every month. Owing to its contents, this magazine has won appreciation from the entire poultry industry. This is the only poultry magazine witnessed so far, which has maximum number of articles to facilitate its readers. The wide circulation in India, SAARC, Gulf and Middle East countries, make it one of the most readable poultry magazines.

Address: Poultry Punch Publications (I) Pvt Ltd, 25, Thyag Raj Nagar Market, New Delhi 110003.

POULTRY REPORTER

Address: 20, Thyag Raj Nagar Market, New Delhi 110003.

POULTRY TIMES OF INDIA AND POULTRY PLANNER

These are official bi-monthly magazines of Pixie Consulting Solutions Ltd. Besides covering important poultry events in the country, these publications also bring out country specific special focus with tremendous success in terms of editorial contents and advertisements. These magazines offer unmatched contents in terms of width and depth of coverage, related to the subjects that are influencing the dynamics of the poultry industry. The aim is to cover news, events, research, innovations, new products and processes and marketing (both national and international) related with poultry.

Address: Ram Bhawan, 1st Floor, 415, Ahimsa Marg, Khar, Mumbai 400052.

POULTRY VOICE

Address: 4-88-1-C, Vikasnagar, Hyderabad 500060.

WORLD POULTRY

For online newsletter and articles on poultry.

Address: PO Box 4, 7000 BA Doetinchem, The Netherlands;

E-mail: info@worldpoultry.net; **Website:** http://www.worldpoultry.net.

WORLD'S POULTRY SCIENCE JOURNAL

The World's Poultry Science Association (WPSA) began publishing this journal in 1928 in the name of International Review of Poultry Science; and in 1945, the journal was renamed as World's Poultry Science Journal (WPSJ). At present, the journal is published quarterly. This journal publishes articles on virtually all aspects of poultry production and poultry science. The WPSJ is published in both a printed and an on-line form by Cambridge University Press. The online publishing agreement for this journal, originally made with CABI Publishing, has now been assigned to Cambridge University Press.

Address: Indian Chapter: Secretary, Dr AL Bhagwat, Flat 3, Chandramapuri, Lane No. 10, Dahanukar Colony, Kothrud, Pune 411038, Maharashtra; **Phone:** +91 20 24270724; **Fax:** +91 20 24270723; **E-mail:** wpsapune@eth.net; **Website:** http://www.wpsa.com.

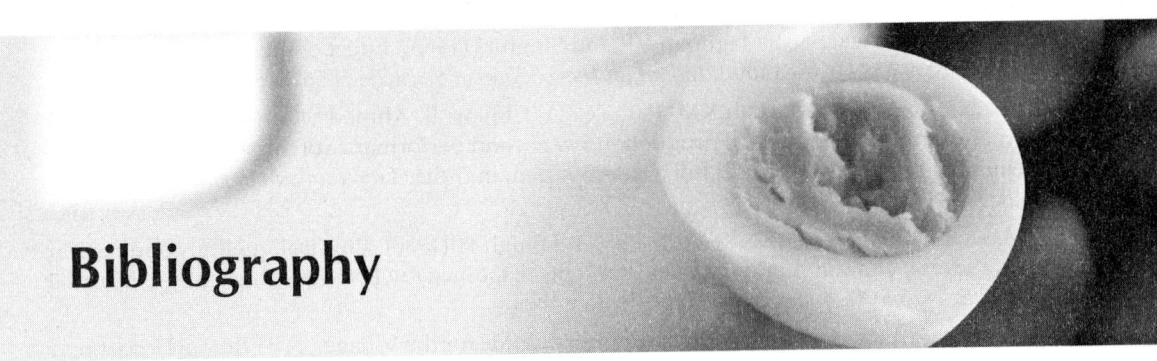

Bibliography

Anonymous (2004). All India Poultry Business Directory (Year Book), 2nd Edition. Sadana Publishers and Distributors, Ghaziabad.

Austic RE and Neshein MC (1990). Poultry Production, 13th Edition. Lea & Febiger, London, UK.

Bandyopadhyay UK and Jana NN (2009). Prospect of Organic Poultry Production in India. Proceedings of National Symposium on 'Organic Livestock farming—Gobal Issues, Trends and Challenges'. West Bengal University of Animal and Fishery Sciences, Kolkata.

Chauhan HVS (1993). Poultry Diseases, Diagnosis and Treatment. Wiley Eastern Limited, New Delhi.

Chauhan PPS and Chauhan RS (2005). Ascites syndrome in broiler birds. Pashudhan, 31(10): 3.

Daghir NJ (2008). Poultry Production in Hot Climates, 2nd Edition. CAB International, Cambridge, USA.

Das SK (1994). Poultry Production, 1st Edition. CBS Publishers & Distributors, Delhi.

FAOSTAT (2005) http://faostat.fao.org/site/340/default.aspex (accessed on 19–22.3.2007).

FAOSTAT (2007) http://faostat.fao.org/site/569/default.aspex (accessed on 14.1.2007).

Ghatnekar GS and Ghatnekar MS (1999). Marketing—A must for poultry. Financial Express, May 3, 1999 (cited from http://www.financialexpress.com).

Gernat A (1914). Poultry Farm Biosecurity Field Manual. Department of Poultry Science, North Carolina State University, USA.

Ghosh N (2008). Animal Production, Diseases and Treatment, 2nd Bengali Edition. Kalyani Publishers, Ludhiana.

Ghosh N (2008). Poultry Farming, 1st Bengali Edition. Kalyani Publishers, Ludhiana.

Ghosh N and Samanta R (2008). Manual on Avian Production and Management. International Book Distributing Co (Publishing Division), Lucknow.

Jacob J and Miles R (2008). Designer and Specialty Eggs. Publication PS51, The Institute of Food and Agricultural Services, University of Florida, Florida.

Jadhav NV and Siddiqui MF (1999). Handbook of Poultry Production and Management, 1st Edition. Jaypee Brothers Medical Publishers (P) Ltd, New Delhi.

Jalaludeen A, Peethambaran PA, Leo Joseph and Manomohanm CB (2004). Duck Production in Kerala. NATP on Ducks, CAS in Poultry Science, KAU, Mannuthy, Trissur, Kerala.

Johari DC, Hazary RC and Sacheti AK (2001). Poultry Production and Breeding. National Council of Educational Research and Training, New Delhi.

Johri TS, Agarwal SK, Sadagopan VR and Singh H (1988). Effect of dietary aflatoxin on the performance of Guinea fowl. *Indian Journal of Animal Sciences*, 58: 673–875.

Kumaresan A, Bujarbaruah KM, Pathak KA, Chhetri B, Ahmed SK and Haunshi S (2008). Analysis of a village chicken production system and performance of improved dual purpose chickens under a subtropical hill agroecosystem in India. *Tropical Animal Health Production*, 40: 395–402.

Mahapatra CM, Pandey NK, Verma SS and Singh H (1986). Physical quality, composition, cholesterol, vitamin A and fatty acid contents of Guinea fowl *vis-a-vis* chicken egg. *Journal of Food Science & Technology*, 24: 168–171.

McArdle AA and Panda JN (1965). A Poultry Guide for the Villager, 3rd Edition. Department of Agriculture, Government of India, New Delhi.

Mehta R, Narrod CA and Tiongco MM (2008). Livestock Industrialisation, Trade and Social-Health-Environment Impacts in Developing Countries: A Case of Indian Poultry Sector, Research and Information System for Developing Countries, New Delhi.

Moregaonkar SD and Patil AD (2006). Gout in broiler: Winter problem—an experience. Pashudhan, 32(1): 3.

Narahari D, Asha Rajini R and Prabaharan R (2000). Poultry Economics and Projects. Tamil Nadu Veterinary & Animal Science University, Chennai.

Panda B and Mahapatra SC (1989). Poultry Production. Indian Council of Agricultural Research, New Delhi.

Prasad J (2000). Poultry Production and Management, 1st Edition. Kalyani Publishers, New Delhi.

Rahman SA (2005). Animal resource development as an alternate source of income generation. Thought—A Sociotechnical Round up, FOSET, 8(3): 24.

Saxena HC and Ketelaars EH (1993). Poultry Production in Hot Climatic Zones. Kalyani Publishers, Ludhiana.

Sharma D, Singh UB, Nayal LMS, Singh S and Singh RV (2000). Carcass characteristics of improved Guinea fowl at different weeks of age. *Indian Journal of Poultry Science*, 35(2): 224–225.

Sharma RP, Chatterjee RN, Rama Rao SV and Sharma SR (2008). Poultry Production in India. Indian Council of Agricultural Research, New Delhi.

Singh KS and Panda B (1988). Poultry Nutrition. Kalyani Publishers, Ludhiana.

Singh RA (1990). Poultry Production, 3rd Edition. Kalyani Publishers, Ludhiana.

Smith TW (1997). Troubleshooting Failures with Egg Incubation. Mississippi State University.

Surai PF and Sparks NHC. Designer EEgg Production and Evaluation. Avian Science Research Centre, Auchincruive, Ayr, KA6 5HW, Scotland, UK.

Vegad JL (2004). Poultry Diseases. A Guide for Farmers and Poultry Professionals, 1st Edition. International Book Distributing Co, Lucknow.

Yadav MP and Kumar D (2008). Poultry—technically the most advanced sector. The Hindu Survey of Indian Agriculture, 93–96.

Index